BC Cancer Agency
Vancouver Cancer Centre
Library
600 West 10th Ave.
Vancouver, B.C. Canada
V5Z 4E6

D0215785

ACOUSTIC TUMORS

Diagnosis and Management

SECOND EDITION

A Singular Audiology Text
Jeffrey L. Danhauer, Ph.D.
Audiology Editor

ACOUSTIC TUMORS

Diagnosis and Management

SECOND EDITION

William F. House, M.D.
Charles M. Luetje, M.D.
Karen Jo Doyle, M.D., Ph.D.

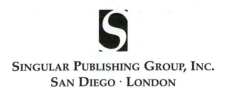

SINGULAR PUBLISHING GROUP, INC.
SAN DIEGO · LONDON

Published by Singular Publishing Group, Inc.
401 West "A" Street, Suite 325
San Diego, California 92101-7904

19 Compton Terrace
London N1 2UN, U.K.

e-mail: singpub@mail.cerfnet.com
Website: http://www.singpub.com

©1997 by Singular Publishing Group, Inc.

Typeset in 10/12 Palatino by So Cal Graphics
Printed in the United States of America by McNaughton & Gunn

All rights, including that of translation, reserved. No part of this publication may be reproduced, stored in a retrieval system or transmitted in any form or by any means, electronic, mechanical, recording, or otherwise, without the prior written permission of the publisher.

Library of Congress Cataloging-in-Publication Data

Acoustic tumors : diagnosis and management / edited by William F.
    House, Charles M. Luetje, and Karen Jo Doyle. —2nd ed.
        p.   cm.
    Includes bibliographical references and index.
    ISBN 1-56593-624-8
    1. Acoustic nerve—Tumors. I. House, William F., 1923–
II. Luetje, Charles M. III. Doyle, Karen Jo.
    [DNLM: 1. Neuroma, Acoustic—diagnosis. 2. Neuroma, Acoustic—
therapy. 3. Ear Neoplasms—diagnosis. 4. Ear Neoplasms—therapy.
WV 250 A185 1996]
RC280.E2A26   1996
616.99'285—dc20
DNLM/DLC   96-26866
for Library of Congress   CIP

CONTENTS

PREFACE to the First Edition

This book begins where "Monograph 11: Acoustic Neuroma," *Archives of Otolaryngology,* December, 1968, ended. It is a definitive study of the diagnosis and management of acoustic tumors. Five hundred patients with unilateral tumors were evaluated and operated on by members of the Otologic Medical Group, Inc., of Los Angeles. The 500 consecutive cases underwent surgery between March 22, 1968, and January 31, 1975. None of these patients had acoustic tumor surgery prior to this time. Monograph II reported on the first 200 cases seen at the Otologic Medical Group, Inc. This series begins with the 201st case and continues through the 700th. During the preparation of this book, the 1000th acoustic tumor patient underwent surgery.

The data used in this book were gathered by careful study of the 500 patient charts from the Otologic Medical Group, Inc., as well as the St. Vincent Medical Center medical records on 251 of the patients. This series of patients consists of 275 females and 225 males. Ages ranged from 9 to 76 years, with a mean age of 47 years. There were 252 cases of left-sided tumors and 248 right-sided tumors. The duration of the first symptom ranged from less than 1 month to 46 years. Tumor size was classified in Monograph II. Only tumors confined to the internal auditory canal were classified as small. Medium tumors were those that protruded into the cerebellopontine angle and did not cause preoperative neurologic symptoms or increased intracranial pressure. Large tumors were those that caused a preoperative neurological sign other than eighth nerve symptoms, or those with increased intracranial pressure or cerebellar ataxia. Occasionally, tumors with associated decreased corneal sensation and measuring 2.5 cm or less would be classified as medium. There were 26 small tumors, 301 medium tumors, and 173 large tumors.

Three surgical approaches were utilized in this series. Translabyrinthine removal was used in 470 cases, transsigmoid in 13 cases, and middle fossa in 17 cases. Total tumor removal was accomplished in 93.4% of all cases. This varied from 100% removal in small tumors to 97.6% in medium tumors, and 85% in large tumors. Operative mortality was 2.6%, case mortality 0.2%; giving a combined mortality of 2.8% (these figures are discussed at length in Volume II, Chapter 11). Results of preservation of facial function and cochlear function are presented in detail in Volume II, Chapters 4 and 2, respectively.

This book is written for the student and practitioner. It is arranged in two volumes so that the reader can sequentially follow the history, pathology, and evaluation of acoustic tumors (in Volume I), and the management of patients with acoustic tumors (in Volume II). It contains specific information regarding each category, which makes the book a reference as well as an instructional text.

The latest data regarding diagnosis of acoustic tumors are included. The major diagnostic advances since the last monograph have been impedance audiometry, computerized cranial tomography, and brainstem electric response audiometry. Each of these topics is discussed in separate chapters.

Other chapters include an outstanding pathology section, divided into pathophysiology and pathology. The dynamic progression of acoustic tumor growth and its effect on the surrounding neural and vascular structures are detailed. More than 1,000 cases have undergone histological review to portray the features of acoustic tumors.

Selected histories and patient reviews have been carefully prepared to provide the reader with the many variations of symptomatic presentation of acoustic tumors. Newer monitoring data and techniques are presented in the chapter on anesthesiology. Definitive eye care for patients after acoustic tumor removal with facial weakness is beautifully detailed. Psychological aspects of acoustic tumor patients have been studied prior to and one year after surgery. In a separate chapter fine detail is given to each fatality.

The cases presented in this book represent the work of many surgeons. Several members of the Otologic Medical Group, Inc., have contributed significant numbers of cases. However, the majority of the cases were operated by Dr. William F. House, teamed with Dr. William E. Hitselberger.

It is app;ropriate to recognize the contribution of Dr. William F. House to the field of acoustic tumor surgery. He introduced the microscope to the field of neurosurgery in the early 1960s. With intense interest in microsurgery for acoustic tumors, Dr. House perfected the techniques for the application of the microscope to this surgery. Later, the field of microsurgery developed.

Acoustic Tumors represents the largest reported series of consecutively operated acouustic tumors in history. It was made possible by the efforts and achievements of Dr. William F. House, who has so rightfully earned the distinct and honored title, the Father of Neuro-otologic Surgery.

Charles M. Luetje

PREFACE to the Second Edition

It is now a century since the first surgical treatment of an acoustic neuroma was reported by Ballance in 1895. The first quarter of the century was dominated by Cushing. His surgical approach was to do a wide bilateral occipital bone removal to allow him to look into both CP angles (preoperatively, they were not sure which side the tumor was on), and not to remove the tumor but to decompress it and give a few years of better life without the blindness from papilledema and ataxia of cerebellar compression. However, Cushing's principal contribution was in the diagnosis of acoustic neuromas. He documented the progression of symptoms from the unilateral hearing loss, which on the average preceded other symptoms by 3 years, to fifth nerve numbness, papilledema, headache, cerebellar ataxia, blindness, and finally death due to respiratory failure. His contributions were the forerunner of the remainder of the century when surgical approaches were constantly leap frogging with improved diagnostic procedures, followed by better surgery, and then better diagnostic procedures.

The next quarter century of the acoustic neuroma saga was dominated by Dandy, Cushing's student. He was able to diagnose tumors much earlier because he could now ask the patient with posterior fossa symptoms which side developed the hearing loss and thus use a more limited unilateral suboccipital approach because he now knew which side to operate on. Temporal bone X-rays were perfected in the 1920s, and Dandy introduced pneumoencephalograms to help visualize the tumor and the ventricles. For a time, the diagnostic advances were ahead of the surgery. Dandy found, by operation on smaller tumors, that if total removal was not done, there was a recurrence within a few years. To remove the tumor completely, he had to take the facial nerve. He popularized the statment: "Loss of the facial nerve is a cheap price to pay for the total removal of an acoustic neuroma."

In the last half of the century, acoustic neuroma surgery has been dominated by microsurgical techniques. Approaches through the temporal bone using the operating microscope, which I pioneered, led to the possibility of totally removing the tumor and at the same time saving the facial nerve. This allowed us to operate on much smaller tumors, because few patients were willing to face a facial nerve paralysis until papilledema, facial numbness, and headache had convinced them something had to be done.

In the 1950s and early 1960s, we were limited by the diagnostic procedures of the 1920s, namely, temporal bone X-rays and pneumoencephalograms. Introduction of pantopaque instead of air into the posterior fossa improved the possibility of early diagnosis. CAT scans soon improved on this, and today MRI is a truly miraculous achievement. Diagnosis has now leapfrogged ahead of surgery.

Today, saving the facial nerve is almost a given. The big challenge now is to save the hearing. Surgical techniques will just have to catch up. This book documents where we are now in the acoustic neuroma saga.

None of us will be around for the next 100 years, but many young surgeons will see amazing developments during the next 50 years that will compare with the advances none of us could have predicted in the second half of this century.

William F. House, M.D.

CONTRIBUTORS

Simón I. Angeli, M.D.
Fellow, House Ear Institute
Los Angeles, California

Pamela S. Bohrer, M.D.
Department of Head and Neck Surgery
Kaiser Permanente Hospital
Santa Rosa, California

Derald E. Brackmann, M.D., F.A.C.S.
Clinical Professor of Otolaryngology—
  Head and Neck Surgery
Clinical Professor of Neurosurgery
University of Southern California,
School of Medicine President,
  House Ear Clinic;
Board of Directors, House Ear Institute
Los Angeles, California

Brett R. Brodersen, M.D.
Saint Vincent Medical Center
Los Angeles, California

Joseph N. Carberry, M.D.
Director, Department of Pathology
Saint Vincent Medical Center
Los Angeles, California

Sujana S. Chandrasekhar, M.D.
Assistant Professor
Section of Otolaryngology
New Jersey Medical School
Newark, New Jersey

C. Y. Joseph Chang, M.D.
Assistant Professor
Department of Otolaryngology—
  Head and Neck Surgery
The University of Texas, Houston
  Medical School
Houston, Texas

Steven W. Cheung, M.D.
Assistant Professor of Otolaryngology
University of California, San Francisco
San Francisco, California

Antonio De la Cruz, M.D.
Director of Education, House Ear Institute
Clinical Professor of Otolaryngology—
  Head and Neck Surgery
University of Southern California,
School of Medicine
Los Angeles, California

Leigh Anne Dew, M.D.
University of Utah
Salt Lake City, Utah

Karen J. Doyle, M.D., Ph.D.
Department of Otolaryngology—Head
  and Neck Surgery
University of California, Irvine, Medical
Center Orange, California

Rick A. Friedman, M.D., Ph.D.
Department of Otolaryngology—
  Head and Neck Surgery
University of Cincinnati
Cincinnati, Ohio

Michael E. Glasscock, III, M.D.
Clinical Professor of Surgery
  (Otology and Neurotology)
Vanderbilt University, School of Medicine
Nashville, Tennessee

Patricia Gentner, R.N.
Otologic Center, Inc.
Kansas City,Missouri

Philip Gruskin, M.D.
Pathologist, Saint Vincent Medical Center
Lynnwood, California
Clinical Laboratory Medical Group
Los Angeles, California

Mary J. Hawkshaw, R.N., B.S.N.
Otologic Nurse Clinician
American Institute for Voice
  and Ear Research
Philadelphia, Pennsylvania

William Hitselberger, M.D.
Department of Neurosurgery
Saint Vincent Medical Center
Los Angeles, California

John W. House, M.D.
House Ear Clinic
Los Angeles, California

William F. House, M.D.
Newport Beach, California

Carol A. Jackson, M.D., P.C.
Hearing and Balance Services
Newport Beach, California

Donald B. Kamerer, M.D.
Professor and Director, Division of
    Otolaryngology
University of Pittsburgh, School of
    Medicine
Pittsburgh, Pennsylvania

Anil K. Lalwani, M.D.
Assistant Professor, Department of
    Otolaryngology—Head and Neck
    Surgery
University of California, San Francisco
San Francisco, California

Robert E. Levine, M.D.
Clinical Professor of Ophthalmology
University of Southern California, School
    of Medicine
Los Angeles, California

William W. M. Lo, M.D.
Clinical Professor of Radiology
University of Southern California
Chief, Neuroradiology Section
Saint Vincent Medical Center
Los Angeles, California

Charles M. Luetje, M.D.
Otologic Center, Inc.
Kansas City, Missouri

William M. Luxford, M.C.
House Ear Clinic
Los Angeles, California

Donald L. Myers, M.D.
Assistant Professor of Neurosurgery
Thomas Jefferson University
Philadelphia, Pennsylvania

Ralph A. Nelson, M.D.
House Ear Clinic
Associate Clinical Professor
University of Southern California (ENT)
University of California, Irvine (ENT)

P. Gerard Reilly, F.R.C.S.Ed. (ORL)
TWJ Fellow
Department of Otolaryngology
University Hospital
Nottingham, England

Robert T. Sataloff, M.D., D.M.A.
Professor of Otolaryngology
Thomas Jefferson University
Philadelphia, Pennsylvania

Clough Shelton, M.D. F.A.C.S.
Associate Professor, Department of
    Otolaryngology
University of Utah, School of Medicine
Salt Lake City, Utah

William H. Slattery, III, M.D.
Director, Clinical Studies
House Ear Clinic/House Ear Institute
Los Angeles, California

Ronald L. Steenerson, M.D.
Atlanta Ear Clinic
Atlanta, Georgia

Charles A. Syms, III, M.D.
Associate Professor of Surgery,
    Uniformed Services
Staff Otologist/Neurotologist
USAF Medical Center
San Antonio, Texas

Debara L. Tucci, M.D.
Division of Otolaryngology—Head and
Neck Surgery
Duke University, Medical Center
Durham, North Carolina

C. Keith Whittaker, M.D.
Clinical Professor of Surgery
University of Kansas, Medical Center
Neurology/Neurosurgery of
    Kansas City, Inc.
Kansas City, Missouri

Charles D. Yingling, Ph.D.
Professor and Director, Neural
    Monitoring
University of California,
    San Francisco
San Francisco, California

CHAPTER 1

A History of Acoustic Tumor Surgery: 1800–1960

William F. House, M.D.

In 1793, John Hunter died in London. As he had insisted, his assistants performed a thorough autopsy, and his remains were buried.

John Hunter's work was to influence greatly the progress of medicine all over the world. His influence was particularly strong in Victorian England during the next 100 years. In fact, a 100 years later, when his remains were discovered in an obscure London church vault, with due pomp and ceremony, they were transferred to Westminster Abby, where his epitaph identifies him as the "Father of Modern Surgery." He was regarded as the greatest comparative anatomist of all time. Although not so recognized during his lifetime, he was London's preeminent surgeon. Most important for the future of medical science, however, was his intellectual legacy, which was passed by his students to succeeding generations of scientists and clinicians. He enjoined them to observe carefully and record their patients' symptoms and correlate these findings with those of thorough autopsy dissection after the patients' deaths.

Hunter's emphasis on the study of anatomy and comparative anatomy through careful clinical observation of function led many of his students to pursue physiology. By the early 1800s, there was intense interest in the function of the various nerves, the central nervous system, and the other organ systems.

In London, Sir Charles Bell was the first to discover the sensory function of the fifth cranial nerve and the motor function of the seventh cranial nerve. In 1806, he published his famous treatise on the anatomy of expression. Several years later, Bell (1830) published an excellent clinical report of an acoustic tumor, giving the clinical findings of the patient and the autopsy report:

> Mrs. F.—The burning sensation commenced on the left side of her tongue, and has gradually increased for twelve months, until now it extends over half the tongue, and mouth, and face, and head. . . .

1

she has lost the sense of taste in the affected side of her tongue . . . Since the age of twenty-one a violent headache had frequently distressed her—accompanied with sickness and vomiting of bile; this headache has continued to return at intervals since the commencement of her present ailment.

[A year later in September, 1828] . . . her speech had become indistinct, her face was drawn to the right side, the masseter and temporal muscles of the left side had ceased to act, the tongue protruded towards the left side, the hearing of the left ear had ceased; . . . she was emaciated and bedridden and complained of great and constant pain at the back part of her head . . . . she seemed to die at length from difficult respiration and want of the power of swallowing.

Post-mortem appearances . . . a tumor containing fluid of the color of urine about the size of a pigeon's egg was discovered. . . on the left side, bounded by the petrous portion of the temporal bone, the pons varolii, and the left lobe of the cerebellum . . . and had by its pressure produced considerable indentation of the left side of the pons . . . the fifth cranial nerve was flattened and thin as if from pressure.... but the seventh, both portio dura [facial nerve] and mollis [acoustic nerve], was completely involved and lost in the tumor from a quarter of an inch from its origin to the meatus internus; and into this foramen . . . could be seen to enter . . . . the membranous portion of the tumor . . . (pp. 194–196, Bell [1830], Plate V, legend on p. 227)

Previously, there were sporadic reports of tumors of the cerebellopontine angle found at autopsy, but they were accompanied by little or no information regarding the clinical findings of the patient. The first of these is probably the case of Sandifort, described in 1777 (as cited in Cushing, 1917). Cruveilhier (1842) gave a remarkable clinical and pathologic report of a 26-year-old patient who died of an acoustic tumor. In this report, he noted that the patient's first symptom was deafness. At autopsy, Cru-

veilhier described the enlarged porus acusticus, the distortion of adjacent cerebral nerves, and the deformation and absorption of the sella turcica.

These reports, of course, were of great clinical interest, but the lesions were beyond any form of treatment available at that time. Developments in bacteriology, asepsis, radiology, anesthesia, clinical diagnosis, medical instrumentation, and related areas were necessary before surgery could become a potent treatment weapon. However, these advances, which were to characterize the nineteenth century as the "Golden Age of Medicine," lay just ahead.

In 1846, Morton successfully demonstrated ether anesthesia during a surgical procedure at Massachusetts General Hospital (as cited in Krumbhaar, 1941). This fantastic discovery eliminated the problem of the surgeon operating on a struggling patient who was being held down by strong assistants. Ether opened up vast new possibilities for remediating the various pathologic lesions that heretofore had been documented only at the autopsy table. It was soon discovered, however, that, even with anesthesia, brain surgery was almost always fatal if the surgeon penetrated past the dura. The reason for the fatality was sepsis. In 1861, Semmelweis, in Vienna, published his discovery that the simple expedient of washing the hands could virtually eliminate puerperal sepsis, but this safeguard was not accepted by learned surgeons of the day (as cited in Krumbhaar, 1941). Pasteur, in his classic experiments from 1857 to 1863, discovered that putrefaction of animal matter was due to the action of microorganisms (as cited in Krumbhaar, 1941). In the early 1860s Pasteur's work came to the attention of a young surgeon named Lister. He recognized the connection between microorganisms and infection and developed the principles of antiseptic surgery. His first publication on this type of surgery appeared in 1867. Medicine had now acquired two essential tools for effective surgical intervention: anesthesia and asepsis.

The 1880s and 1890s saw an intense interest in neurology. Such great names as Hughlings Jackson, Oppenheim, Babinski, and many others established neurology as a medical specialty in major medical centers. From 1890 to 1900, the experimental work of Luciani, Russell, Ferrier, and Turner delineated that homolateral disturbances in the cerebellum led to trunk and limb coordination disorders that were designated variously by the terms ataxia, dysmetria, astasia, dystonia, and asynergia (Ferrier & Turner, 1984; Luciani, 1891; Russell, 1894, 1895, 1896). Another important development regarding brain tumors was the ophthalmoscope, invented in 1850 by Helmholtz. It was introduced into neurology by von Graefe, who first recognized papilledema and its relationship to intracranial tumors.

Thus, in the 1890s, two great disciplines within the field of medicine, neurology and surgery, seemed ready to converge. By this time, neurologists could recognize a patient with an intracranial tumor because of headaches and papilledema, and they usually were able to localize the tumor as being either above or below the tentorium, if the patient had cerebellar ataxia. Neurologists were beginning to think in terms of surgical removal of intracranial tumors. In 1893, on the basis of postmortem studies, a New York neurologist estimated that 7% of all intracranial tumors were considered operable (Starr, 1893). This neurologist teamed up with the famous New York surgeon, McBurney, for whom an abdominal incision is named (McBurney & Starr, 1893). In 1891, they unsuccessfully explored the posterior fossa for an acoustic tumor.

At this time, undoubtedly, there were unsuccessful cases in various large clinics around the world, but they were not reported. The following year, Ballance, in London, operated for the neurologist Beevor with a successful result (Ballance, 1907):

Operation, November 19, 1894. Scalp flap thrown down and right occipital region and bone removed toward the external occipital protuberance and exostosis was discovered and removed. The exostosis presented toward the dura as well as externally. The inward projection had occluded the lateral sinus. When therefore the exostosis was removed the sinus filled up causing a considerable alteration in venous circulation. The result was the patient collapsed and respiration ceased. The patient was revived with much diffculty.

Operation, November 26, 1894. Flap thrown down and the dural flap thrown down. Solid tumor attached to the dura over the inner aspect of the posterior surface of the petrous somewhat firmly fixed. A finger had to be insinuated between the pons and the tumor to get it away. The patient after somewhat protracted convalescence recovered. The fifth and seventh cranial nerves were injured at the operation and the right eye ulcerated and had to be removed. The optic neuritis of the left eye cleared up with recovery of good eyesight. Some trophic ulceration of the angle of the mouth and the right ala nasi. This ultimately healed.

September, 1906. The patient is alive and well. He has right facial palsy and anesthesia corresponding to the fifth nerve. (pp. 112–114).

There was some speculation about whether this was an acoustic tumor or a meningioma. Nevertheless, this discussion testifies that it was possible, even at that time, to successfully enter the posterior fossa for surgical removal of a tumor.

In his later years, and following the publication of his excellent book on intracranial tumors (Ballance, 1907), Ballance became more associated with otologic surgery. He published an excellent two-volume work on the surgical management of temporal bone infections extending into the central nervous system (Balance, 1919). Other neurologists became interested in surgery. Sir Victor Horsley and Stewart and Holmes (1904) were but a few. Horsley may have been the first true neurologic surgeon.

Details of various surgeons' attempts at removal of acoustic tumors during the late nineteenth century were meager and sketchy. In the opening years of the twentieth century, neurologic localization had progressed to the point that posterior fossa tumors causing elevated intracranial pressure could be diagnosed during the patient's lifetime. Neurologists seeing these patients had induced a few of their surgical colleagues to attempt surgical relief of this lesion. A few successes were reported.

The beginning of the twentieth century was the turning point in the story of the acoustic tumor. By now, the principles of John Hunter had paid off handsomely. Clinical observation of the signs and symptoms of posterior fossa lesions, along with careful autopsy dissection, made diagnosis of these lesions possible during the patient's lifetime. A few successful surgeries by Ballance, Horsley, and others had confirmed the hope that surgery might avert the horrible suffering and death that these lesions caused. The next 15 years provided a tremendous interest in the study of these tumors and trials of a number of different surgical approaches to remove them successfully. In Baltimore, Harvey Cushing, 33 years old in 1902 and the most notable name among young surgeons devoted to the treatment of acoustic tumors, stepped into medical history (Cushing, 1917). Halsted trained Cushing as a general surgeon and encouraged him to follow his interest in brain tumors. From 1902 to 1917, when he served in the war in France, Cushing observed 784 brain tumor cases. Thirty of these proved to be tumors of the nervus acusticus. They became the basis of his classic 1917 monograph. In the preface to this monograph, Cushing sets out his important work hypothesis, which enabled him to accomplish much in the treatment of brain tumors in general and acoustic tumors in particular:

Most of the publications on the topic of brain tumors attempt to cover the entire subject from one aspect or another, but time is ripe for special studies of special tumors in special localities, particularly if the surgical treatment of these difficult lesions is to be perfected. (p. v).

In 1902, diagnosis had progressed to the point where patients with particular symptoms were found definitively to have a brain tumor. Usually, tumors from above the tentorium could be separated from those below the tentorium. However, usually it was not possible to determine whether the posterior fossa lesion was cerebellar or extracerebellar. If the determination of extracerebellar could be made, it could not be said on which side of the posterior fossa the tumor had arisen. Obviously, if surgery was to be successful, more accurate diagnosis was necessary. A recognition of differences in tumors arising within the posterior fossa developed. Henneberg and Koch (1902) introduced the term "cerebellopontine angle tumor" (*Kleinhirnbruckenwinkeltumor*). Their paper emphasized the growing recognition that references to tumors should indicate an anatomical region rather than a point of origin.

Virchow's great work in cellular pathology in the 1850s and 1860s emphasized the histologic study as an adjunct to gross pathology (e.g., Virchow, 1858). In the first decade of the twentieth century, Verocay (1910), in a special study of acoustic tumors, emphasized their benign histologic nature and studied their probable points of origin.

A good picture of the evaluation and surgery of acoustic tumors in the early 1900s can be gained by reading the first two case reports of Cushing's 1917 monograph on the subject. Both cases were operated within 3 months of each other in 1906. In the first case, Cushing describes his problems operating on these patients in the prone position. Within 3 months, he had developed what he called the "outrigger," a better support for the patient's shoulders and a headrest that extended beyond the table. The anesthesia used in these cases was ether, delivered by mask to the patient. (Bennett had developed the gas machine in

1895.) Endotracheal anesthesia was available at this time, but the prone position minimized the problem of the tongue falling back. Apparently, for this reason, Cushing never used endotracheal anesthesia during the period of his monograph (before 1917).

Halsted introduced rubber gloves in 1890. Acoustic tumor operations were carried out at Halsted's clinic at Johns Hopkins Hospital in Baltimore. Notable in the evaluations of these patients is the lack of vestibular findings or x-rays, which were not used at this time in acoustic tumor evaluation.

The following is a quote regarding Cushing's (1917) first two cases:

> The first patient was operated upon eleven years ago with a resultant fatality due to pneumonia. The operation was abandoned in the hope of completing it at a second session. For the situation, as now recalled, brings up a picture of the patient's head insecurely held by an assistant, the anesthesia awkwardly administered to a subject having respiratory embarrassment, and an inexperienced operator attempting to expose the cerebellum in a wobbly and bloody field.

CASE 1

J.H.H. Surg. No. 18640. A right acoustic neuroma (variously diagnosed) producing cerebellopontile symptoms. Post-operative fatality from pneumonia after a first-stage operation. Autopsy.

Jan. 12,1906. Admission of Henry S., age 43, an asylum superintendent, referred by Dr. J. T. McPherson of College Point, N.Y., with the complaint of headaches.

Chronology of symptoms.—For many years deafness in right ear (character of onset not inquired into but supposed to be due to chronic middle-ear disease). For three years attacks of sudden intense suboccipital pain, occasionally radiating through to orbit and accompanied by a sensation of weakness in the legs, so that he would sink to his knees. These paroxysms have recurred at irregular intervals; they are of variable duration. They usual-

ly provoke yawning, which appears to relieve the attack. For some time neuralgic pain in the left infra-orbital region, for which teeth have been extracted without relief. There has been increasing unsteadiness of gait and he observed that as long as he was moving forward he did fairly well, but on stopping or turning he would have to sit down else he would fall. For some months progressive failure of vision, some mental impairment, thickness of speech. No history of vomiting. For past month too unsteady to rise from bed.

Positive neurological findings.— (A) *General pressure.* Bilateral choked disc with secondary atrophy nearly complete on right, where light reaction practically lost. Relative anosmia. No x-ray studies. Deep reflexes exaggerated and equal. (B) *Localizing.* (1) *Cerebellar.* Nystagmus produced. Gait very unsteady; especial disability of right side. Romberg positive: falls backward. Coarse ataxia right hand and foot. (2) *Extracerebellar. Cerebral nerves.* Vth—Hypaesthesia to all forms of sensation on right (no note on corneal reflex). Jaw deflects to right. VIth—Internal squint on right. VIIth—No evident motor involvement: some loss of taste on right anterior two-thirds of tongue. VIIIth—Complete deafness on right to all forks (AC and BC) and voice sounds, but middle tones of Galton whistle can be heard. No x-ray porus. IXth, Xth, XIth—Dysarthria and right ageusia. XIIth—Tongue protrudes to right (probably motor Vth— cf. position of jaw).

Clinical diagnosis.—Cerebellar tumor. Presumable site not noted.

Jan. 18, 1906. Operation.—Attempted suboccipital exploration. The anesthetic was badly taken: irregular and labored respiration with cyanosis was present from the outset. This forced an abandonment of the procedure before the exposure of the cerebellum had been completed. He succumbed to a post-operative pneumonia on the third day.

Autopsy.—Anatomical diagnosis: Pneumonia and cerebellopontile tumor. The brain, removed after fixation *in situ*, shows a marked foraminal pressure cone. No note concerning the condition of the porus acusticus. An enucleable tumor in the right lateral recess. Relation of tumor to nerves not particularly noted. The growth has produced a marked secondary hydrops ventriculorum. Histological report (Mallory): "Dural endothelioma; dense and slowly growing." From another section a diagnosis was made of "glioma," as structures suggesting glia fibrils were observed. Still another section examined elsewhere was regarded as "fibroma." A re-examination of the tumor at the present time shows no evidence on its surface of a defect corresponding with a broken attachment in the auditory meatus. The tumor has rather an unusual shape with a central groove. It measures 4 by 4 by 3½ cm. The sections show most beautifully the palisade or regimental alignment of the nuclei in the fibrous zones. In many areas there are whorl arrangements of the cells. The tissue in some sections is almost entirely fibrous, but in others a reticular tissue with occasional round cells predominates. There are swollen cells filled with a lipoid substance and the fibrous bands show some oedema.

Diagnosis (1916).—A typical acoustic neurofibroma.

Comment.—From our present standards, the clinical notes on this case are very incomplete, and it is only incidentally mentioned, in connection with the examination of the cerebellar nerves, that the right ear had been deaf for many years. There is no note as to the presence or absence of tinnitus or possible vertiginous attacks, but it is of interest that deafness was not absolute. Of course, this was before the days of satisfactory labyrinthine tests. The general symptoms were very advanced, with pronounced secondary pressure manifestations. As was the case for patients with brain tumors a decade ago, near blindness had supervened before surgical intervention was contemplated.

This was my first surgical experience with a recess tumor and, indeed, one of the first with a cerebellar exposure for any purpose and the outcome was not encouraging, for the difficulties of position, anesthesia, or both seemed almost insurmountable. The experience proved a

valuable one, however, for it led to the development of the outrigger with shoulder supports, which has since been utilized in all subsequent posterior operations, as will be told in a later chapter.

From our present vantage point, the confusions relating to the histology of the lesion are interesting to look back upon, particularly as the characteristic nuclear arrangements in this tumor are so striking. The designation of fibroma was a most natural one.

The following case, likewise, is far advanced, and the patient had been subjected before admission to various so-called decompressive cranial procedures in the hope of checking the progressive loss of vision.

CASE 2

J.H.H. Surg. No. 18939. A left acoustic tumor with an advanced local syndrome and general pressure disturbances which had progressed to blindness. Three previous decompressive operations. Partial removal of tumor. Survival three years, eight months.

Mar. 25, 1906. Admission of Albert H. F., age 25, a salesman, recommended by Dr. Frederick Greenbaum of West Frankfort, Illinois., with the complaint of "brain tumor." Trauma eight years or more ago; a fall striking left occiput producing a superficial scalp wound; no serious after-effects.

Chronology of symptoms.—For several years defective hearing in the left ear (significance not appreciated). First symptoms associated with existing malady began nine months ago, with dizziness and a sense of rotation, and ringing noises with pulsation in the left ear. He soon noticed a difficulty in climbing stairs and that he "could not walk straight." This was followed by a marked unsteadiness of gait, ascribed to weakness of the left leg. Soon the left arm and hand became involved. Some suboccipital headaches; never severe: subsiding under iodides. Periods of diplopia, and for past month rapid failure of vision, with complete blindness five days before admission.

Treatment before admission.—A prolonged course of iodides. On *February 10* a trephine opening over left cerebellar hemisphere without incision of the dura; no relief. On *March 7* another opening over right cerebellar hemisphere with dura unopened. On *March 17* an osteoplastic flap over right cerebellar region with puncture and withdrawal of fluid: dura intact. On same day a small subtemporal decompression with incision of dura: wound not completely healed.

Positive neurological findings.—(A) *General pressure.* Optic atrophy with blindness secondary to choked disc. Protrusion of recent small subtemporal decompression. No present headaches or vomiting. No x-ray studies. Deep reflexes exaggerated with possible increase in left over right: superficial plantar normal. (B) *Localizing.* (1) *Cerebellar.* Nystagmus, coarser excursions to left. Conjugate movements to either side poorly sustained. A coarse ataxia of entire left side of astonishing degree. Gait and station impossible to test. (2) *Extracerebellar. Cerebral nerves.* Vth—Hypaesthesia over entire left trigeminal field: areflexa cornealis. Jaw deflects to the left. VIth—Negative: history of diplopia. VIIth—Weakness of expressional movements on left: imperfect winking reflex. Taste not tested. VIIIth—Complete left deafness. No x-ray; no caloric tests. IXth. Xth, XIth,—Considerable dysarthria. XIIth—Tongue protrudes to left (probably from trigeminal motor palsy and deflection of jaw).

Clinical diagnosis.—Tumor of left lateral recess.

April 3, 1906. Operation.—Through a "cross-bow" incision giving a bilateral exposure with chief removal of bone on the left, the angle was well exposed. The growth, together with the cerebellar hemisphere, which had been covered by a protecting pledget of cotton, were both retracted to the right side so that the lesion, which at first was completely overlooked, was not seen until the search, which had been carried nearly to the auditory meatus, was about to be abandoned. A nodular, encapsulated, movable growth was finally disclosed. In the attempt to enucleate it intact, it was broken in two and possibly only about its lower half was removed. The upper fragment was left in place.

Post-operative notes.—The patient made a good surgical recovery despite a temporary increase in his dysarthria with some difficulty in swallowing. There was otherwise no change in the local neurological findings. The wound healed *per primam*. He was discharged *April 26, 1906.*

Pathologic note.—Sections of the tissue show for the most part a fibrous basis with some tendency in places to palisade and whorl formation. There are large areas of sparse round cells in a reticular meshwork. Many of these cells are large with abundant protoplasm containing a large nucleus, and they suggest ganglion cells.

Subsequent notes.—The patient was lost track of until the appearance of a paper by Dr. Julius Grinker in 1910, in which his case was reported. His death occurred suddenly while conversing over the telephone on Dec. 2, 1909, three years and eight months after the operation. "He had a peculiar seizure, in which he fell backward, striking the ground with his head and becoming unconscious." Coma supervened and he died two hours later. Postmortem examination showed a recent hemorrhage filling the subarachnoid cyst around a large growth, obviously, from the photograph, an acoustic tumor. The growth was reported to be a "glioma."

Comment.—This is one of the few cases in which there was a definite history of local injury. In this respect, the acoustic tumors differ from many other forms of intracranial tumor, particularly the endotheliomata, in which trauma so frequently figures as an apparent predisposing cause. The significance of the initial auditory disturbances was not appreciated when this patient was seen, and it is not improbable that they were of long standing and accompanied by vertiginous attacks. These matters were not investigated thoroughly, and the fact that his unilateral deafness was mentioned only casually among the notes of the physical examination

With our present experience, it is quite possible that a total enucleation of this favorable tumor might have been accomplished. (pp. 18–25)

Thus, it can be seen that Cushing's first two cases were one fatality and one survival. The operative mortality rate in acoustic tumors reported by leading European surgeons of the time ran from 70% to 90%. Why, with this shocking mortality, were not all further attempts at acoustic tumor surgery abandoned? Why not let the patient live the remaining months or years before inevitable, sudden respiratory failure and death? Why perform a surgery with an 80% chance that the patient would not live more than a few days?

Insight into the answers to these questions is given by Cushing in his discussion of his third acoustic tumor, operated in September, 1906. The patient was a 42-year-old woman with a 4-year history of deafness and a 3-year history of severe cerebellar ataxia, which made her bedridden. She had severe occipital headaches with marked suboccipital pain and tenderness. The patient had been given antiluetic treatment. Two years before surgery, she began developing vision loss and blind spells. A year before surgery, she had become completely blind and had lost most of her hearing, apparently due to pressure on the eighth nerve opposite the site of the lesion. A bilateral suboccipital craniotomy was done with intracapsular removal of a large portion of her tumor. She made a good postoperative recovery, with marked lessening of headache and even some improvement in vision. The ataxia subsided, enabling her to walk about without assistance. Three years later, she developed difficulty swallowing and died suddenly, apparently from respiratory failure. Cushing commented:

In view of the advanced symptoms the results in this case were as good as might be expected—with three and a half years of fairly comfortable life. Had the operation been carried out a year before, when the diagnosis was first made, or even a few months earlier, so that the unfortunate woman might have enjoyed life with vision, the results would have been still more gratifying. (p. 26)

From this description, we can conclude that patients with acoustic tumors in the early 1900s were not properly diagnosed until they were extremely far advanced. Their suffering was intense, including headache, blindness, vomiting, dizziness, and ataxia. Only very few of these patients found their way to a medical center where a diagnosis of posterior fossa lesion could be established. The popular diagnosis at the time for any illness that the doctor could not explain was syphilis, since the Wasserman test had not yet been developed. In most instances, patients were kept comfortable until death by the use of opiates (e.g., laudanum), which were readily available over the counter. The first drug laws regulating narcotics did not come into being in the United States until 1914. These medications must have further depressed respiratory function, mercifully hastening death, due to pneumonia or respiratory failure.

Unless this bleak picture of the patient with an acoustic tumor is kept in mind, the brilliant contributions of Cushing and others cannot be appreciated adequately. Cushing's surgical approach at this time was purely palliative. He attempted to decrease the elevated intracranial pressure by decompression of the suboccipital area by partial removal of the tumor.

Eleven years after he had treated Case No. 3, he stated in his monograph:

It has taken many years and much insistance to make the profession appreciate that a choked disc is a mechanical process due to tension which can be surgically relieved even though a localizing diagnosis cannot be made. It will doubtless take many years more to make them feel that it is somewhat disgraceful under these circumstances to permit a patient to become blind or even to allow the process to advance to such a stage that vision becomes impaired. (p. 275)

Thus, even in his early years, Cushing was thinking about better diagnosis and increasing the awareness of doctors of acoustic tumors so that these patients could be referred for surgical relief at a much earlier stage. In addition, he and surgeons all over the world were thinking of better surgical techniques to lower the mortality of patients who presented for treatment. More on the diagnostic aspects later. Now, let us examine the surgical ideas of the day.

In the early 1900s, the radical mastoid operation had been perfected. A number of surgeons confined their activities to aural surgery. They also were involved with the management of draining abscesses that had spread to the middle or posterior cranial fossa from the mastoid and with the management of lateral and sigmoid sinus thrombosis. It was only natural that neurologists enlisted the aid of these surgeons in surgical treatment of patients diagnosed with a posterior fossa tumor. The earliest attempts at tumor removal had been made through the Krause approach, which was a unilateral suboccipital approach, but it produced high mortality (Krause, 1903). Panse (1904) reasoned that a more direct approach would be through the temporal bone. This operation was termed a translabyrinthine operation. Apparently, it was a radical mastoidectomy with removal of all of the labyrinth, the cochlea, and the facial nerve. Also apparently, only a few of these procedures were performed, with high mortality due to hemorrhage from the venous sinuses surrounding the temporal bone or due to cerebrospinal leak through the mastoid cavity. This leak was extremely difficult to control with the the iodoform gauze packing that was used at that time. In 1911, Quix, of Utrecht, excised a small tumor. The patient, who died 6 months later, was found to have only a partial removal of the tumor (Quix, 1915). However, Zange (1915) and Schmiegelow (1915) had performed more operations with the translabyrinthine approach and were recommending its use.

Later, the translabyrinthine approach was combined with the suboccipital approach and, in a few cases, the sigmoid sinus also was ligated. In 1913, Marx was able to find a record of only five combined translabyrinthine-suboccipital approaches. One of the main causes of death of these patients was meningitis from the cerebrospinal fluid fistula through the radical mastoid cavity (Marx, 1913). The few patients who survived had partial removals, with little relief of increased intracranial pressure symptoms due to lack of decompression of the posterior fossa. These patients had facial paralysis that did not result from the partial suboccipital removal.

Cushing, in his description of the various procedures used at the time, prophetically stated:

> It is, however, within the realm of possibility that in the case of a very early and minute tumor largely limited to the internal canal the translabyrinthine operation may in time become the operation of choice, but this will necessitate far more precocious and more exact diagnosis than we as yet are capable of. (p. 249)

Over the years, then, Cushing developed and standardized his bilateral suboccipital exposure, combined with partial removal of the acoustic tumor. Cushing summarized the advantage of the operation as he perfected it:

> From the outset this operation has seemed to possess certain advantages which are lacking in those heretofore described. Briefly, they lie in the wide bilateral exposure of the posterior surface of the cerebellum, and this, combined with the early evacuation of the cerebrospinal fluid, serves to promptly relieve the intracranial tension which in turn permits of sufficient dislocation of the hemispheres to expose the recess without jeopardizing the medullary centers or traumatizing the adjacent cerebellar lobe. Moreover, carefully planned haemostasis not only makes it possible to carry the procedure through in one session, but justifed an exact reapproximation of the divided tissues in layers without drainage, thereby greatly lessening the risk of postoperative complications

as well as giving the patient a sound and presentable neck. The large cranial opening, furthermore, serves as an effective palliative measure not only against the possible early edema but as a future decompression in view of almost inevitable continuance of the growth. Some of the imperfections of the operation, as it has been outlined, lie in its magnitude, the expenditure of time,—for one could hardly undertake two such procedures in a day,—and the fact that a partial intracapsular enucleation is advocated at the present time rather than an attempted complete extirpation. These, however, are drawbacks which must necessarily characterize all operations for tumors in this difficult region if they are undertaken with due precautions and respect for life. (pp. 272–273)

Most attempts at total enucleation of the tumor at this time were done by inserting a finger through the suboccipital area and attempting to pull the tumor out piecemeal or totally. Bleeding from branches of the basilar artery often was profuse, leading to immediate fatality. If the patient did survive, a facial paralysis and involvement of the ninth, tenth, eleventh, and twelfth cranial nerves resulted. Therefore, Cushing abandoned early attempts at total removal. He simply scooped out the center of the tumor with a curette, then placed Zinker's solution in the interior of the tumor to stop bleeding.

In 1911, Cushing developed silver clips. obviously, these were a major advance in the control of intracranial bleeding (Cushing, 1911). However, what was done in the first 17 years of the twentieth century to achieve better diagnosis of these tumors? A review of the case histories and findings of 30 verified and 3 unverified acoustic tumors in Cushing's book reveals that these patients presented at the Hopkins and Harvard clinics in the last stages of brain tumor development. Most patients had dysarthria; many had mental dullness that comes with elevated intracranial pressure. Soon after being seen, these patients be-

came comatose. Most patients were so ataxic that they were bedridden, able to stand only with assistance. They had severe headaches, suboccipital discomfort, and impaired vision. Several were totally blind from elevated intracranial pressure. Cushing also mentioned cerebellar crises that were "paroxysm of a most extreme and agonizing type, with retraction of the neck and back, respiratory difficulties, and altered pulse, a sense of impending death and often with loss of consciousness" (p. 231).

One can imagine Cushing at the bedside of these horribly ill patients. He must have been tempted to take a brief history from a relative about the duration of the headache and ataxia, examine the opti fundi (the ophthalmoscope had been made portable and electric by Dennett in the early 1900s), then proceed with a general neurologic examination to determine the "localizing signs," which were recorded as cerebellar and extracerebellar in nature. These measures obviously would have been enough to place the lesion in the posterior fossa and probably determine the side of the lesion. However, he criticized himself for his poor evaluation of Case 1, for which, under clinical diagnosis, he states simply, "cerebellar tumor, presumable site not noted."

In reading Cushing's case histories, we see more and more careful documentation of the development of the patient's symptoms and more increasingly detailed neurologic evaluation. As new clinical tests became available, they were evaluated carefully and applied. Hearing tests were more than just a whisper in each ear; the tuning fork test and the Galto whistle test were used. The problems of masking in unilateral hearing losses obviously were appreciated and were discussed in his book:

> In reviewing the records it has been of interest to find that the first observer in going over the cerebral nerves has sometimes been confused regarding the question of deafness, and in a number of patients it was thought that bone conduc-

tion was present and, in some instances, air conduction also, when both were subsequently disproved. The absence of the latter, indeed, has only been absolutely certified in some patients by the complete deafness to external sounds which ensues when the unaffected ear is being irrigated in the course of the caloric tests. As Grey points out, the perception of after tones and the transmission of tones of the fork in the opposite ear somewhat interfere with the Rinne test and not infrequently, even with acoustic tumors of large size, the tones perceived by the unaffected ear are referred by the patient in part to the diseased side. (p. 154)

Early in the twentieth century, Barany published many articles on caloric testing (Barany, 1906, 1908, 1910a, 1910b, 1913). His work won him the Nobel prize in 1914. Cushing described the first use of caloric tests in his Case 8, of September, 1910. The differentiation between labyrinthine unsteadiness and cerebella ataxia was an important topic in neurologic circles of the day and was discussed fully by Wilson and Pike (1915b). X-rays had been discovered by Roentgen in 1895. Its first successful use in disclosing an intracranial tumor was in 1897, when Oppenheim detected the absence of the landmarks of the sella turcica and correctly diagnosed a tumor of the pituitary body. It was not until 1912, however, that Henschen reasoned from his study of autopsy cases of acoustic tumors that the dilated porus acusticus should be visible by X-ray (Henschen, 1912). Schuller, in a book on X-ray findings in patients with intracranial tumors, emphasized widening of the sinusoidal grooves and dilation of the siploetic vessels. The book described a lateral projection of the temporal bones, called the Schuller position. This position was used to attempt to visualize the dilated porus acusticus. However, confusion often resulted because of superimposition of the external auditory canal and the internal auditory canal. Nevertheless, in 1913, in Case 12 of his monograph, Cushing mentioned

that X-rays of the porus acusticus were not conclusive. It was to be many years before X-ray techniques would be perfected to be of real value.

Over a period of 15 years, Cushing questioned not only his patients, but also, their relatives, I am sure. He carefully recorded all of the myriads of details obtained—some relevant, some irrelevant. He did this not only for acoustic tumors, but for all tumors he found in his large, clinical practice. Gradually, the chronology of the symptoms of acoustic tumors began to form in Cushing's mind. His methods and conclusions were clinical research at its finest. At the end of his chapter on symptomatology he discussed his conclusions in brilliant simplicity:

> From the above group analyses of the individual symptoms, as well as from the story connected with the case histories, it can be gathered that the symptomatic progress of the average acoustic tumor occurs more or less in the following stages: First, the auditory and labyrinthine manifestations; second, the occipitofrontal pains with suboccipital discomforts; third, the incoordination and instability of cerebellar origin; fourth, the evidences of involvement of adjacent cerebral nerves; fifth, the indications of increase in intracranial tension with a choked disc and its consequences; sixth, dysarthria, dysphagia, and finally cerebellar crises and respiratory difficulties. (p. 158)

In several other places of the monograph, Cushing emphasized that unilateral hearing loss is the first symptom of an acoustic tumor, and that it is a symptom about which the patient must be carefully questioned:

> The chronology of symptoms in the foregoing series of cases makes it clear that the clinical diagnosis of an acoustic tumor can be made with reasonable assurance only when auditory manifestations definitely precede the evidences of involvement of other structures in the cerebellopontine angle.

It would appear that patients rarely call attention to the premonitory auditory symptoms, which are either forgotten or are not associated with the subsequent and more incapacitating phenomena, and it is equally certain that the sequence is apt to be slighted by the questioner. On the other hand, a progressive unilateral loss of hearing, if unattended by tinnitus, may not be observed by the patient, and it is interesting to note how often, when it is observed, attention is called to the fact by disability in use of the telephone (cf. Cases XX, XXIV, XXV, and XXVIII). (p. 152)

Today, some 60 years later, it is unfortunate that we still see patients who have noted a difficulty in one ear while using the telephone and who, at that point, are not evaluated carefully for an acoustic tumor.

Thus, Cushing made great contributions to the early diagnosis of acoustic tumors. It was not until publication of his book in 1917 that his better diagnosis was appreciated by others in the medical profession. Cushing did not have the advantage that the next generation of surgeons was to have: referral at a less advanced stage in the development of the acoustic tumor. Therefore, during these years, his attempts to lower the morbidity and mortality of this condition concentrated on improved surgical technique. His summary of the analysis of mortality with these cases is a masterpiece:

(1) *The operative mortality*. This in the case of cerebellopontile-angle tumors, the majority of them as we have seen being acoustic tumors, has been variously estimated—though always high. This is so both for the cases assembled from miscellaneous reports in the literature as well as from the reports from individual clinics.

Henschen in 1910 collected 43 cases with partial tumor removal of which only 8 lived for any length of time. Leischner's statistics gathered in 1911, including 10 cases from Eiselberg's clinic, gave a mortality of 70 per cent. According to Fumarola, Krause had only 4 recoveries in a series of 30 angle tumors (86.6 per cent mortality) and Eiselberg in 1912, 4 recoveries in 12 cases (66.6 per cent mortality). Tooth's statistics of the operations with removal, complete or partial, of extracerebellar tumors during the years 1902 to 1912 at the National Hospital gave 24 cases with 17 deaths attributed to the operation (70.8 per cent), whereas 11 out of 12 cases succumbed after a mere suboccipital decompression for tumor (91.6 per cent). In the 70 cases of which Henschen found record between 1910 and 1915 there was a 68.7 per cent mortality.

Shocking as these figures are and desperate as the condition must be which justifies operation attended with such high risks, it must be acknowledged that they represent the experience of surgeons who at the time of their report had had but few cases, and whose later records would have been far better. After the first operation the surgical mortality in the writer's series of acoustic tumors was 100 per cent. After the first 10 cases it was lowered to 40 per cent, after 15 cases it had dropped to 33.3 per cent, after 20 cases to 30 per cent, after 25 cases to 24 per cent, and after 30 cases to 20 per cent; and it must continue to fall until it drops to 10 or 5 per cent or better, even though the total figures must carry the burden of early inexperience. (p. 274)

In his first chapter, Cushing (1917) summarized the great difference between his era and the first era of acoustic tumor history, the nineteenth century, which was dominated by the principle of clinical observation and autopsy findings, as outlined by John Hunter. The second era or, as I like to call it, the Cushing era, saw a transition to the ability to study surgical pathology, rather than autopsy pathology:

Whereas formerly occasional examples of the various types of tumor might have been made the subject of study, the opportunity of investigating the lesion except at autopsy was rarely given and then only as a terminal condition after the clinical picture had become more or less confused. Today the opportunity is given of verifying the lesion in an increasing number of cases at a much more early stage than has heretofore been possible, and the operating room has largely supplanted the postmortem laboratory as the source of material for study. This is merely a repetition of the story concerning lesions in many other parts of the body. (pp. 1–2)

The most important legacy of the Cushing era was the elucidation of the chronology of the development of symptoms of patients with acoustic tumors. The speciality of neurosurgery was established firmly during this time, and the concepts and techniques of intracranial surgery were improved vastly. All over the world, great teachers of neurosurgery now were indoctrinating the next generation of surgeons. They were able to spend their entire careers in the field of neurosurgery, starting at the level of expertise at which their teachers left off.

The next era of the acoustic tumor was to last from the beginning of World War I until after the end of World War II, when microsurgical techniques were introduced. During this time, there were no dominating Cushings. Instead, many individuals contributed to the step-by-step progress in diagnosis and surgery that steadily improved the outlook of patients with acoustic tumors.

By the beginning of World War I, all of the important elements in the management of acoustic tumors had come into being. Cushing had elucidated brilliantly the progression of symptoms of these lesions, from the earliest unilateral hearing loss to death some years later caused by respiratory failure due to elevated intracranial pressure. Systematic neurologic examinations and the hearing and vestibular tests of the day were applied to these patients. Subjecting the temporal bone to X rays had begun.

On the surgical side, anesthesia had improved steadily since its discovery 75 years previously. The antiseptic principles of Lister, which made brain surgery possible, were being replaced gradually by the concepts of aseptic surgery. Decompression of increased intracranial pressure, introduced

by Cottrell (1899), was fairly well understood. The methods of handling brain tissues and controlling hemorrhage by the use of Horsley's bone wax and Cushing's clips now were widespread knowledge. Most importantly, neurosurgery now had become a specialty, so that diagnosis was linked to surgery and surgery to diagnosis, each putting pressure on the other for constant improvement. This era of the acoustic tumor saga was to last 40 years, until the introduction of microsurgery techniques. It was to see the shift away from mere alleviation of symptoms and prolongation of life to an attempt, in almost all cases, to cure the acoustic tumor.

The next dominant figure to emerge on the pages of this history is Walter Dandy. He was a student of Cushing and, after Cushing left for Harvard, he remained at Johns Hopkins Hospital. If Dandy's writings are any indication, he was brilliant, innovative, and very opinionated. Probably one of the greatest neurosurgical technicians of all time, he was able to accomplish surgical results far beyond those of his contemporaries. He lacked the painstaking clinical observation of Cushing, but he made up for this in brilliant surgical observation and innovation. For reasons now somewhat obscured by time, these two men came into conflict, failing to recognize the great synergism of their contributions. Because of Cushing's careful documentation and widespread publication of the symptoms of acoustic tumors, these lesions were being recognized universally at a much earlier stage in their development. Recognition and proper diagnosis of acoustic tumors—in some cases, before any evidence of increased intracranial pressure had occurred—made it necessary to modify the entire thinking regarding the surgical approach to these lesions. Dandy's (1918) first great contribution was the introduction of cerebral pneumography, which, of course, was of great importance in the localization and preoperative assessment of all intracranial masses.

By 1925, most acoustic tumors were diagnosed when symptoms included unilateral progressive hearing loss, fifth nerve numbness, and elevated intracranial pressure. However, they were rarely in the extremes of Cushing's cases. Obviously, an operation designed to decompress the posterior fossa and partially remove the tumor in order to give a few years of more comfortable life was inappropriate for these cases. Dandy correctly recognized that, if surgery were to be undertaken at this stage in the development of the acoustic tumor, the object of the surgery must be to cure the patient of his tumor and not merely to palliate his symptoms.

In 1915, when Dandy saw his first two cases, he apparently tried surgical decompression, which consisted of bilateral cerebellar exposure and opening of the posterior fossa dura (Dandy, 1925). Both patients died within 12 hr. Both had elevated intracranial pressure but were conscious and in good physical condition at the time of the operation. He reasoned that the problem was the shift of both of the cerebellar hemispheres and the brainstem away from the tumor and, in addition, the pressure downward on the tentorium by the elevated intracranial pressure due to hydrocephalus. He recognized the block of the aqueduct of Sylvius, but he did not indicate whether he used a ventricular tap during this procedure. His article reveals him to be aware of this procedure:

> Krause (1903) introduced a very useful procedure to reduce the excessive pressure which was nearly always present with cerebellopontile tumors. A trocar was passed through the tentorium into the lateral ventricle permitting the evacuation of its fluid. This procedure (ventricular puncture), in much more refined form, has come to be a most important item in all operations for tumors below the tentorium. (p. 132)

Cushing, in his 1917 monograph, also recommended this procedure in all of his surgical cases. Dandy continued:

> In desperation, our next effort, total extirpation with the finger at one stage, then seemed the only alternative. It was, of course, merely a reversion to the well tried and fruitless method of Horsley, Krause, Eiselsberg and others. Nor was there reason to expect better results. After two initial successes, four deaths in succession showed the futility of further attempts. (p. 134)

Sudden traumatic removal of the tumor by this method resulted in what he called an "excessive bleeding," controlled by packing with cotton, then attempting to find the bleeders to clip. He also placed small bits of muscle over the bleeders, as had been recommended many years previously by Horsley.

Next, he tried Cushing's intracapsular enucleation on three cases, resulting in one recovery and two later fatalities from meningitis, one on the fourth postoperative day and one on the forty-sixth day:

> Despite enthusiastic hopes (for intracapsular enucleation as introduced by Cushing), however, our first experiences with intracapsular enucleation were unfortunate in being less satisfactory than had been anticipated. Following an uneventful and quick recovery from the effects of the operation, the first patient 7 days later became listless and drowsy; vomiting, dysphagia and dysarthria appeared; and during the succeeding 3 days all symptoms became progressively worse and finally alarming. The late appearance of these symptoms seemed to exclude the postoperative complications which might have been expected, hemorrhage or infection, and suggested that in some way the reaction about the stump of tumor which remained was responsible for the condition. The wound was reopened and the shell of the tumor extirpated with the index finger. There was surprisingly little hemorrhage, which was readily controlled. The patient's condition then steadily improved. Diminished drowsiness was at once apparent, the vomiting at once ceased, and 5 days later she was able to

swallow. From the result of this case it seemed logical to infer that if the shell of the tumor could in some way be removed at the first operation, this stormy and dangerous course following subtotal removal might be avoided. (p. 134)

Apparently, two more cases then were done in two stages, the second stage being the finger enucleation. This was followed by combining intracapsular enucleation with a finger enucleation of the partially removed tumor at one stage. Dandy now recognized that the finger enucleation was far too unreliable and often traumatic. Therefore, he developed a very painstaking removal of the capsule following extensive enucleation of the interior of the tumor. He describes it this way:

> The contents of the tumor are then curetted with the brainstem and cerebellum always fully exposed. Continuing this method, the capsule gradually becomes thinner and when drawn forward permits inspection of the cleavage line between the brainstem and capsule of the tumor. When the poles of the tumor have invaded the middle cranial fossa and the spinal canal, removal of their interior allows them to be easily withdrawn into the posterior fossa; such polar extensions of the tumor are least adherent to the brainstem. Gradually in this way the entire capsule is separated from the brainstem. As the capsule is cautiously retracted, several small blood vessels crossing from the brainstem or cerebellum are brought into view and double 'clipped' and the vessel divided. Practically all bleeding can be forstalled in this way. Removal of the capsule of the tumor in this way is necessarily very tedious and time consuming. The method employed is but the application of the fundamental surgical teachings of my former chief, the late Professor Halsted. By this great master every operation, whether unusual or commonplace, was performed with the utmost care. All tissues were handled with the greatest gentleness, the field unstained with blood, and a step was never taken blindly. Always his work was painstaking, the field of operation immaculate, and hemorrhage minimal. Time of operation was always subordinate to accurate and thorough performance. (p. 137)

By 1925, 9 years after he had entered practice, Dandy had treated 23 acoustic tumors. He had been able to cure surgically five successive patients. This was a truly monumental achievement. Dandy's next contribution was to modify the surgical approach to a unilateral cerebellar approach by gaining exposure through an incision of the outer cap of the cerebellum. This approach became the standard method of removal of acoustic tumors until the advent of microsurgery in 1961, and it is well illustrated in Dandy's 1940 article (Dandy, 1969).

Dandy's techniques obviously were brilliant, because they lowered operative mortality and, at the same time, affected a cure. However, they resulted in total loss of facial nerve function in virtually every case. In years to come, there were attempts, especially by Olivecrona (1967a, 1967b), to save facial nerve function by using Dandy's techniques.

Over the years, as diagnoses were made earlier, many more tumors were seen before an elevated intracranial pressure had occurred. It became recognized universally and accepted that, in operating on smaller tumors, the operative mortality was much decreased. At first, this was believed to be the case simply because these patients had less preoperative edema of the brain, since they did not have elevated intracranial pressure and, therefore, postoperative brainstem infarction was reduced greatly. Dandy (1969) recommended clipping and cauterizing the vessels surrounding the tumor. Apparently, there was no appreciation of the end-artery status of the anterior-inferior cerebellar artery.

Atkinson (1949) published a careful study documenting his discovery that occlusion of the anterior-inferior cerebellar artery is the principal cause of operative fatality in acoustic neuroma surgery. Previously, brainstem infarction and cerebellar edema seen at the autopsy of patients shortly after acoustic tumor surgery were believed to be due to excessive manipulation of these structures during the surgical procedure. The condition of brainstem infarction and cerebellar edema was called malacia pontis. Atkinson reviewed the postoperative course of six patients who died within several days following removal of acoustic neuromas. In each case, either a thrombosis or surgical division of the anterior-inferior cerebellar artery was found. In one of the cases, the tumor was small, its size approximating a pigeon's egg. The anterior-inferior cerebellar artery was torn as it went across the inferior surface of the tumor. Atkinson noted necrosis of the pons and cerebellar peduncles in the area of distribution of the anterior-inferior cerebellar artery in each of these cases. Atkinson's observations explained a major cause of operative mortality, but they did not result in changes in surgical technique, because magnification was not being used and because once an artery—the anterior-inferior cerebellar or any other—was torn, it had to be controlled by clipping or cautery.

Until now, we have been telling the story of the acoustic tumor from the perspectives of the pioneers who were contributing to its management. Let us now diverge to a description of the treatment of a typical acoustic tumor diagnosed during the time from the end of World War II until the advent of the microsurgical treatment in 1961.

World War II had stimulated great interest in neurosurgery, with a large number of well-trained young neurosurgeons entering practice between 1945 and 1950. Almost all hospitals had a staff neurosurgeon who was considered capable of management of all neurosurgical problems, including cerebellopontine angle tumors. These specialists, who might have seen only two or three acoustic tumors in their practice, usually proceeded with surgical management upon presentation of a case. Twenty years earlier, when there were few neurosurgical clinics,

a surgeon saw more cases and, thus, became more skilled in the techniques that had been standardized so beautifully by Dandy. It became widely recognized that the average neurosurgeon treated brain tumors, especially acoustic neuromas, with a higher morbidity and mortality rate than did the neurosurgeon who had gained great experience in large teaching centers.

After World War II, most acoustic tumors were diagnosed by otologists. The surgical treatment of otosclerosis, so firmly established by Lempert in the late 1930s, had spurred careful evaluation of patients with hearing loss. Vestibular studies now were being used commonly in the evaluation of patients with dizziness. X rays of the petrous pyramids, pioneered by Hinchen and perfected by Towne and others in the 1920s, now had become a standard practice. Unilateral hearing loss combined with facial numbness now equaled the diagnosis of acoustic neuroma in the minds of all otolaryngologists. These patients routinely were referred for surgical evaluation. In a growing number of cases, patients with unilateral hearing loss were evaluated carefully by X-ray and vestibular studies, enabling the discovery of tumors, the symptoms of which still were confined to the eighth nerve. It was at this point that a great dilemma arose: Should the patient be subjected to surgery immediately, trading partial hearing loss for total hearing loss and facing a facial paralysis and a significant fatality risk from the surgery, or should the patient be observed for a few more years, and allowed to enjoy a normal life without facial paralysis until more symptoms develop due to a larger tumor? At the later time of surgery, the patient not only would suffer postoperative facial paralysis, but there he also would be a much higher risk of operative mortality and morbidity due to the larger size of the tumor. In many cases, the patient was observed for a few years until marked fifth nerve paresthesia and, usually, early papilledema presented. Watchful expectation was championed by Pennybacker and Cairnes (1950); immediate surgery was championed by Dandy (1925).

If all surgeons could have duplicated the 2.4% mortality that Dandy encountered in a particularly good run of 41 cases, then the early surgery demanded by otologists and neurosurgeons would have been justified. However, Dandy's lifetime mortality was 22.1% (Revilla, 1948). Mortality figures for acoustic tumors for most surgeons at this time varied quite widely, seemingly in relation to the experience of the surgeon. When the results of a number of surgeons who were not doing a significant volume of tumors were compiled, the mortality figures were higher, as pointed out by Bloch and Nathanson (1963) in the Mount Sinai Hospital series. Their series of 64 cases had an overall mortality of 31%. Figures presented by the California Tumor Registry about this time were discouraging. They showed that, from 1942 to 1962, various neurosurgeons in reporting hospitals operated on 85 patients. Thirty-one patients died within 1 month of surgery, representing a mortality of 36.5%. Another six patients died within 1 year, representing a mortality of 43.5%.

Pool (1966), an experienced neurosurgeon, reported an operative mortality of 12.5% for 72 cases operated between 1950 and 1965. Olivecrona, who reported a total of 415 acoustic neuromas operated between 1931 and 1960, obviously was the world's most experienced operator at that time. His overall mortality was 19.2% (Olivecrona, 1967a). Olivecrona (1967a) conclusively pointed out that his mortality was almost five times as high for large tumors as it was for the group he considered to include small tumors or as he described them, "hazel nut size." The difference was 4.5% for in the small tumors and 22.5% mortality for the large tumors.

The mortality, however, was not the only issue to be considered. In many cases, a complete disabling due to severe ataxia and sometimes contralateral paresis made the patient incapable of self-care. This disabling occurred in 18% of survivors in a study compiled of 125 cases from the Ricks Hospital in Copenhagen (Thomsen, 1976).

Thus, in 1960, 60 years after the beginning of active interest in the diagnosis and surgery of acoustic tumors, it was clear that definitive diagnosis was far more advanced than definitive surgical treatment. The challenge was obvious. New surgical methods would have to be found that would allow us to take advantage of the low surgical mortality of operating on small tumors and, at the same time, preserve facial nerve function. This challenge was met in the next era of the history of the acoustic tumor by the applications of microsurgical techniques.

REFERENCES

Atkinson, W. J. (1949). Anterior-inferior cerebellar artery. *Journal of Neurology, Neurosurgery, and Psychiatry, 12*, 137–151.

Ballance, C. (1907). *Some points in the surgery of the brain and its membranes* (p. 276). London: Macmillan.

Ballance, C. (1919). *Essays on the surgery of the temporal bone.* London: Macmillan.

Barany, R. (1906). Untersuchungen uber den vom Vestibularapparat des Ohres reflektorisch ausgeosten rhythmischen Nystagmus und seine Begleiterscheinungen. *Montsschr. Ohrenh. 11*, 193–297.

Barany, R. (1908). Operationsmethode zur Entfernung von Akustikustumoren. *Z. Ohrenh. 4*, 414-415.

Barany, R. (1910a). Die nervosen Storungen des Cochlear- und Vestibularapparates. In V. Lewandowski, *Handbuch der Neurologie,* (Vol. 1, pp. 919–958). Berlin.

Barany, R. (1910b). Spezielle Pathologie der Erkrankungen des Cochlear- und Vestibularapparates. In V. Lewandowski, *Handbuch der Neurologie,* (Vol. 1, pp. 811–873). Berlin.

Barany, R. (1913). Die Ausfuhrung der vestibularen Kleinhirnprufung. *Trans. Int. Cong. Med. (Lond.),* Sec. 11, 53–54.

Bell, C. (1830). The nervous system of the body, Appendix of cases (pp. 112–114). London.

Bloch, J. M., & Nathanson, M. (1963). Results in acoustic neuroma surgery. *Journal of the Sinai Hospital, 30*, 217–227.

Cottrell, B. (1899). Remarks on surgical aspects of a case of cerebellopontine tumor. *Trans. Med. Chir. Soc.* (Edinb.), *18*, 215.

Cruveilhier, J. (1842). *Anatomie pathologique du corps humain,* (Vol. 11, Part 26, pp. 1–8). Paris.

Cushing, H. (1911). The control of bleeding in operations for brain tumors, with the description of silver "clips" for the occlusion of vessels inaccessible to the ligature. *Annals of Surgery,* 4, 1–19.

Cushing, H. (1917). *Tumors of the nervous acusticus and the syndrome of cerebellopontile angle,* (2nd ed.). New York: Hafner Publishing. Reprinted 1967 by W. B. Saunders.

Dandy, W. E. (1918). Ventriculography following the injection of air into the cerebral ventricles. *Annals of Surgery, 68,* 5.

Dandy, W. E. (1925). An operation for the total removal of cerebellopontile angle (acoustic) tumors. *Surgery, Gynecology, and Obstetrics, 41,* 129-148.

Dandy, W. E. (1969). The brain. In *Lewis' Practice of surgery* (p. 527). New York Harper and Row.

Ferrier, D., & Turner, W. (1894). A record of experiments, illustrative of the symptomatology and degenerations following lesions of the cerebellum, etc. *Phil. Tr. Lond. 174,* 476.

Henneberg, & Koch. (1902). Über "centrale" Neurofibromatose und die Geschwulste des Kleinhirnbruckenwinkels (Acusticusneurome). *Arch. F. Psychiat. 36,* 251–304.

Henschen, F. (1912). Die Akustikustumoren, eine neue Gruppe radiographisch darstellbarer Hirntumoren. *Fortschr. a. d. Geb. d. Rontgenstrahlen, 18,* 207–216.

Krause, F. (1903). Zur Freilegung der hinteren Felsenbeinflache und des Kleinhirns. *Beitr. Klin. Chir., 37,* 728–764.

Krumbhaar, E. B. (1941). *A history of medicine.* New York: Alfred A. Knopf.

Luciani, L. (1891). *Il Cerevelletto.* Firenze: R. Instituto di Studi Superiori.

Marx, H. (1913). Zur Chirurgie der Kleinhirnbruckenwinkeltumoren. *Mitt. a. d. Grenzgeb. d. Med. u. Chir., 24,* 117–134.

McBurney, C., & Starr, M. (1893). A contribution to cerebral surgery: Diagnosis, localization and operation for removal of three tumors of the brain, with some comments upon the surgical treatment of brain tumors. *American Journal of the Medical Sciences, 24,* 361–387.

Olivecrona, H. (1967a). Acoustic tumors. *Journal of Neurosurgery, 26,* 6–13.

Olivecrona, H. (1967). The removal of acoustic neurinomas. *Journal of Neurosurgery, 26,* 100–103.

Panse, R. (1904). Ein Gliom des Akustikus. *Arch. Ohrenh., 11,* 251–255.

Pennybacker, J. B., & Cairnes, H. (1950). Results in 130 cases of acoustic neurinoma. *Journal of Neurology, Neurosurgery, and Psychiatry, 13(1),* 272–277.

Pool, J. L. (1966). Sub-occipital surgery for acoustic neuromas: Advantages and disadvantages. *Journal of Neurosurgery, 24,* 483-492.

Quix, F. (1915). Ein Fall von operierter Acusticus-Geschwulst mSt Darstellung mikrophotographischer Lichtbilder und Besprechung der Operationstechnik. *Monatsschr. Ohrenh.* 49, 717–718.

Revilla, A. (1948). Neuromas of the cerebellopontine recess: Clinical study of 160 cases including operative mortality and end results. *Bulletin of the Johns Hopkins Hospital, 83,* 47.

Russell, J. S. R. (1894). Experimental research into the functions of the cerebellum. *Phil. Tr., Lond., 75,* 109.

Russell, J. S. R. (1895). The values of experimental evidence in the diagnosis of diseases of the cerebellum. *British Medical Journal, 2,* 1079.

Russell, J. S. R. (1896). The effects of interrupting afferent and efferent tracts of the cerebellum. *British Medical Journal, 2,* 914.

Schmiegelow, E. (1915). Beitrag zur translabyrintharen Entfernung der Akustikustumoren. *Z. Ohrenh, 23,* 1–21.

Starr, M. (1893). *Brain surgery.* New York: W. Wood & Co.

Stewart, T., & Holmes, G. (1904). Symptomatology of cerebellar tumors: A study of forty cases. *Brain 27,* 522–591.

Thomsen, J. (1976). Sub-occipital removal of acoustic neuromas: Results of 125 operations. *Acta Otolaryngologica, 81,* 406-414.

Towne, E. D. 1926. Erosion of the petrous bone by acoustic nerve tumor. *Archives of Otolaryngology, 4,* 515-519.

Verocay, J. (1910). Zur Kenntnis der "Neurofibrome." *Beitr. Pathol. Anat. Allg. Pathol., 18,* 1–68.

Virchow, R. (1858). Das wahre Neurom. *Arch. f. Path. Anat., 13,* 256–265.

Wilson, J., & Pike, F. (1915a). The differential diagnosis of lesions of the labyrinth and of the cerebellum. *Journal of the American Medical Association, 15,* 2156–2161.

Wilson, J., & Pike, F. (1915b). Vertigo. *Journal of the American Medical Association, 14,* 561-564.

Zange, J. (1915). Translabyrinthare Operationen von Acusticus- und Kleinhirnbruckenwinkeltumoren. *Berl. Klin. Wochenschr., 3,* 1334.

CHAPTER 2

A History of Acoustic Tumor Surgery: 1961–Present

Michael E. Glasscock, III, M.D.
Pamela S. Bohrer, M.D.
Ronald L. Steenerson, M.D.

In the preceding chapter of this book, William F. House provides the reader with a fascinating account of the early history of acoustic tumor diagnosis and surgery. This chapter continues the account, encompassing the time from 1961 to the present.

The three giants in the field of acoustic tumor surgery in this century have been Harvey Cushing, Walter Dandy, and William House, the last of whom is the leading authority on acoustic tumor surgery today. House's personal series is the largest ever accumulated; he has firmly established his place in medical history.

When a person has attained worldwide fame, the success often is seen as an overnight phenomenon resulting from an abundance of luck. In truth, most success stories are founded on hard work and years of preparation and sacrifice. Many times, the individual has had to stand alone and be the recipient of criticism, jealousy and, often, open hostility. New ideas in medicine traditionally have met great resistance. For William House, the early years were not easy ones. This modern era of acoustic tumor surgery began in 1956, when Dr. House made the diagnosis of a tumor in a young Los Angeles fireman. The man had very few symptoms, predominantly unilateral hearing loss and tinnitus. He was referred to a local neurosurgeon for definitive treatment. At that time, neurosurgeons did not operate upon cerebellopontine angle tumors unless symptoms included cranial nerve deficit (exclusive of the eighth cranial nerve), ataxia, or papilledema. The rationale pertained to the high morbidity and mortality rates associated with posterior fossa surgery as it was performed in the 1950s. Most surgeons would wait until the tumors were large and life-threatening before attempting to remove them. The young fireman was observed for 1 year following his diagnosis. At that time, he developed fifth cranial nerve findings, headaches, and papilledema. Surgery was performed by means of the suboccipital route without the benefit of microsurgical technique. The patient died on the third postoperative day.

During the next year, Dr. House diagnosed two additional tumors. These patients survived surgery, but both were left with major neurological deficits. Simultaneously, Dr. House was in the process of developing the middle fossa approach to the contents of the internal auditory canal (House, 1961). He had used this procedure to section the vestibular nerve and to decompress the facial nerve. It occurred to Dr. House that he might be able to approach an acoustic tumor through the middle fossa and identify the facial nerve in the internal auditory canal. His plan was to trace the nerve into the posterior fossa, then remove the remainder of the tumor from the suboccipital route. With these thoughts in mind, Dr. House contacted Dr. John B. Doyle, a Los Angeles neurosurgeon, and formed a surgical team. They aimed at developing a new technique for the removal of acoustic tumors that would lower morbidity and mortality.

The classic middle fossa approach, as employed by neurosurgeons, had been performed always with the surgeon in a seated position. Therefore, Doyle and House made some modifications to the Zeiss operating microscope and asked Mr. Jack Urban of the Urban Engineering Company to design a chair that would provide the surgeon with armrests while operating. The first microsurgical removal of an acoustic tumor was performed on February 15, 1961. As a matter of fact, this was the first use of microsurgical technique in neurosurgery. A partial removal of the tumor was accomplished, and the patient later died in 1967 after two subsequent suboccipital procedures (House, 1977).

The initial eight cases in Dr. House's series were performed through the middle fossa between the dates of February 1961 and May 1962 (House, 1964). At that time, House and Doyle were removing a large part of the labyrinth to expose the posterior fossa. The main reason for choosing the middle fossa route was to be able to identify the facial nerve in the lateral extent of the internal auditory canal, where there were bony landmarks. It soon became apparent that the procedure was unsatisfactory, because very few of the tumors could be removed totally. It occurred to Dr. House that a direct approach through the mastoid and labyrinth might be a better choice, particularly since he and Doyle already were destroying the labyrinth.

Panse (1904) had approached the cerebellopontine angle through the mastoid in the early 1900s but lacked the aid of microsurgical technique and adequate instrumentation. In his procedure a radical mastoidectomy was performed, and the facial nerve was removed. As one would expect, there was a great deal of difficulty with postoperative cerebrospinal fluid leak. Having become interested in the possibility of this approach, Dr. House performed a series of cadaver dissections in order to work out a method of exposing the internal auditory canal and cerebellopontine angle through the labyrinth. With the aid of magnification, the dental drill, and irrigation/suction, he was able to devise this method, as well as preserve the posterior canal wall, tympanic membrane, and facial nerve.

With the development of the translabyrinthine approach, a difference of opinion ensued between the two surgeons. This philosophical separation of ideas was the beginning of a long and continuing controversy concerning the best method of dealing with cerebellopontine angle lesions. House's first translabyrinthine procedure was performed without the assistance of Doyle. In fact, there was a heated argument concerning the case just prior to surgery. However, House and Doyle continued to work together during this time period and performed some surgical cases as one-stage, some as two-stage, and a few from the suboccipital route using the microscope.

Obviously, at this point, there was some question about whether the technique could be employed for the removal of larger tumors. In 1963, House and Doyle no longer could agree upon basic techniques. In July of that year, Dr. William Hitselberger began to work with Dr. House, and they became a unique surgical team. After further cadaver dissections, they began to employ the translabyrinthine procedure on a routine basis for tumors of all sizes. Dr. House's first 53 cases, most of which had been performed with Dr. Hitselberger, were reported in 1964. Many of these cases were subtotal; as the surgeons gained experience, however, this percentage dropped (House, 1968).

Dr. Hitselberger worked diligently to learn temporal bone anatomy and surgical technique. He mastered the microscope and dental drill and became the first neurosurgeon to perform mastoidectomy and labyrinthectomy surgery routinely. His association with Dr. House and the translabyrinthine procedure, however, did not make him popular with his neurosurgical colleagues. During their pioneering year, House and Hitselberger underwent close scrutiny by the Los Angeles neurosurgical community. At St. Vincent's Hospital, interdepartmental bickering and politics became a very real issue. At one point, the administrator of the hospital had to lock Dr. House's charts in her personal office to keep them from hostile surgical committee members.

At national meetings, translabyrinthine adversaries lambasted House and Hitselberger for their work. The neurosurgical community as a whole continued over the next few years to disagree vehemently with translabyrinthine surgery. Slowly, however, House and Hitselberger were able to win over a few neurosurgeons. One of these was a leading Los Angeles neurosurgeon, Dr. Henry Dodge. He reviewed their cases and helped them obtain credibility.

Other neurosurgeons across the country began to lessen the intensity of their attack, but they continued to disapprove of transtemporal bone removal of acoustic tumors. In 1963, Dr. House offered a small, informal course on the diagnosis and surgical management of these lesions and, in 1965, he sponsored a large international symposium on acoustic tumor diagnosis and treatment. Leading neurosurgeons, otologists, neurologists, and audiologists attended the 1965 meeting. For 5 days, the subject was covered thoroughly by a wide range of disciplines. One of the most important aspects of that meeting was the overall summary of the advances that had been made in early diagnosis. The first monograph (House, 1964) had been published the preceding December, setting forth a logical, step-by-step method for early detection of acoustic tumors for the first time.

Over the next 30 years, it has come to be recognized that all three approaches (suboccipital, middle fossa, and translabyrinthine) are valuable. Dr. House has trained many young disciples, and these surgeons, in turn, have trained others, refining and improving upon basic techniques. The extended middle fossa (House, Hitselberger, & Horn, 1986) and trans-cochlear (House & Hitselberger, 1976) approaches are the latest additions to the surgical repertoire. Well-rounded surgeons specializing in acoustic neuroma removal now have a variety of techniques in their armamentarium and use them to tailor the treatment for each patient. In order to choose an approach, the surgeon must know the size and location of the lesion, the preoperative hearing status, and the patient's general health status.

The most recent addition to the operating room of the acoustic surgeon is the facial nerve monitor (Dickins & Graham, 1991). Dr. House developed a method for identifying the facial nerve anatomically, and the microscope and microsurgical instrumentation help the surgeon to leave it intact. Particularly, as smaller and smaller tumors have been encountered, facial nerve preservation has become an expected outcome. The facial nerve monitor serves as an educational instrument. It notifies the surgeon immediately when damage is occurring, and it allows modification of technique to minimize trauma. The facial nerve can be preserved in most smaller lesions; large tumors still present a challenge in effective management.

As Dr. House developed surgical techniques that allowed removal of acoustic neuromas with low mortality and ever decreasing morbidity, a need arose for earlier, more accurate diagnosis of cerebellopontine lesions. Cushing (1963) had been the first clinician to recognize and accurately describe the natural history of a cerebellopontine angle tumor. He noted that the most common initial symptoms were hearing loss and tinnitus. Lempert (1963), who had popularized the use of the audiometer, probably was the father of modern otology due to his many innovative surgical techniques. House, with the advantage of sophisticated audiometric studies, pioneered the concept of a neurotologic evaluation for all patients presented with unilateral tinnitus, unilateral hearing loss, or any form of spatial disorientation.

The neurotologic evaluation has become increasingly sophisticated. Two branches of diagnostic testing have evolved, including the audiologic/electrodiagnostic tests and the radiographic evaluations. Audiologic testing became more important in the 1960s, because early diagnosis meant improved surgical outcome. Through the contributions of Raymond Carhart (1957), James Jerger (1960), and others (Jerger, Shedd, & Harford, 1959), pure tone threshold testing was followed by the rapid development of other techniques that were designed to differentiate between cochlear and retrocochlear hearing loss. By the mid-1970s, there was a battery of tests (Sanders, Josey, & Glasscock, 1974) that were used to identify retrocochlear pathology. This test battery consisted of pure tone audiometry, speech discrimination assessment, tests for recruitment (including the Short Increment Sensitivity Index, SISI, the Alternate Binaural Loudness Balance Test, ABLB, and the stapedial reflex), and tests for adaptation (including Bekesy audiometry and assessments of tone decay and stapedial reflex decay). Electronystagmography (ENG) also was popularized because patients with

acoustic neuromas often had subtle vestibular dysfunction. This battery of tests had the advantage of being completely noninvasive, but the predictive value was only 82% for acoustic neuromas.

In 1976, Seltzer and Brackmann (1977) described the application of auditory brainstem response (ABR) testing for diagnosing retrocochlear disease, including the characteristic findings of interaural latency differences and poor waveform morphology. The use of ABR blossomed, and long-term studies have shown it to be better than 90% sensitive for even small lesions. The modern test battery includes the ABR, as well as pure tone audiometry, speech discrimination with rollover, and acoustic reflexes testing. Unfortunately, tiny tumors can be missed, even with the combined use of these techniques. Room still exists for an inexpensive, noninvasive, office-based, diagnostic procedure that is highly sensitive and specific.

Of all the diagnostic techniques available to the otologist, X-rays have become the most valuable and accurate. Compere (1964) advocated X-rays of the internal auditory canal performed with a special head unit that could be used in the physician's office. Throughout the 1960s, plain film expertise improved until almost any tumor that was large enough to expand the porus acousticus could be identified (Valvassori, 1969).

Dr. Robert Scanlan, a radiologist at St. Vincent's Hospital in Los Angeles, was responsible for the development of posterior fossa myelography as a means of detecting acoustic tumors. On a visit to the Mayo Clinic, he observed a posterior fossa study being performed and noticed that the internal auditory canal filled easily with iophendylate (Pantopaque). It occurred to Dr. Scanlan (1964) that it might be possible to outline a tumor at the internal auditory canal by this method. Upon returning to Los Angeles, he discussed this possibility with Dr. House, and they began using the procedure on a routine basis. Later,

Dr. House was to combine this study with yet another new X-ray advancement, polytomography. Known as the polytome Pantopaque procedure (Glasscock, Overfield, & Miller, 1976), it involved a small amount (1 cc) of dye placed in the subarachnoid space, then maneuvered into the internal auditory canal without fluoroscopic guidance. The accuracy of the polytomograph made the diagnosis of small tumors extremely precise. Polytomography also had the advantage of being performed as an outpatient procedure. Angiography became popular (Valvassori, 1969) and was helpful if the surrounding vasculature was distorted by the tumor mass.

The early 1970s saw the advent of computerized tomographic (CT) scanning. This was an exciting era in radiology, opening visual doors that heretofore had been closed. With the use of intravenous contrast, most lesions with cerebellopontine angle extension could be identified (Scott, Davis, Trevor, & Schneer, 1977). However, small tumors, especially when confined to the internal auditory canal, could not be visualized even with enhanced CT. Opaque cisternography with Metrizamide or Pantopaque was attempted but was not particularly helpful. In 1978, Sortland (1979) described CT combined with air-contrast meatography. This was the magic combination. Even small intracanalicular tumors could be visualized reliably. For about a decade, air-contrast CT scanning was the gold standard for acoustic neuroma diagnosis. It generally was well-tolerated by patients, and the most common side effect was headache. However, by nature it was an invasive procedure, and sometimes results were inconclusive if air could not be diverted into the internal auditory canal.

The last great event in the radiologic diagnosis of acoustic neuroma was the introduction of magnetic resonance imaging (MRI) in the mid-1980s. When it was first introduced, MRI was not much better than CT scanning for looking at the cerebello-

pontine angle. It was the FDA approval of intravenous gadolinium contrast in June of 1988 that changed the face of acoustic neuroma diagnosis (Stack et al., 1988). On T_1 weighted images, gadolinium markedly increases the signal intensity of acoustic neuromas, bringing them into stark contrast with the surrounding tissues. It is possible to identify tiny tumors, on the order of a few millimeters, with impressive accuracy. MRI scanning does not expose the patient to ionizing radiation, and gadolinium does not incite an allergic reaction, as traditional intravenous contrast materials do. The strength of MRI is the delineation of soft tissue detail. Over the years, the resolution of MRI has continued to improve so that structural details such as cystic degeneration, have become readily discernible. MRI has become the gold standard for acoustic neuroma diagnosis, and a good quality scan is nearly 100% sensitive.

The era of Dr. William House has brought advances that the early fathers of acoustic neuroma surgery could only dream about. It is now possible to diagnose a tumor the size of a pinhead before any symptoms, even hearing loss, have occurred. The tumor then can be removed, leaving the patient with little more than a surgical scar to testify to the surgical intervention. Where to go from here?

Future progress can be made in nonsurgical treatment of tumors and hearing preservation. Radiosurgical techniques, such as the gamma knife, have shown promise (Noren, Greitz, Hirsch, & Lax, 1983). Short-term results are reported in terms of decreasing size and cessation of growth of tumors. These statistics are not satisfactory for proponents of surgical cure. More long-term follow-up is eagerly awaited to assess the efficacy of radiosurgery.

As morbidity and mortality have improved, preservation of hearing has become an increasingly desirable outcome. The suboccipital and middle fossa routes are touted for use in these situations but, in most series, hearing conservation is successful only 35% of the time (Glasscock, McKennan, & Levine, 1987). Perhaps the next great surgeon in acoustic tumor history will teach us how to achieve this goal. There is ample opportunity for the giants of the future to join the ranks of Cushing, Dandy, and House and make a brighter future for patients with acoustic neuromas.

REFERENCES

Carhart, R. (1957). Clinical determination of abnormal auditory adaptation. *Archives of Otolaryngology, 65*, 32–39.

Compere, W.E. (1964). The radiographic examination of the petrous portion of the temporal bone. In *Radiograpic Atlas of the Temporal Bone, Book I* (1st ed.). St. Paul, MN. American Academy of Ophthalmology and Otolaryngology.

Cushing, H. (1963). *Tumors of the Nervus Acusticus and the Syndrome of the Cerebellopontine Angle* (2nd ed.). New York: Hafner Publishing.

Dickins, J.R.E., & Graham, S.S. (1991). A comparison of facial nerve monitoring systems in cerebellopontine angle surgery. *American Journal of Otology, 12*, 1–6.

Glasscock, M.E., McKennan, K.X., & Levine, S.C. (1987). Acoustic neuroma surgery: The results of hearing conservation surgery. *Laryngoscope, 97*, 785–789.

Glasscock, M.E., Overfield, R.E., & Miller, G.W. (1976). Polytomography in an otologic practice. *Southern Medical Journal, 69*, 1433.

House, W.F. (1961). Surgical exposure of the internal auditory canal and its contents through the middle cranial fossa. *Laryngoscope, 71*, 1363–1385.

House, W.F. (1964). Report of cases: Transtemporal bone microsurgical removal of acoustic neuromas (Monograph). *Archives of Otolaryngology, 80*, 617–667.

House, W.F. (1968). Partial tumor removal and recurrence in acoustic tumor surgery. *Archives of Otolaryngology, 88(Suppl.)*, 86–106.

House, W.F. (1977). History of the development of the translabyrinthine approach. In H. Silverstein & H. Norrell (Eds.), *Neurological surgery of the ear* (pp. 235–238). Birmingham: Aesculapius Publishing Company.

House, W.F., & Hitselberger, W.E. (1976). The transcochlear approach to the skull base. *Archives of Otolaryngology, 102, 334*–342.

House, W.F., Hitselberger, W.E., & Horn, K.L. (1986). The middle fossa transpetrous approach to the anterior-superior cerebellopontine angle. *The American Journal of Otology, 7*, 1–4.

Jerger, J.F. (1960). Bekesy audiometry in analysis of audiometric disorders. *Journal of Speech and Hearing Research, 3*, 275–287.

Jerger, J., Shedd, J., & Harford, E.R. (1959). On the detection of extremely small changes in sound intensity. *Archives of Otolaryngology, 69*, 200–211.

Lempert, J. (1963). Improvement of hearing in cases of otosclerosis: New one stage surgical technique. *Archives of Otolaryngology, 67*, 233–258.

Noren, G., Greitz, D., Hirsch, A., & Lax, I. (1993). Gamma knife surgery in acoustic tumors. *Acta Neurochirurigca, 58(Suppl.)*, 104–107.

Panse, R. (1904). Ein Gliom des Akusticus. *Archiv für Ohrenheilkunde, 61*, 251–255.

Sanders, J.W., Josey, A.F., & Glasscock, M.E. (1974). Audiologic evaluation in cochlear and eighth nerve disorders. *Archives of Otolaryngology, 100*, 283–289.

Scanlan, R.L. (1964). Positive contrast medium (iophendylate) in diagnosis of acoustic neuroma. *Archives of Otolaryngology, 80*, 698–706.

Scott, W.R., Davis, K.R., Trevor, R.P., & Schneer, J.A. (1977). Computerized tomography of the cerebellopontine angle. In H. Silverstein & H. Norrell (Eds.), *Neurological surgery of the ear* (pp. 206–215). Birmingham: Aesculapius Publishing.

Selters, W.A., & Brackmann, D.E. (1977). Acoustic tumor detection with electric response audiometry. *Archives of Otolaryngology—Head and Neck Surgery, 103*, 181–187.

Sortland, O. (1979). Computed tomography combined with gas CT cisternography for the diagnosis of expanding lesions of the cerebellopontine angle. *Neuroradiology, 18*, 19–22.

Stack, J.P., Ramsden, R.T., Antoun, N.M., Lye, R.M., Isherwood, I., & Jenkins, J.P.R. (1988). Magnetic resonance imaging of acoustic neuromas: The role of gadolinium—DTPA. *British Journal of Radiology, 61*, 800–805.

Valvassori, G.E. (1969). The abnormal internal auditory canal: The diagnosis of acoustic neuroma. *Radiology, 92*, 449–459.

CHAPTER 3

Pathology of Acoustic Tumors

Philip Gruskin, M.D.
Joseph N. Carberry, M.D.
Sujana S. Chandrasekhar, M.D.

The acoustic tumor is one of the more common intracranial tumors, after the various gliomas and meningiomas. Multiple studies have shown approximately similar incidence—acoustic tumors representing 8.7% of over 2,000 intracranial tumors in one series (Cushing, 1932) and 11.5% of 642 cases in another (Walshe, 1931). "Neurinomas" accounted for 7.6% of 6,000 brain tumors (Zulch, 1957) and 8% of 5,250 verified brain tumors in Olivecrona's series (Hoessly & Olivecrona, 1955). The overwhelming majority of intracranial schwannomas originate from the acoustic nerve, particularly the vestibular branch (see "Site of Origin"), while other cranial nerves account for a small fraction. "Neurinomas" are approximately 78% of tumors in the cerebellopontine angle (Revilla, 1948). About 5% of acoustic tumors are bilateral (Pool, Pava, & Greenfield, 1970).

Sandifort in 1777 (as cited in Cushing, 1917/1963, and Information Center for Hearing, 1971) is credited with the original postmortem description of what presumably was an acoustic tumor. Later (1810), Leveque-Lasource (as cited in Cushing, 1917/1963) correlated the postmortem findings of a probable acoustic tumor with clinical findings. (Cushing [1917/1963] believed, however, that these two cases may have been meningiomas, rather than acoustic tumors.) In Charles Bell's 1830 monograph is his sketch of an acoustic tumor showing cystic degeneration (as cited in Cushing, 1917/1963). Subsequently, the acoustic tumor became a more recognized entity, both clinically and pathologically.

ANATOMICAL CONSIDERATIONS

The gross anatomy of the eighth cranial nerve is well known. Each of the two components (cochlear and vestibular) of the eighth nerve is approximately 17–20 mm in length (Pool et al., 1970). The neuroglial-neurolemmal (glial-Schwann cell) junction is 10–13 mm distal to the brainstem in the male and 7–10 mm distal to the brainstem in the female. This junction frequently is more distal in the vestibular branch than it is in the cochlear component (Schuknecht, 1974).

Much of the overall microscopic anatomy is demonstrated in Figures 3–1, 3–2, and 3–3.[1] As the nerve emerges from the brain, it resembles bundle-like extensions of the central nervous system. Initially, it does not contain Schwann cells but, rather, neuroglial cells. The glial-Schwann cell junction often is relatively distinct, but not always sharp. Occasionally, islands of glial cells are distal to this junction. In most instances, the glial-Schwann cell junction is within the region of the acoustic meatus. However, there is variation in this position; sometimes it is more proximal, and sometimes it is more distal. The distal part of the nerve lies in the internal auditory canal and is invested by Schwann cells.

SITE OF ORIGIN

In most cases, the tumor arises in the region of the internal acoustic meatus. However, the tumor may arise in any area of the nerve covered by Schwann cells, i.e., the more distal part. As stated above, the glial-Schwann cell junction usually lies in the region of the internal acoustic meatus, but it may be more central, outside the temporal bone, or it may be more distal. Schuknecht (1974) states there is no evidence to support the contention that schwannomas arise predominantly at the glial-Schwann cell junction; they may arise anywhere between this junction and the cribrose area. There were no reports of primary tumors occurring in the neuroglial portion (Information Center for Hearing, Speech, and Disorders of Human Communication, 1971).

Most tumors originate from the vestibular branch, but some can originate from the cochlear nerve. The classic study of Skinner (1929), with reference to Henschen, might explain why these tumors are much more apt to occur in the vestibular division and distal segment, and why this tumor, common in this nerve, is most uncommon in other cranial nerves. It was determined that the vestibular ganglion, as opposed to others, has an increased number of cells, between the ganglion cells, and these cells have a disordered appearance. This may predispose the vestibular nerve to develop tumors.

Various temporal bone studies have disclosed small asymptomatic schwannomas and have demonstrated their early features, including site of origin. The Hardy and Crowe study (1936) of temporal bones in 250 cases disclosed acoustic tumors in 6 of these cases. Later, Leonard and Talbot (1970) reviewed the original Hardy and Crow series and added additional cases. They accepted only three of the original six cases as being "neurilemmomas" and added one more (totaling 4 cases of early asymptomatic "neurilemmomas" in 883 temporal bones). These four tumors arose from the vestibular nerve or between the vestibular nerve and cochlear nerve. Another series of 893 temporal bones revealed 5 occult vestibular schwannomas (Stewart, Liland, & Schuknecht, 1975). Gussen (1971) described an acoustic tumor limited to the modiolus. There was no evidence of tumor extending into the modiolus from the internal auditory canal, and the tumor appeared to arise from the portion of the nerve peripheral to the spiral ganglion. A tumor apparently arising in the vestibule was presented by Wanamaker (1972), who felt that tumors could develop from the nerves to either the saccule or utricle. Naunton and Petasnick (1970) encountered six acoustic tumors in which the internal auditory meatus was normal or without significant asymmetry, yet the tumors were large and predominantly in the cerebellopontine angle, with extension into the internal auditory meatus. Their impression was that these tumors arose from a portion of the nerve trunk central to the internal auditory meatus. Medi-

---

[1] Figures reprinted from *Acoustic Tumors: Volume 1. Diagnosis* (pp. 85–148), by W.F. House and C.M. Luetje (Eds.), 1979, Baltimore: University Park Press. Copyright 1985 by the House Ear Institute. Reprinted with permission.

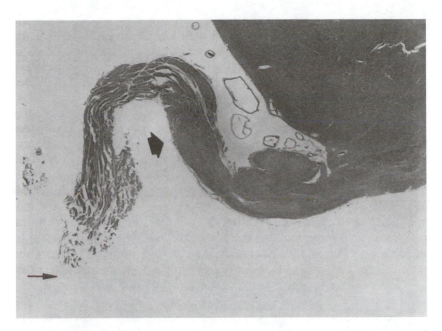

Figure 3–1. Normal anatomy of the eighth cranial nerve. Glial-Schwann cell junction (*broad arrow*), nerve entering brain (*upper right*), and region of Scarpa's ganglion (*small arrow*). (Ganglion not seen in this section—see Figure 3–3.) Routine autopsy specimen. (H & E × 9)

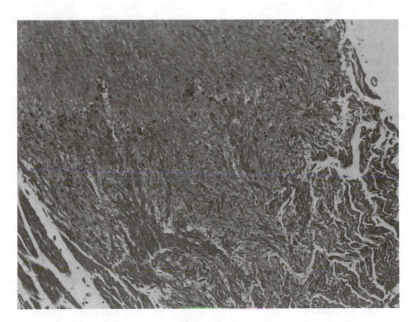

Figure 3–2. Higher power of Figure 3–1: glial-Schwann cell junction. Lighter area (*top half*) glial portion with calcospherites. Myelinated fibers covered by Schwann cells (*lower half*). (H & E × 90)

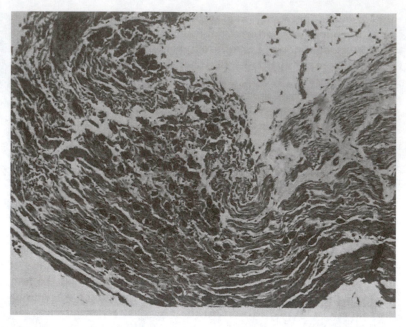

Figure 3–3. Deeper section of nerve in Figure 3–1 (in region of small arrow in Figure 3–1) to show Scarpa's ganglion. (H & E × 90)

ally-arising acoustic neuromas are described in another study (Tos, Drozdziewicz, & Thomsen, 1992).

It now is evident that acoustic tumors may arise from either branch of the eighth nerve and anywhere between the glial-Schwann cell junction and the origin of the nerves in the labyrinth (Stewart et al., 1975). An extensive schwannoma with intracranial spread and lateral extension to the external auditory canal has been reported (Woolford, Birzgalis, and Ramsden, 1994), as well as an external ear canal schwannoma (Wu et al., 1993).

Multiple schwannomas occurring at almost any site usually are considered part of von Recklinghausen's disease.

TERMINOLOGY AND CELL OF ORIGIN

To date, numerous names (more than 25) have been applied to eighth nerve tumors. The multitude of names stems from the con-

fusion regarding the cell of origin, with the name of the tumor based on the presumed cell of origin. Names for eighth nerve tumors have included acoustic nerve tumor, acoustic neuroma, angioneurofibroma, false neuroma, fibroglioma, fibromyxoma, glioma, myoschwannoma, neurilemoblastoma (Geschickter), neurinoma, neurofibromyxoma, neurilemmoma, neurolemmoma, neuroma fibrillare, peripheral glioma, perineural fibroblastoma, perineural glioma, schwannoglioma, and schwannoma (Stout, 1949). Additional terms have included neurofibroma, fibroma of the eighth nerve, lemmoma, lemmoblastoma, cerebellopontine tumor, acoustic tumor, tumor of acoustic nerve, and recess tumor (Pool et al., 1970). Other names have been used.

The neuroectodermal origin from Schwann cells first was suggested in 1908 by Verocay (as cited in Pool et al., 1970), who expressed the opinion that the tumor arose from "nerve fiber cells" that he thought were capable of producing nerve fibers. The term "neurinoma," meaning nerve fiber tumor, therefore was suggested. Mallory (1919) believed that the common tumor of the nervus acusticus and other central nerves was a perineurial fibroblastoma, while Antoni (as cited in Pool et al., 1970) maintained that the tumors originated from the cells of Schwann (lemmoblasts) and, thus, suggested the name "lemmoma," or "lemmoblastoma." It was Masson's thought (as cited in Pool et al., 1970) that the tumors arose from the sheath of Schwann and, thus, the tumor was termed a "schwannoma." To Stout (1935), the previous terms were not totally acceptable as indicating the cell of origin. Therefore, he took the phrase "nerve sheath tumor," which was descriptive as far as a cellular origin from fibroblast or Schwann cell, and constructed a new term, "neurilemmoma." Friedmann (1974) used the term "Schwann cell tumor of the ear."

Before continuing the discussion of cell of origin and terminology of eighth nerve tumors, a definition of solitary schwannoma and solitary neurofibromas is appropriate. A solitary schwannoma is a benign, slowly growing, encapsulated neoplasm that originates in a nerve and is composed of Schwann cells in a collagenous matrix (Harkin & Reed, 1969). A solitary neurofibroma is a benign, slowly growing, relatively circumscribed but nonencapsulated neoplasm originating in a nerve and composed principally of Schwann cells. The intercellular matrix contains collagen fibrils in a nonorganized mucoid or myxomatous component (Harkin & Reed, 1969). The neurofibroma has a different appearance and natural history from that of schwannoma. The neurofibroma is formed by a combined proliferation of all the elements of the peripheral nerve—Schwann cells, neurites, fibroblasts and, probably, perineurial cells. Schwann cells usually predominate (Ackerman, 1974).

Peripheral nerves contain axons, Schwann cells, fibroblasts of the endoneurium, and epineurium and perineurial cells. Ordinary fibroblasts, such as those found in the endoneurium, have no basement membrane

and, since the tumor cells are surrounded by basement membrane (see "Electron Microscopy"), fibroblasts are not thought to be the cell of origin. Also, nerve fibers themselves do not proliferate in acoustic tumors and, therefore, are not thought to be the cell of origin. The term "neurinoma" therefore is not correct.

Some of the debate regarding the cell of origin revolved around the Schwann cell and perineurial cell. Harkin and Reed (1969) felt that the two cell types could not be distinguished by any techniques then in use, including histochemistry, electron microscopy, or tissue culture. They postulated that it may arise from either or both cell types. There is not general acceptance that the Schwann cell and perineurial cell are identical. Perineurial cells also have a basement membrane, like Schwann cells, but unlike Schwann cells, perineurial cells contain large numbers of micropinocytotic vesicles (Russell & Rubinstein, 1977) and terminal bars (Cravioto, 1969).

Most electron microscopists and others feel that the tumors are derived from Schwann cells, while others considered that perineurial cells may be the cells of origin (Cravioto, 1969; Rubinstein, 1972; Russell & Rubinstein, 1977). Ultrastructural study indicates a tumor of Schwann cell origin (Silverberg, 1983) (see also "Electron Microscopy" section).

In addition to the predominant tumor cell, acoustic tumors contain connective tissue fibers, collagen, and reticulum. Schwann cells may be able to produce collagen (Harkin & Reed, 1969; Murray & Stout, 1940). Silver reticulum stains on acoustic tumors often show abundant argyrophilic fiber (see "Microscopic Pathology" section).

Pineda and Feder (1967) discuss the term "acoustic neuroma" and feel it may be misleading. True neuroma should be composed of nerve cells and nerve fibers, while a false neuroma is a tumor of nerve sheath without neoplastic proliferation of genuine nerve cells. Therefore, acoustic nerve neoplasms more properly should be called "false neuromas." The term "neurolemmoma," although it reflects the cell of origin more accurately (sheath of Schwann, or neurolemma), too often is confused with the term neurilemmoma (neurilemma: a thin outer covering, not properly the Schwann or sheath cell). Therefore, they suggested that neoplasms of the acoustic nerve be called schwannomas.

In conclusion, most authorities feel that the Schwann cell is the cell of origin. The term neurofibroma does not seem appropriate. Acoustic tumor, acoustic neuroma, neuroma, neurilemmoma, and neurolemmoma all are terms in general use but, with regard to the aforementioned discussion, we feel that schwannoma is the most acceptable term at this time.

GROSS PATHOLOGY

The schwannoma is considered one of the few, truly encapsulated neoplasms, with the capsule formed by the perineurium. In practice, however, the capsule is difficult to identify in surgical material of acoustic tumors. The nerve of origin may be demonstrated at the periphery, flattened along the edge of the tumor.

The acoustic tumor may vary considerably in size, from a microscopic tumor to one that is quite large. We have received specimens up to 5 or 6 cm in diameter and weighing up to 30 g or more. Some of these have been tumors only partially removed, either in a first-stage operation or for other reasons and, therefore, may have been even larger.

The shape of the tumor may depend on its location. Those originating in the internal auditory canal usually are round or oval, as are tumors that originate central to the internal auditory meatus and, therefore, are primarily in the cerebellopontine angle. Externally, tumors are relatively smooth and lobulated.

Classically, however, most tumors originate in the region of the internal auditory meatus and, as they grow, they enlarge the meatus and extend into the cerebellopontine angle. Expansion of the meatus causes the classic funnel-shaped appearance. When they reach the cerebellopontine angle, they may attain considerable size. Therefore, many tumors consist of two portions: a stalk within the meatus and a larger extratemporal portion, the overall configuration resembling a mushroom.

An arachnoidal cyst containing xanthochromic or clear fluid may overlay the dorsolateral aspect of the tumor (Pool et al., 1970).

The color and consistency, in our experience, often depend on the size of the tumor and the degree of degenerative change. Small tumors (less than 15 mm) may be yellow or pink to pink-grey and have a rubbery consistency. On cut section, they have a semi-translucent appearance and are solid (Figure 3–4). Medium-size tumors have the gross appearance of schwannomas seen elsewhere in the body, with a pale yellow color. Usually firm to rubbery, they are glistening on cut section and usually are solid (Figure 3–5).

The larger tumors (Figure 3–6) have a much more varied gross appearance, due to degenerative changes. The color is more mottled, with the most consistent finding being a bright yellow (predominantly from histiocytes) to yellow-tan color, which is opaque, rather than semi-translucent on section. Areas of acute or recent hemorrhage appear red, while older hemorrhage appears brown. Fibrosis is more grey. The larger tumors may be solid, but often are not, and cystic change can be prominent. The consistency also is quite variable. There may be areas that are rubbery, edematous, soft, or fibrous. Some tumors represent all these characteristics in one part or another, while others are predominantly one type.

From a practical standpoint regarding the biopsy material received from surgery, the color alone often is a clue to the diagnosis. Yellow tissue (Figure 3–7), even in small biopsy fragments, usually is indicative of schwannoma, while white or grey fragments often are meningiomas. However,

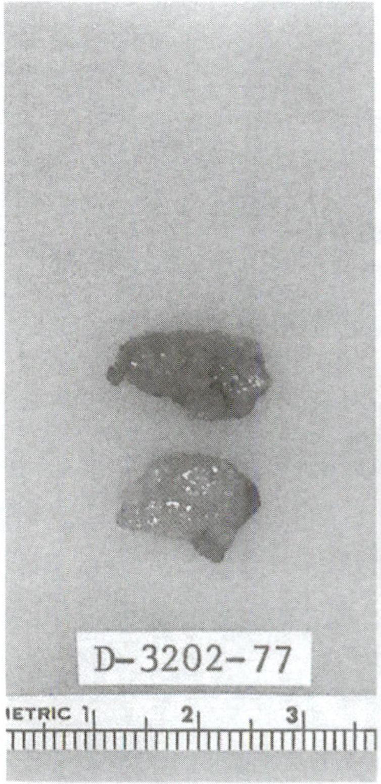

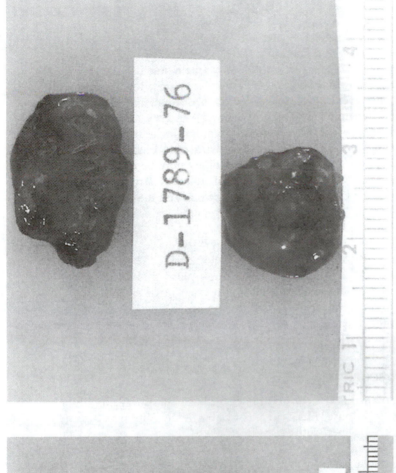

Figure 3–4. (left) Small acoustic schwannomas, bisected. External surface (*top*) and cut surface (*bottom*).

Figure 3–5. (right) Medium size schwannoma, bisected. Cut surface (*top*) shows solid tumor with focal hemorrhage. External surface (*bottom*) is lobulated.

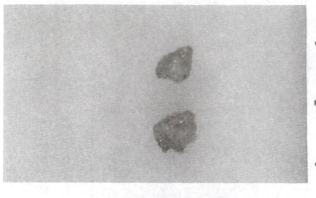

D-2585-77

Figure 3-7. (*right*) Typical biopsy specimen of acoustic schwannoma. Yellow color and glistening surface are characteristic.

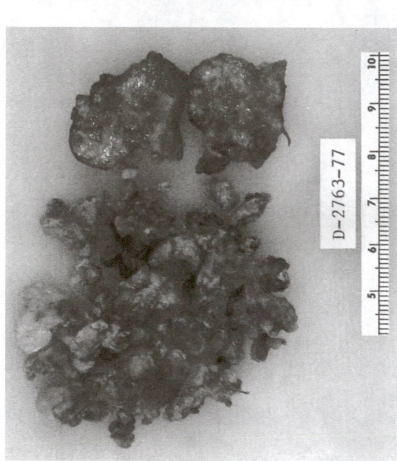

D-2763-77

Figure 3-6. (*left*) Large acoustic schwannoma, as often received in multiple pieces. Variegated appearance with bright yellow areas and hemorrhage.

this is not absolute, as we have encountered a few biopsies of yellow meningiomas (see Figure 3–75) (see "Differential Diagnosis" section) and white or grey schwannomas.

The gross features of acoustic tumors, including the relationship to the surrounding structures, are demonstrated in Figure 3–8 and 3–9.

Some of the clinical symptomatology may be explained by changes in the tumor and by involvement of adjacent structures. Hemorrhage may produce enlargement, as may edema. The tumor may shrink again when the edema disappears. Occasionally, degenerative change with fibrosis actually may shrink the tumor.

As the lesion grows, it destroys its nerve and ganglia, with a resultant loss of vestibular function and hearing. The facial nerve, which is in proximity to the eighth nerve, also may be affected. The internal auditory and other arteries, for example, the anterior inferior cerebellar, may be compressed, with resultant dysfunction and degenerative changes. When the tumor extends into the cerebellopontine recess, symptoms may be those of a classic mass lesion in this area, and even death may result.

MICROSCOPIC PATHOLOGY

More than 4,000 acoustic tumors have been removed surgically by the House Ear Clinic. Most of the available microscopic sections have been reviewed. Although any tumor may have the "classic" pattern of a schwannoma in a given area, any one may manifest myriad patterns, particularly in a localized area. There probably are more variations in histologic patterns in acoustic tumors than in many other tumors.

Figures 3–10 through 3–13 demonstrate the overall relationship of a typical acoustic tumor to its nerve of origin. Figures 3–14 through 3–19 also show the nerve of origin in relation to the tumor. Often, the nerve is compressed at the periphery (Figure 3–14), or the nerve may be split partially by the tu-

mor (Figures 3–15 and 3–16). Ganglion cells may be noted in the nerve. Sometimes, fibrous tissue of perineurium is included; this tissue forms the capsule of these tumors, although we often find this difficult to demonstrate. The nerve may be surrounded by the tumor, rather than compressed along an edge (Figure 3–17), and ganglion cells may be intermixed with the tumor cells (Figures 3–18 and 3–19).

The classic description of a schwannoma is a tumor composed of Antoni type A and type B tissue. Type A is composed of more compact tissue, with elongated spindle cells, in irregular streams and with a tendency to palisading. Type B tissue, often intermingled with type A, is characterized by a loose texture, often with sponginess and cyst formation.

Figures 3–20 through 3–24 show typical acoustic tumors with Antoni A and B areas. Much of the tumor is composed of bundles of interlacing eosinophilic spindle cells, with a moderate degree of cellularity. There is mild nuclear pleomorphism. Most acoustic tumors are predominantly type A tissue.

The various patterns found in acoustic schwannomas may be either focal or diffuse. The following descriptions cover the vast array of patterns. Although patterns may be of more importance to the pathologist, the surgeon should be aware of these possibilities, particularly as they relate to diagnosis of small biopsies and frozen sections. If the entire tumor were submitted, most tumors could be diagnosed by the surgical pathologist. However, the routine biopsy material of 5 mm or less may create problems in diagnosis, because only a small area is seen. Even when an entire tumor is available, a rare one will be difficult to diagnose.

Various patterns and changes may occur in the tumors because of compression of vessels, compression against bone, degeneration, inherent nature of the tumor, hemorrhage, and other factors.

In more compact areas, spindle cells can vary in arrangement, including typical interlacing bundles (Figure 3–21), herring-

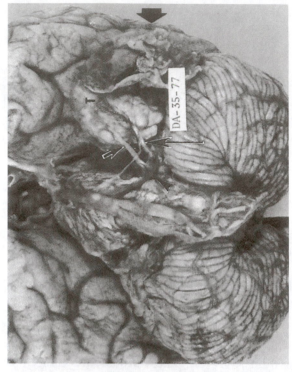

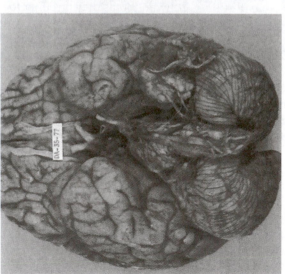

Figure 3–8. (*left*) Brain from a patient with NF-2 disease and bilateral acoustic tumors. (Right tumor previously surgically removed.)

Figure 3–9. (*right*) Same specimen as in Figure 3–8. The tumor (*T*) is 3.4 cm in diameter and originates from the eighth cranial nerve (*long arrow*). The seventh cranial nerve (*short arrow*) is stretched over the tumor. Crossing these two nerves is the small internal auditory artery arising from the basilar artery. The anterior inferior cerebellar artery (*arrowhead*) is compressed between tumor and cerebellum. The temporal bone (*broad arrow*) is removed en bloc with the tumor.

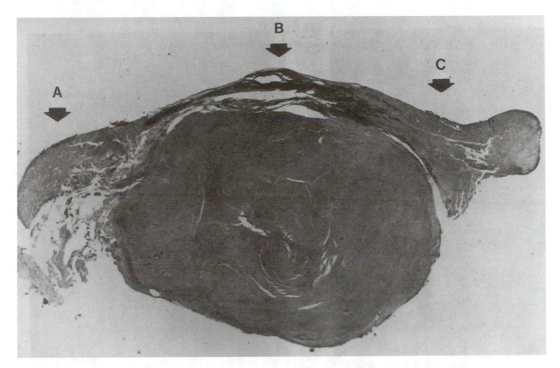

Figure 3–10. An acoustic schwannoma and its nerve origin. Scarpa's ganglion (*arrow A* and Figure 3–11), compressed nerve with hemorrhage (*arrow B* and Figure 3–12) and glial–Schwann cell junction (*arrow C* and Figure 3–13). (H & E × 14).

bone pattern (Figure 3–25), whorled bundles resembling meningioma (Figures 3–26 and 3–27), parallel fibers (Figure 3–28), bundles or cords (Figure 3–29), or small bundles resembling neurofibroma (Figure 3–30).

Schwannomas also are well noted for their various patterns of palisading. A large part of a tumor may show palisading of cells, such as that in Figure 3–31. Other patterns (Figure 3–32) may be seen focally. Sometimes there is palisading of nuclei with more central eosinophilic fibrillar material, as illustrated in Figure 3–33. Palisading structures resembling tactile corpuscles are called Verocay bodies. However, the term "Verocay body" has been used by many to mean any body-like configuration of tumor cells. It has been our experience that palisading and Verocay bodies frequently are absent in many acoustic tumors. In addition, palisading is a phenomenon that is not limited to schwannomas and can be found in other tumors, for example, leiomyomas, leiomyosarcomas, and those of fibrous tissue origin.

Looser areas may have a myxoid pattern (Figure 3–34) with acid mucopolysaccharide material in the intercellular space (confirmed by Alcian blue stain).

Foamy histiocytes vary tremendously in number and may be localized or diffuse (Figure 3–35). These impart the bright yellow color often seen grossly. They may or may not be seen in a region of acute or old hemorrhage. Characteristically, they are part of Antoni B areas, but they may be present in Antoni A tissue.

The prominent vascular pattern is one of the most consistent histologic findings. Almost all tumors are predominantly vascular, both in the Antoni-A and Antoni-B areas. The blood vessels, however, show considerable variation, not only from tumor to tumor, but within any given tumor.

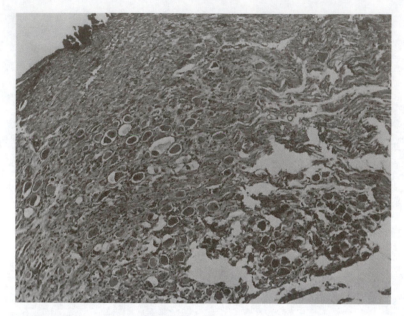

Figure 3–11. Same specimen as Figure 3–10 (at *arrow A*). Scarpa's ganglion. (H & E × 90)

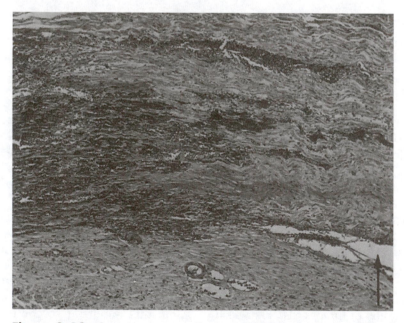

Figure 3–12. Same specimen as Figure 3–10 (*at arrow B*). Compressed nerve with hemorrhage (*top*) is separated (*arrow*) from tumor (*bottom*). (H & E × 90).

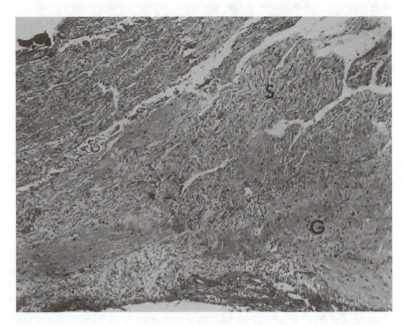

Figure 3-13. Same specimen as Figure 3-10 (*at arrow* C). Glial (G) and Schwann cell (S) junction. (H & E × 90)

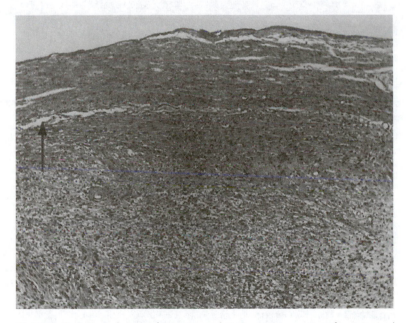

Figure 3-14. Relation of acoustic schwannoma to nerve of origin and ganglion cells (Figures 3-14 through 3-19). Compressed nerve (top) separated (*arrow*) from tumor (*bottom*). (H & E × 108)

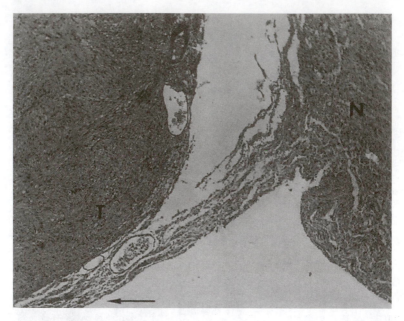

Figure 3–15. Nerve (*N*) partially split by tumor (*T*). Ganglion cells in the nerve (*arrow*). (H & E × 90)

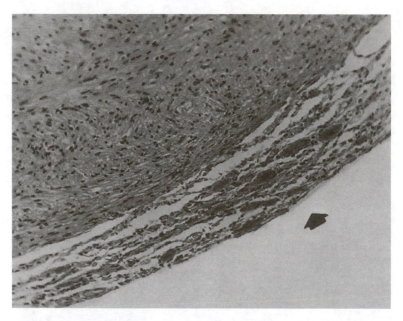

Figure 3–16. Higher power of Figure 3–15. Ganglion cells (*arrow*). (H & E × 216)

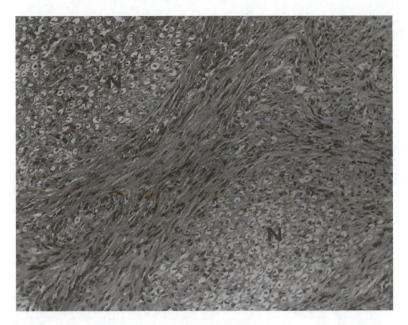

Figure 3–17. Nerves (*N*) are seen on end are surrounded by tumor. (H & E × 180)

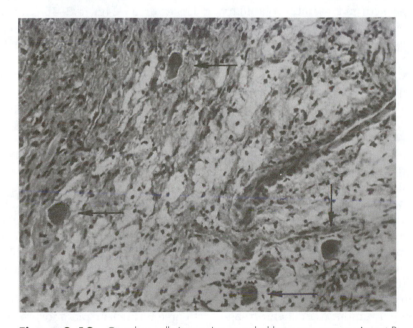

Figure 3–18. Ganglion cells (*arrows*) surrounded by tumor, near an Antoni B area with histiocytes. (H & E × 288)

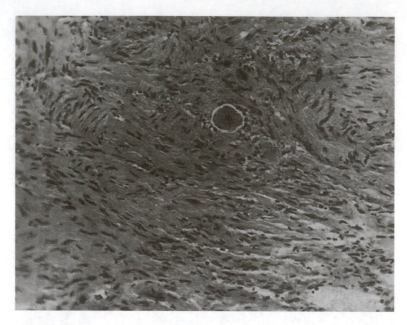

Figure 3–19. Ganglion cell entrapped in neoplasm (Antoni A area). (H & E × 216)

Vessels can be of relatively small diameter, closely packed, and resemble a capillary hemangioma, glomus tumor, or other vascular tumor (Figures 3–36 and 3–37). Occasionally, one encounters a localized area with quite dilated, thin-walled blood vessels, resembling cavernous hemangioma (Figure 3–38). Usually, vessels are of moderate size (Figure 3–39), and they may contain thrombi (Figure 3–40). Other areas may contain irregularly dilated vessels with hyalinized walls (Figure 3–41). Not infrequently, there is bright eosinophilic material, probably fibrin, in the walls of some vessels (Figure 3–42). Other vessels, individually or in groups, may have intensely hyalinized walls (Figure 3–43). Hemorrhage and hemosiderin deposits often are found in the region of thrombi (Figure 3–44). Hemorrhage of varying ages is a fairly consistent finding in larger tumors. Acute hemorrhage easily can be recognized, but often cannot be distinguished from surgical artifact. Slightly older hemorrhage with hematoidin pigment can be found, but hemosiderin pigment is the more usual finding.

Necrosis occurs microscopically and in larger areas. Figure 3–45 shows a microscopic area of necrosis with an associated thrombus in a vessel. Often such a thrombus is not seen.

Cellularity also can vary considerably. Average cellularity is as previously shown (Figure 3–22), but some areas can be sparsely cellular and some intensely cellular (Figure 3–46). Fibrosis ranges from focal to broad areas composed almost entirely of hyalinized tissue (Figure 3–47). Some fibrosis may be old healing from ischemic necrosis. However, fiberosis is not always an inherent part of the tumor and may be related to previous operation. Rarely, microscopic islands of hyalinized fibrous tissue, probably not blood vessels, are encountered (Figure 3–48).

Another feature of acoustic schwannoma, or any schwannoma, is the type and degree of nuclear pleomorphism. An ordinary acoustic tumor (Figure 3–22) may have mild nuclear pleomorphism. The degree of pleomorphism can be more marked, such as that seen in Figure 3–49, and multinucleation is possible (Figure 3–50). Some-

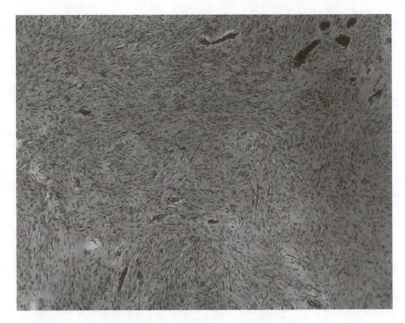

Figure 3–20. Typical acoustic schwannoma (Antoni A area) composed of irregular interlacing bundles of spindle cells. (H & E × 57.6)

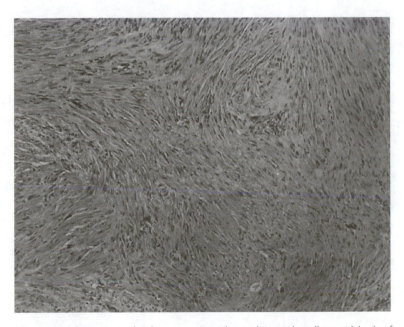

Figure 3–21. Typical schwannoma with interlacing bundles and lack of palisading. Same case as Figure 3–10. (H & E × 90)

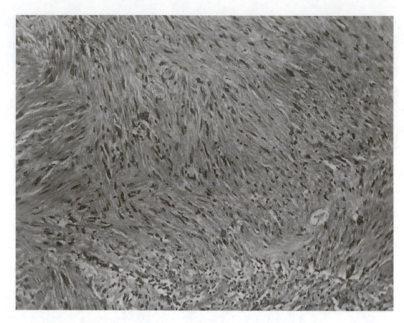

Figure 3–22. Higher power of Figure 3–21. Spindle cells with mild nuclear pleomorphism and average degree of cellularity. (H & E × 144)

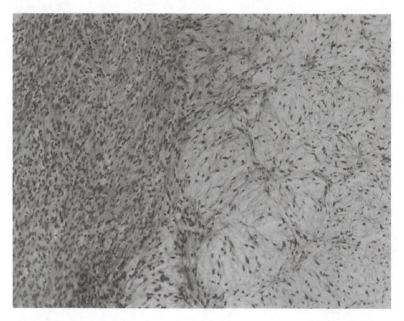

Figure 3–23. Acoustic schwannoma showing junction of Antoni A tissue (*left*) and Antoni B tissue (*right*). (H & E × 144)

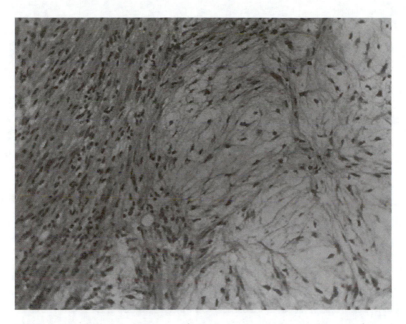

Figure 3–24. Higher power of Figure 3–23. Antoni A tissue (*left*) and Antoni B tissue (*right*). H & E × 288)

times, pleomorphism is seen in areas of necrosis (Figure 3–51) or adjacent to thrombi (Figure 3–52). Some feel that pleomorphism is a degenerative change, but often there is no necrosis or obvious degenerative change associated with it. To the unwary, pleomorphism may imply malignancy. In our experience, however, pleomorphism alone should not raise a suspicion of malignancy.

Although mitotic figures occasionally may be identified in schwannomas in other locations, it is only in rare acoustic schwannomas that we have been able to demonstrate them.

Cystic change usually is seen in larger tumors. Figure 3–53 shows microcystic areas developing in Antoni B tissue. Occasionally, schwannomas may contain small or large cysts, such as those in Figure 3–54. In this type, there usually is no specific cellular lining of the cyst but, sometimes, there may be a layer of flattened cells.

Inflammatory changes, such as focal lymphocyte collections (Figure 3–55) and densely packed plasma cells, are seen occasionally (Figures 3–56 and 3–57). Neutrophils may be present, of course, for various reasons.

There is a wide range of patterns of calcifications that can occur in, or be related to, acoustic tumors. The internal auditory canal is lined by dura, which may contain psammoma bodies. Psammoma bodies can be present, therefore, along the edge of an acoustic tumor (Figure 3–58). Although psammoma bodies characteristically occur in meningiomas and some papillary tumors, in rare instances, true laminated psammoma bodies can be identified in the substance of an acoustic tumor (Figures 3–59 and 3–60). Additionally, irregular calcifications may occur along the edges of the tumor (Figure 3–61). Some of these probably are bone fragments from the auditory canal, but similar irregular calcifications may occur within the tumor, away from the edges. Other patterns are seen, such as those depicted in Figure 3–62, with broader and finely stippled calcifications. A calcified tumor is reported with calcification as a dominant characteristic (Thomsen, Klinken, & Tos, 1984). Even os-

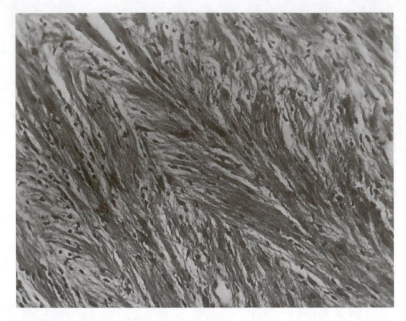

Figure 3–25. Spindle cell pattern in acoustic schwannomas (Figures 3–25 through 3–30). Herringbone pattern. (H & E × 225)

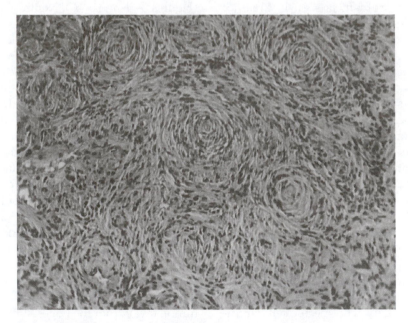

Figure 3–26. Meningioma-like whorls. (H & E × 216).

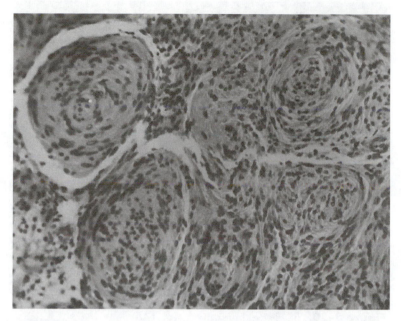

Figure 3–27. Meningioma-like whorls (different case than Figure 3–26).
(H & E × 252)

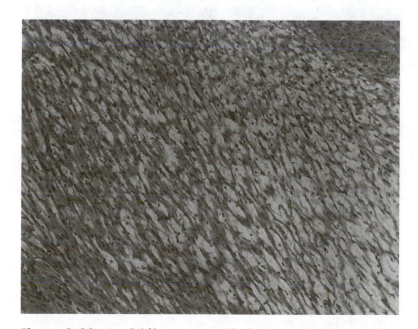

Figure 3–28. Parallel fibers separated by histiocytes. (H & E × 144)

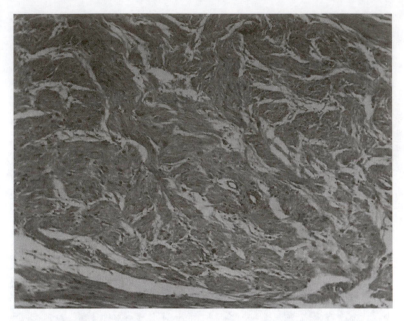

Figure 3–29. Bundles or cords. (H & E × 144)

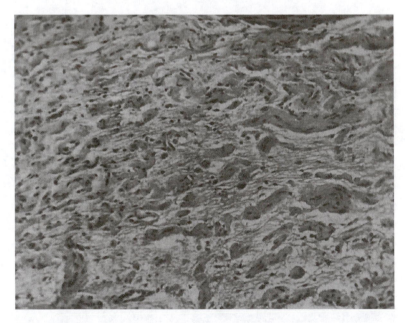

Figure 3–30. Neurofibroma-like area. (H & E × 216).

Figure 3–31. Prominent palisading pattern composes most of this schwannoma. (H & E × 126)

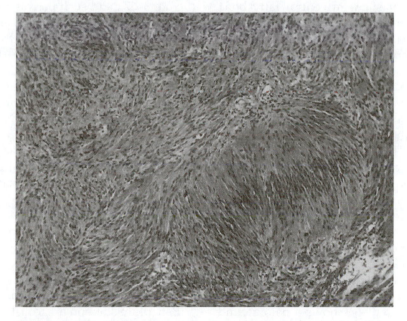

Figure 3–32. Schwannoma with organoid pattern of palisading (*lower right*). (H & E × 126)

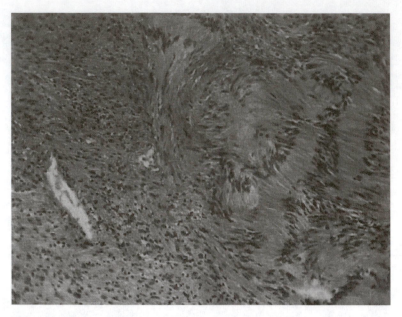

Figure 3–33. Palisading in acoustic schwannoma-columns of nuclei separated by anucleate eosinophilic fibrillar material. (H & E × 180)

seous metaplasia with central fatty bone marrow is possible (Figure 3–63).

We have not observed tumors with melanin deposits, but such have been described (Dastur, Sihn, & Pandya, 1967; Miller, Sarikaya, & Sos, 1986). We have experienced two tumors presented clinically as acoustic neuromas that were diagnosed as malignant melanoma. One was in a 43-year-male. This was presumably primary at least in the area of acoustic nerve (cerebellopontine angle) and no other tumor or history of melanoma was identified. We have not diagnosed any melanotic schwannoma but such have been described (Dastur et al., 1967; Miller et al., 1986).

Focally, acoustic tumors may have an appearance resembling primary brain tumors, that is, various gliomas, as well as meningiomas. Figure 3–64 shows a halo around cells in the tumor resembling oligodendroglioma. The patterns in Figures 3–65 and 3–66 certainly resemble low grade gliomas. An otherwise typical schwannoma may have areas of palisading around blood vessels

(Figure 3–67), and such perivascular cuffing is reminiscent of glioblastoma, ependymoma, and oligodendroglioma. In other instances, a schwannoma resembles the fibroblastic or transitional types of meningioma.

Tumors in neurofibromatosis type 2 (NF-2) may have special features and also are discussed separately (see "Neurofibromatosis 2 and Multiplicity").

Schwannomas do not show a proliferation of nerve fibers as an actual part of the tumor. The acoustic (or other) nerve often is stretched over the tumor. Some twigs of the nerve may enter the tumor, as can be seen on Bodian stain. Fibers of the nerve of origin may be in the deeper aspect of the tumor, but they are not thought to be actually part of the neoplastic process and may have grown in from another location.

Reticulum stain on an acoustic tumor often demonstrates numerous argyrophilic delicate fibers parallel to the long axis of the tumor cell (Figure 3–68). The nature of these argyrophilic fibers has been in question, and possibly basement membrane material

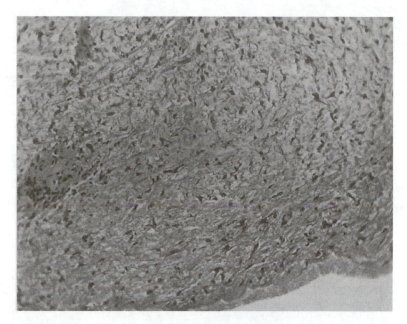

Figure 3–34. Myxoid area of schwannoma (Antoni B area). (H & E × 252)

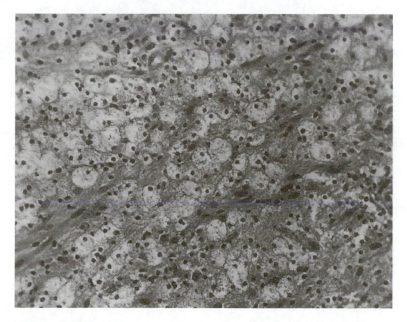

Figure 3–35. Histiocytes in acoustic schwannoma. (H & E × 288)

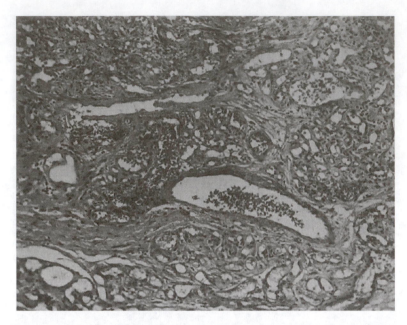

Figure 3–36. Vascular patterns in acoustic schwannomas (Figures 3–36 through 3–44). Small vessel proliferation is so marked it obscures the underlying schwannoma. (H & E × 144).

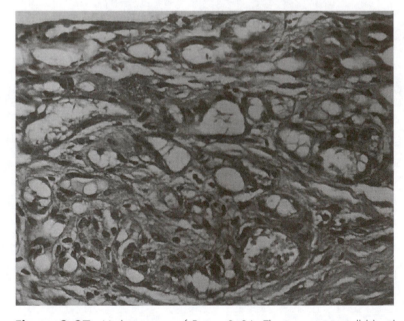

Figure 3–37. Higher power of Figure 3–36. The numerous small blood vessels mimic capillary hemangioma. (H & E × 378)

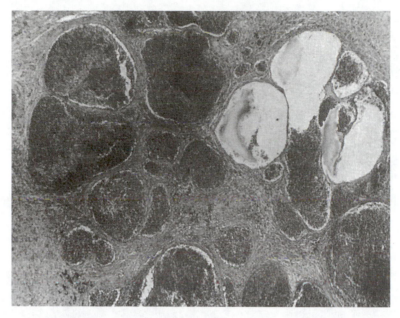

Figure 3–38. Numerous dilated thin-walled blood vessels resembling cavernous hemangioma. (H & E × 90)

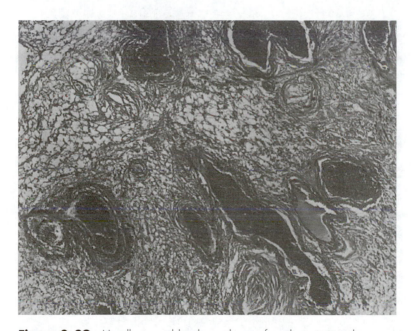

Figure 3–39. Usually, tumor blood vessels are of medium size, as these are. (H & E × 90)

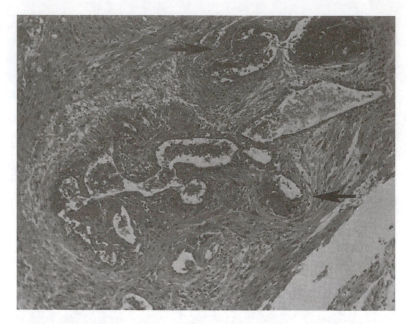

Figure 3–40. Thrombi (*arrows*) in various stages of organization. (H & E × 144)

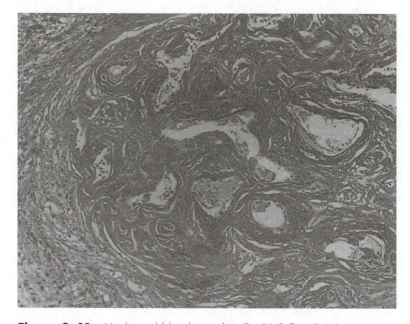

Figure 3–41. Hyalinized blood vessel walls. (H & E × 144)

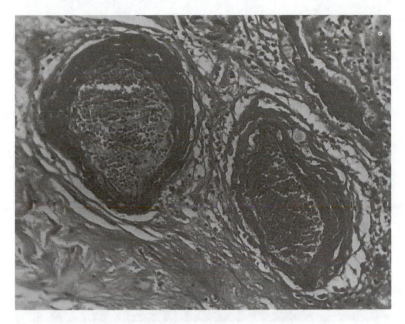

Figure 3–42. Bright eosinophilic appearance of vessel walls, apparently from fibrin, is typical of schwannomas. (H & E × 216).

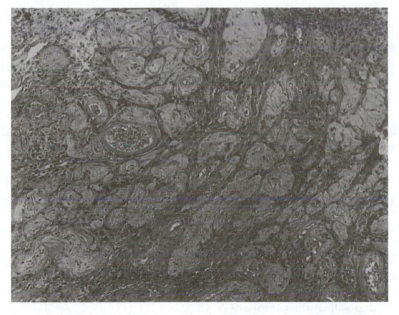

Figure 3–43. Hyalinized blood vessels barely recognizable as vessels. (H & E × 144)

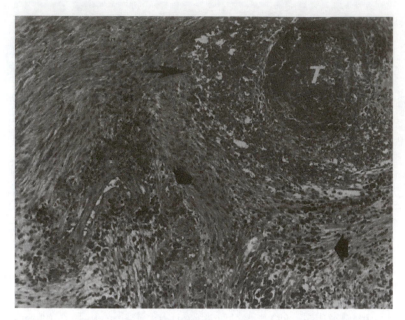

Figure 3–44. Thrombus (T) with associated hemorrhage (*long arrow*). Hemosiderin deposits (dark material, *short arrows*). (H & E × 144)

plays a role in this staining (Rubinstein, 1972). Not all areas of the tumor will show reticulum on silver stain.

IMMUNOHISTOCHEMISTRY

Immunohistochemical procedures are not performed routinely on schwannomas but, in selective cases, they may be helpful in distinguishing schwannoma from spindle cell meningioma. Meningiomas demonstrate mesenchymal and epithelial differentiation and are reported to have consistent and reliable histochemical positivity for both epithelial membrane antigen (EMA) and vimentin. For EMA, meningioma tumor cell staining usually is diffuse and appears in linear deposits at the periphery of the cell. Cytokeratin has been reported in a small percentage of meningiomas, as well as the presence of progesterone receptors (Taylor & Cote, 1994). We have not used these markers to help distinguish between

the two tumors or when the two tumors are admixed in NF-2 patients.

The S100 protein is a reliable marker for Schwann cells and is positive, in our experience, in all schwannomas. Reactivity is found in the cytoplasm and nuclei and is more prominent in the Antoni A areas. S100 also can be positive in meningiomas, but reactivity is focal and predominantly cytoplasmic. Vimentin is positive in both tumors and is mostly used to establish the immunoreactivity of the tumor (Taylor & Cote, 1994). Glial fibrillary acid protein (GFAP) has not been helpful in distinguishing between schwannoma and meningioma.

ELECTRON MICROSCOPY

Electron microscopy studies of these tumors reveal some characteristic ultrastructural features.

The principal cell (Figures 3–69 and 3–70) in these tumors is an elongated cell with the

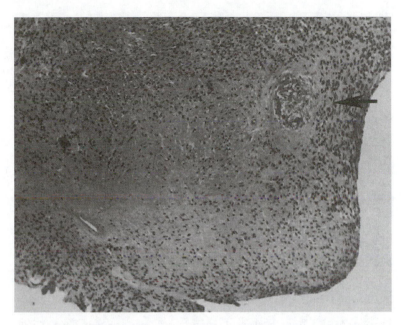

Figure 3–45. Micronecrosis with associated organizing thrombus (*arrow*) in acoustic schwannoma. (H & E × 162)

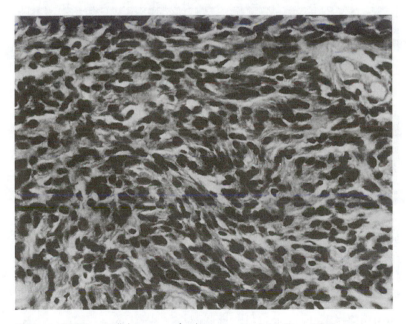

Figure 3–46. Cellular area of schwannoma. (H & E × 576)

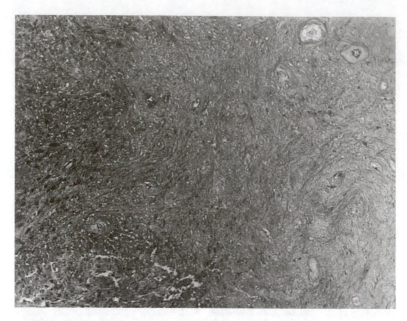

Figure 3–47. Large hyalinized area (*right*) of schwannoma. Junction with more cellular component (*left*). (H & E × 144)

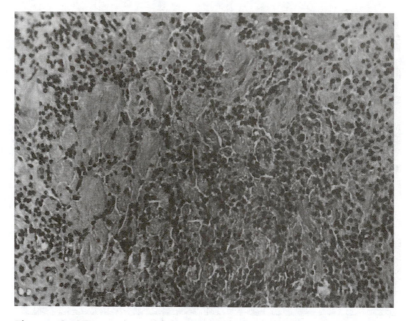

Figure 3–48. Hyalinized foci, probably not blood vessels, in a schwannoma. (H & E × 288)

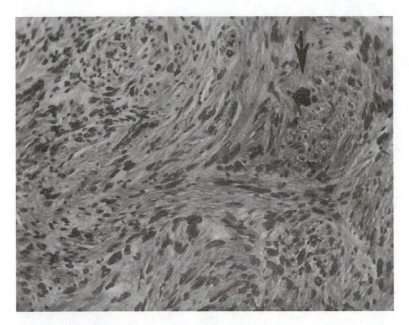

Figure 3–49. Nuclear pleomorphism in acoustic schwannomas (Figures 3–49 through 3–52). Prominent nuclear pleomorphism. Multinucleate cell (*arrow*). (H & E × 216

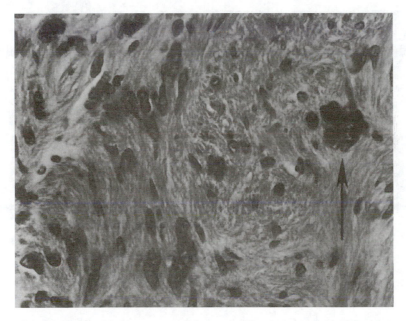

Figure 3–50. Higher power of Figure 3–49, showing the multinucleate cell (*arrow*). (H & E × 576)

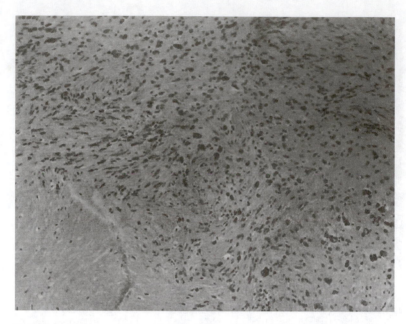

Figure 3–51. Moderate nuclear pleomorphism adjacent to necrosis (*bottom left*). (H & E × 162)

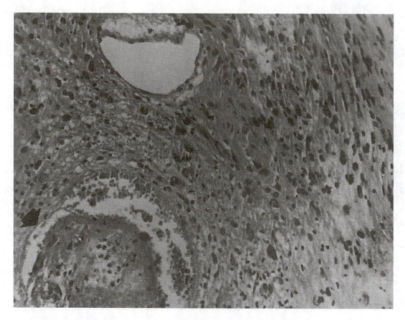

Figure 3–52. Moderate nuclear pleomorphism adjacent to thrombus (*arrow*). Same case as Figure 3–51. (H & E × 288)

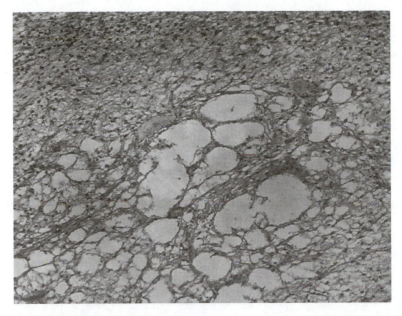

Figure 3–53. Microcystic change developing in Antoni B area of schwannoma. (H & E × 144).

morphologic features of a Schwann cell, forming extremely thin, interdigitating cell processes. Basement membrane material covers the cell and its processes and coats the plasmalemma (cell membrane) (Rubinstein, 1972). The cytoplasm contains fine filaments and glycogen particles among the other cell organelles. In schwannomas, basement membrane surrounds tumor cells and their processes. In gliomas, basement membrane has not been demonstrated. Meningiomas have basement membrane, but the membrane envelops the surface of groups of cells, rather than individual tumor cells, as in the schwannoma (Pool et al., 1970).

The Antoni B cell is a basement membrane coated cell, but it contains large numbers of organelles, mitochondria and dense bodies, and vacuoles. This is compatible with a high degree of metabolic activity (Russell & Rubinstein, 1977) (Figure 3–71).

The intercellular areas of these tumors are another region of note. The extracellular space may contain some bundles of collagen fibrils. Normal collagen has cross-stria-

tion periodicity of 700 Å (range 640–710 Å) (Harkin & Reed, 1969). There is also fine granular and filamentous material.

A characteristic finding in these tumors is the banded fusiform fibers identified in the intercellular spaces. Described by Luse (1960) as pointed at each end with cross-banding between 1200–1500 Å they are now referred to as Luse bodies (Figures 3–69, 3–71 and 3–72). These structures also are well described by Friedmann (1974).

Cravioto's ultrastructural study (1969) of 50 acoustic tumors showed these banded fusiform fibers, with 1200-Å repeating macroperiods in the extracellular space of the dense areas of every tumor studied. These fibers probably represent a form of long spacing collagen (Cravioto, 1969; Cravioto & Lockwood, 1968). Cravioto and Lockwood (1968) further described these as averaging 3 μm. in length and 0.5 μm in diameter, with two distinct cross-striated lines (narrower dense line, 300 Å, and a less dense line, 500 Å). The main periodicity (between dense bands) ranged from 550 Å to 1400 Å.

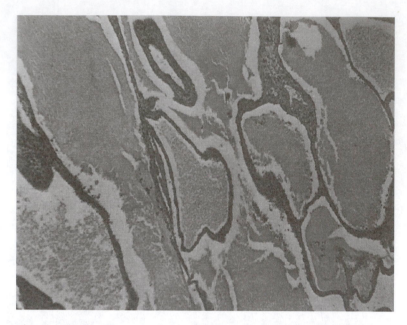

Figure 3–54. Acoustic schwannoma. Large cysts of this type are uncommon. (H & E × 72)

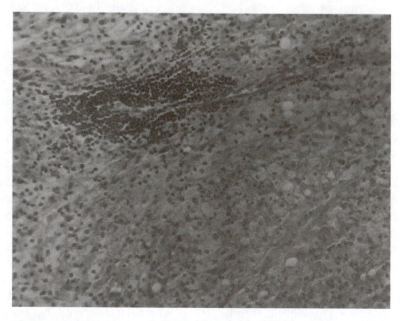

Figure 3–55. Focal collection of lymphocytes (*upper left*) in acoustic tumor. (H & E × 252)

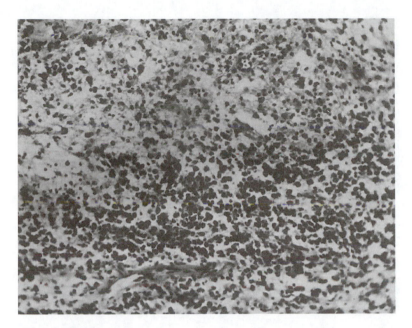

Figure 3–56. Densely packed plasma cells (*bottom*) in acoustic tumor. (H & E × 225)

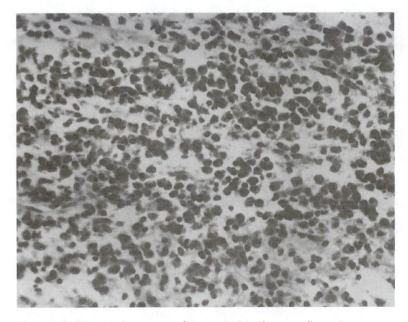

Figure 3–57. Higher power of Figure 3–56. Plasma cells appear mature. (H & E × 432)

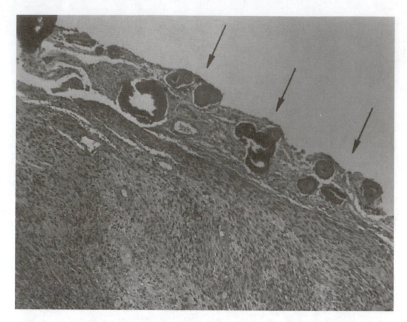

Figure 3–58. Patterns of calcification in acoustic schwannomas (Figures 3–58 through 3–63). Numerous psammoma bodies (*arrows*) (from dural lining of internal auditory canal) along edge of acoustic tumor (*bottom*). (H & E × 117)

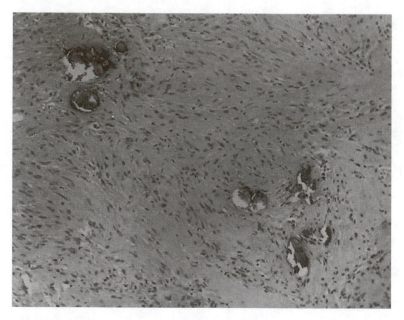

Figure 3–59. True psammoma bodies in acoustic schwannoma. (H & E × 144)

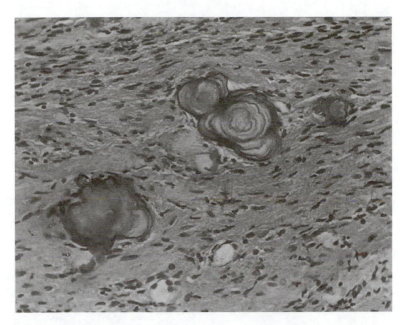

Figure 3–60. Higher power of Figure 3–59, after decalcification. Concentric laminations of psammoma bodies. (H & E × 288)

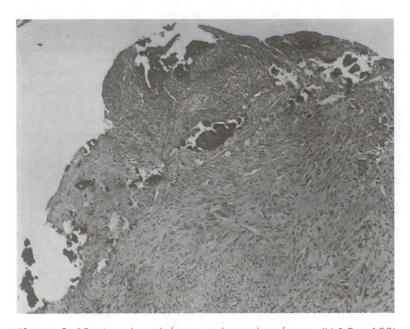

Figure 3–61. Irregular calcifications along edge of tumor. (H & E × 108)

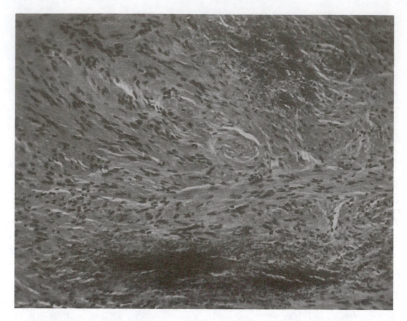

Figure 3–62. Broader and finely stippled calcification (*top and bottom*). (H & E × 117)

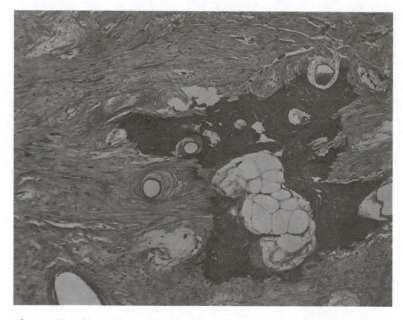

Figure 3–63. Osseous metaplasia with fatty bone marrow. (H & E × 72)

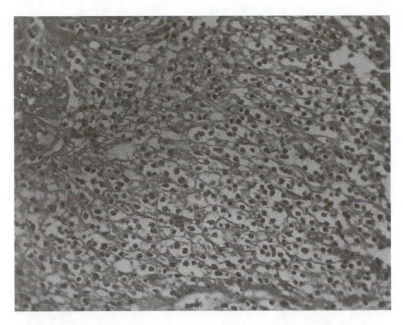

Figure 3–64. Patterns of acoustic schwannoma resembling primary brain tumors (Figures 3–64 through 3–67). Halo around small cells resembling oligodendroglioma. (H & E × 288)

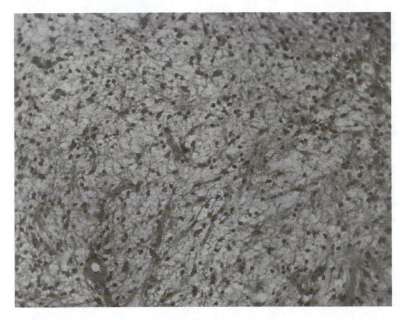

Figure 3–65. This area resembles low grade glioma. (H & E × 270)

Figures 3–66. Same case as Figure 3–65, different area, also resembling low grade glioma. (H & E × 216)

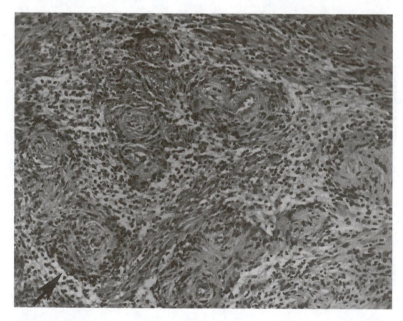

Figure 3–67. Perivascular cuffing (*arrow*) mimics glioblastoma multiforme, ependymoma, and oligodendroglioma. (H & E × 225)

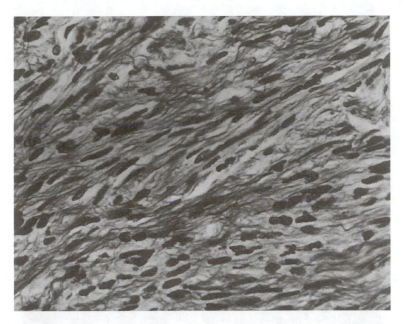

Figure 3–68. Silver reticulum stain of acoustic schwannoma. Numerous argyrophilic fibers parallel to the spindle cells of the tumor. (× 576).

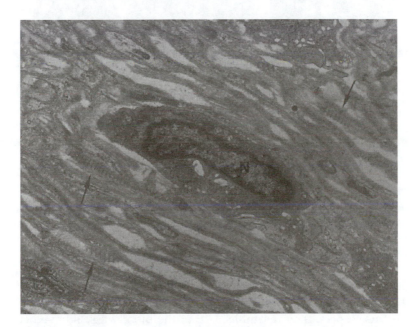

Figure 3–69. Antoni A area of acoustic schwannoma, electron micrograph. Numerous elongated cells and processes, with nucleus (N) of one cell in center. Many intercellular Luse bodies present, some of which are indicated (*arrows*). (× 7,380) (Tissue in Figures 3–69 through 3–72 fixed in 2% buffered glutaraldehyde and stained with uranyl acetate and lead citrate.)

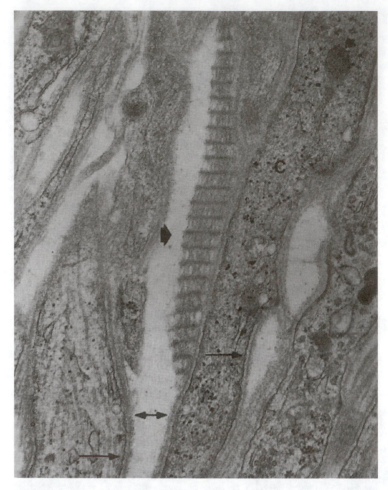

Figure 3–70. Electron micrograph, Antoni A area of acoustic schwannoma. Elongated cell (C), Luse body (*short arrow*) blending into basement membrane (*double-headed arrow*), and plasmalemma (*long arrows*). (× 30,000)

Basement membrane material could be followed into the banded structures and was thought to be forming part of it.

It has been stated that "neurilemmoma" cells lack what is probably the only pathognomonic feature of normal Schwann cells: mesoaxons. In this respect, they resemble the perineurial cell (Ackerman, 1974). We have seen a few probable mesoaxons in our electron micrographs of acoustic tumors.

Ultrastructural study shows that the tumor consists largely of cells lined by contin-

uous basal laminas and forming pseudomesoaxons. The cells do not invest axons. These findings indicate a tumor of differentiated Schwann cells (Mangham, Carberry, & Brackmann, 1981).

An interesting feature in schwannomas is that the blood vessels have been found to be of fenestrated type (Hirano, Dembitzer, & Zimmerman, 1972). Possibly, this may explain the findings seen in radiologic studies (tumors blush on angiography or contrast enchancement of the tumor on computed

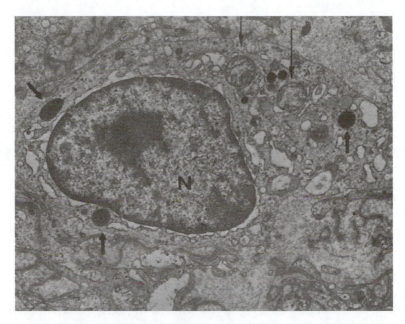

Figure 3–71. Electron micrograph showing cytoplasmic features of Antoni B cell. Nucleus (N), dense bodies (*short arrows*), and mitochondria (*long arrows*). (× 7,560)

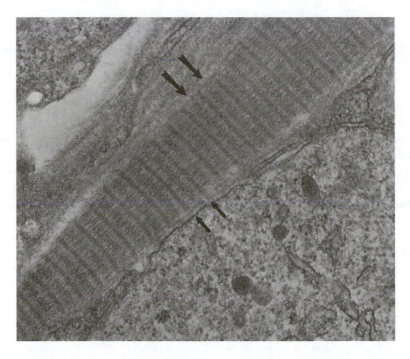

Figure 3–72. Portion of Luse body, electron micrograph. Narrow, dense cross bands (*small arrows*) and wider, less dense cross bands (*large arrows*). (× 40,890)

tomography). Also, the role of fenestrae, as related to the elevated spinal fluid protein associated with these tumors, is worth considering (Hirano et al., 1972).

TISSUE CULTURE

The classic study of Murray and Stout (1940) showed that distinctive types of Schwann cell could be cultured from type A and type B areas of human schwannomas. The cells from type A and B areas each had different growth characteristics, but both were regarded as having the same cellular origin—Schwann cells. Those derived from type B tissue had a more pronounced liquefactive action on culture media than did those of type A. This may have some bearing on the disposition of type B tissue to undergo cystic degeneration. Previously, type B was thought to be a degenerative phase of type A, yet, when cultivated in vitro, the cells did not die but, in fact, were highly active metabolically (Murray & Stout, 1940). Murray and Stout also concluded that the "neurilemmoma" is of Schwann cell origin, and no typical fibroblasts appeared in the outgrowths. The collagen and reticulum in these tumors, therefore, presumably are formed under Schwann cell influence. After Murray and Stout's original report in 1940, the similar in vitro behavior of two examples of cerebellopontine angle tumor was confirmed (Murray, 1942), including production of reticulum in the vicinity of Schwann cells, not fibroblasts.

Cravioto and Lockwood (1969) studied 50 acoustic tumors in tissue culture with observance of four main cell types. No conclusion could be reached regarding the origin of the collagen and reticulum fibers. Their ultrastructural study of acoustic tumors (1968) showed that in vivo and in vitro cell processes frequently were surrounded by basement membrane, and there was formation of fusiform banded fibers (Luse bodies).

Tissue cultures of 12 acoustic schwannomas (Lumsden, 1971) yielded two tumor cell types, frequently bridged by transitional forms. One cell type in culture corresponded to Antoni type B and the other to Antoni type A. Also emphasized in this study was the ability of the Schwann cell in vitro to become a macrophage with phagocytic properties.

Therefore, tissue culture, as well as electron microscopic findings of Antoni B type cells, tends to disprove the previous impression that Antoni B tissue is merely a degenerative form of type A.

MALIGNANT TUMORS

Malignant schwannomas of the eight nerve must be extremely rare. In review of most of the microscopic sections of over 4,000 acoustic tumors, none have been diagnosed as malignant, nor in subsequent follow-up have any proven to be malignant.

Since the terminology of malignant tumors arising in nerve is somewhat confusing, a definition of malignant schwannoma seems justified.

A malignant schwannoma was defined previously as a malignant neoplasm of nerve sheath origin, thought to be of Schwann cell origin that locally infiltrates and also metastasizes (Harkin & Reed, 1969). An erroneous diagnosis of malignant schwannoma can be made either by calling a benign schwannoma malignant or by mistaking other neoplasms, for example, fibrosarcoma or leiomyosarcoma, for nerve sheath neoplasms (Harkin & Reed, 1969). The term malignant schwannoma is acceptable if its use is restricted to those variants of malignant nerve sheath tumor that show distinctive features of Schwann cell differentiation. If the term is restricted in that sense, it seldom will be used (Harkin & Reed, 1969). Microscopically, malignant schwannomas are composed of spindle cells, mitoses are present and may be numerous, nuclei are hyperchromatic, there is increased cellularity, and areas of necrosis may occur.

The term malignant peripheral nerve sheath tumor (MPNST) has been used for a malignant neoplasm arising from supportive non-neuronal components of peripheral nerves (Burger & Scheithauer, 1994). This expresses the uncertainty regarding the nature of the cells and is a less committal term (Burger & Scheithauer, 1994; Burger, Scheithauer, & Vogel, 1991). Actual established Schwann cell origin is not always the case (Burger et al., 1991). There is association with von Recklinghausen's disease (Burger et al., 1991; Ducatman et al., 1986) and also with radiation (Ducatman et al., 1986). They may have herringbone patterns similar to fibrosarcoma or storiform patterns resembling malignant fibrous histiocytoma (Burger et al., 1991). In addition, approximately 10% demonstrate "metaplastic" elements, including heterologous elements, such as skeletal muscle, bone, cartilage, and epithelial tissues (Burger et al., 1991).

The term "malignant triton tumor" is applied to malignant schwannomas with rhabdomyoblastic differentiation (Han et al., 1992).

Ash (1960) stated that malignant deterioration of the acoustic nerve tumor occurs occasionally, and malignant melanoma has been reported as arising from the melanoblasts that occasionally are included in the tumor.

Malignant transformation of a vestibular schwannoma in a 9-year-old girl was described by Schuknecht (1974). In that case, a schwannoma of the vestibular nerve was in continuity with a malignant tumor that had invaded the petrous bone and destroyed part of the internal auditory canal. The tumor was described as being highly cellular with hyperchromatic nuclei and numerous mitotic figures.

A malignant nerve sheath tumor of the acoustic nerve was reported in a 54-year-old man, without stigmata of von Recklinghausen's disease (Kudo, Matsumoto, & Terao, 1983) and another case was described as malignant acoustic schwannoma, with no stigmata of neurofibromatosis (Mrak, Ranigan, & Collins, 1994). Still another case was reported as the recurrence of acoustic neu-

rilemoma as a malignant spindle cell neoplasm that was thought to be malignant progression from a benign acoustic neurilemoma, an unusual occurrence in a patient without stigmata of von Recklinghausen's disease (McLean et al., 1990).

A malignant triton tumor of the acoustic nerve that probably arose from a pre-existing acoustic schwannoma was reported (Han et al., 1992), as well as a malignant triton tumor in the cerebellopontine angle that appeared to arise from the eighth nerve sheath (Best, 1987).

Finally, a lesion interpreted as malignant melanotic schwannoma of the eighth cranial nerve was reported in a 77-year-old man (Earls et al., 1994).

DIFFERENTIAL DIAGNOSIS

Acoustic tumors are the most frequent tumors of the cerebellopontine angle. Gonzalez Revilla (1948) reviewed 205 tumors in the cerebellopontine recess and found that 78% were "neurinomas" (eighth nerve tumors, except for a few), 6.3% meningiomas, 6.3% cholesteatomas, 5.9% gliomas, and the remaining 3.5% abscesses and miscellaneous tumors. However, there are numerous tumors and pathological conditions that may occur in or near that region and pose a problem in differential diagnosis. Most of these are mentioned as space-occupying lesions, but they may be distinguished by clinical means, grossly or microscopically and, therefore, do not present real diagnostic problems. Those that are of special interest are discussed subsequently (*vide infra*).

Space-occupying angle lesions would include cholesteatomas (primary cholesteatomas more often simulate acoustic tumors than do the secondary), dermoids, teratomas, chordoma, and choroid plexus tumor. Metastatic malignant neoplasm is always a possibility. On review of the previously published reports of secondary malignant tumors of the temporal bone, Schuknecht found the most common primary sites of origin, in order of frequency, to be breast, kidney, lung, stomach, larynx, prostate, and thyroid gland (Schuknecht, Allam, & Murakami, 1968). Leukemias and lymphomas can involve this area, as can tumors from adjacent areas, for example, lymphoepitheliomas. Neoplasm to neoplasm metastasis is possible, for example, bronchogenic carcinoma metastasizing to an acoustic "neurinoma" (LeBlanc, 1974).

We have encountered five cases of lipomas of the eighth nerve (Figure 3–73). Histologically, there is no problem in distinguishing schwannomas from lipomas. Lipomas can be diagnosed or suspected by their MRI findings (see Chapter 6, "Radiologic Findings in Acoustic Tumors").

Vascular lesions may affect the eighth nerve, including aneurysms, compression of nerve by a crossing artery, and AV malformation. We have encountered several cases of a peculiar lesion composed of numerous irregular vascular channels with thick walls (Figure 3–74). These lesions have been up to 1 cm in diameter and have been located in or near the internal auditory canal. The exact classification is as yet undetermined, but the possibilities considered are cavernous hemangiomas and vascular hamartoma or malformation. We currently refer to these vascular lesions as benign vascular tumors. They may be of dural sinus origin. Clinically, they present as acoustic tumors (or as seventh nerve tumors with facial weakness). Grossly, they are red-pink and spongy, which is unlike a schwannoma. (Lo et al., 1989; Mangham, Carberry, & Brackmann, 1981). Other lesions may simulate cerebellopontine angle tumor, such as arachnoiditis, abscesses, arachnoid cysts, granulomas, tuberculosis, parasites, and hematomas. Histologically, leiomyomas may resemble schwannomas, but a leiomyoma in this location would be extremely unusual. Rarely, a melanotic schwannoma can occur (Dastur et al., 1967; Miller et al., 1986). Schwann cells are derived from the neural

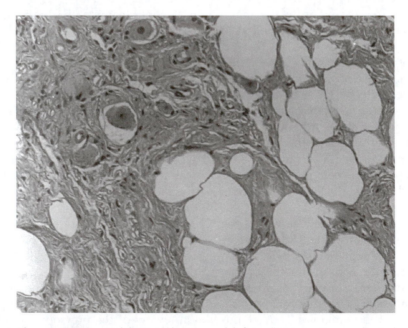

Figure 3–73. Eighth nerve lipoma, adult fat cells separating myelinated nerve fibers and ganglion cells. (H & E × 216)

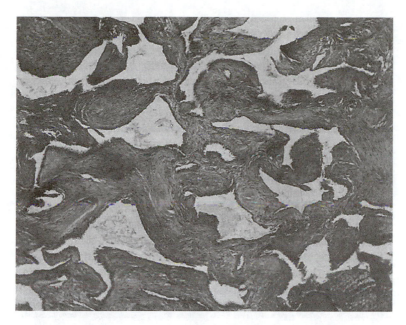

Figure 3–74. Cavernous hemangioma, or vascular hamartoma or malformation, composed of numerous irregular dilated channels with thick walls (see text). This is not a schwannoma. (H & E × 61.2)

crest and probably bring melanoblasts with them. Therefore, if one encounters a tumor with melanotic cells, a primary as well as metastatic tumor should be considered.

By far the most practical problem in differential diagnosis (in terms of frequency of occurrence and gross and microscopic appearance) is differentiating meningioma from acoustic schwannoma. Although small biopsies of acoustic tumors received from surgery are characteristic 90% to 95% of the time (Figure 3–7), meningiomas may have the same pale yellow semi-translucent appearance. Meningiomas may even be bright yellow (Figure 3–75), as one would expect more typically from a histocytic area of acoustic tumor. Later, the larger gross specimen of acoustic tumor is usually typical, but it can be more tan-white and rubbery, like meningioma, and meningioma can resemble typical acoustic tumor. Microscopically, meningiomas may have numerous patterns. The meningothelial or psammomatous menin-

giomas usually are easy to recognize microscopically, but the fibrous and transitional types may be difficult to distinguish from schwannoma. This may be especially true on frozen section or particularly when only small fragments of tissue are received. Schwannomas can have whorls mimicking meningioma (Figures 3–26 and 3–27). When the entire tumor becomes available, the problem usually is resolved.

Various gliomas may occur in this region and may even extend from the brainstem along the eighth nerve and present as an eighth nerve tumor. Since a portion of an acoustic tumor may resemble a glioma (Figures 3–64 through 3–67), this again may be a problem, especially on frozen section or in a small biopsy. Areas of schwannomas may have vascular patterns resembling capillary hemangioma, glomus tumor, or cavernous hemangioma (Figures 3–36, 3–37, and 3–38).

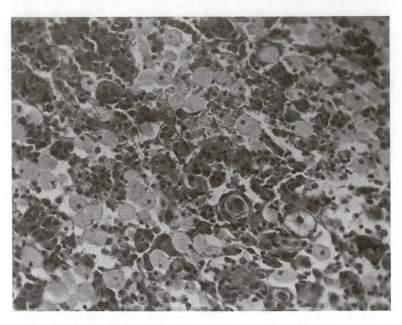

Figure 3–75. Meningioma containing histiocytes, specimen grossly yellow. (H & E × 288)

NEUROFIBROMATOSIS 2 AND MULTIPLICITY

Von Recklinghausen's disease presents three forms that appear relatively distinct: a central form, (neurofibromatosis 2, or NF-2) with multiple intracranial and intraspinal tumors; a peripheral form (NF-1) that is associated with café au lait patches; and a visceral form. Of course, there may be some overlap (Rubinstein, 1972).

The earliest recorded examples of bilateral recess tumors in association with central neurofibromatosis appear to have been those of Wishart in 1822 and Knoblauch (as cited in Cushing, 1917/1963). Gardner and Turner (1940) studied a family in which von Recklinghausen's disease in the form of bilateral acoustic tumors had been transmitted through generations. It was assumed that all family members who were deaf, or deaf and blind, had bilateral acoustic tumors. In the six members on whom operation or necropsy was performed, this assumption was proved correct.

Figures 3–8 and 3–9 show the specimen from a 53-year-old man with bilateral acoustic tumors (right previously operated). After complete autopsy, the only other indications of neurofibromatosis 2 were a small schwannoma in a nerve near the temporal bone and multiple small schwannomas in the cauda equina and in a few of the cervical spinal roots, so that the main manifestation of the disease was bilateral acoustic schwannomas. We have not been able to appreciate any gross difference in appearance between the unilateral and bilateral tumor as they are received from surgery.

One of the interesting phenomena, however, in NF-2 is that there may be one or multiple schwannomas involving an individual nerve or any of numerous nerves, as well as one or multiple meningiomas. Schwannomas and meningiomas may be present in the same surgical specimen as collision tumors or as separate individual lesions. One may or may not be able to distinguish the two grossly.

Microscopically, in most cases of NF-2 the acoustic schwannoma is identical on routine H & E stain to any of the usual unilateral tumors. Occasionally, however, tumors in NF-2 may show areas that appear to be intermediate in pattern between meningioma and schwannoma (Figures 3-76 through 3-79). Actually, this is not surprising, since the cells in both schwannomas and meningiomas originate from the neural crest. Occasionally, in some cases of otherwise typical unilateral schwannomas, there are areas that have cross features between meningioma and schwannoma. Whether in these cases this is part of NF-2 or just variance in microscopic pattern is only a matter of speculation. However, it is always possible that there is a small, as yet undetected, contralateral schwannoma.

The other common feature in NF-2 is the multiplicity of meningiomas. Often these are tiny or microscopic and may be considered focal meningeal proliferations or "micromeningiomas." They often occur at the edge of an otherwise typical example of schwannoma (Figures 3–80 and 3–81). Meningiomas may be microscopically intermixed with schwannoma (Figures 3–82 and 3–83). Of course, the meningiomas can be large.

On routine H & E stain in NF-2, the acoustic tumor appears similar to that in the unilateral case.

Some authors claim that they can distinguish the schwannomas of patients with NF-2 from those of patients who do not have NF-2 (Sobel, 1993). We have reviewed these findings, and the changes outlined in this paper as occurring in NF-2 tumors also

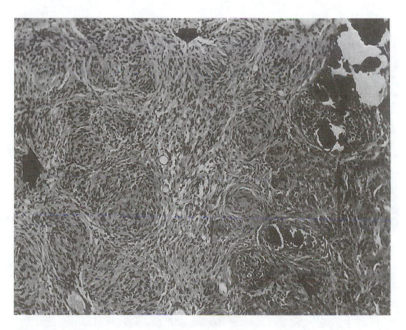

Figure 3–76. Acoustic tumors and meningiomas in NF-2 (Figures 3–76 through 3–83). One of multiple pieces of tissue received during acoustic tumor surgery. Nests of meningiothelial cells with psammoma bodies (*long arrows*), mixed with whorled areas (*large broad arrow*), probably meningioma, and other areas (*small broad arrow*) in the center which are difficult to distinguish from schwannoma. (H & E × 135)

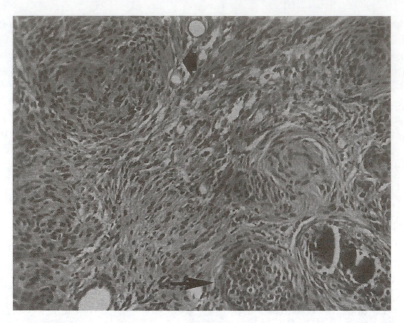

Figure 3–77. Higher power of Figure 3–76. Meningiothelial nests (*long arrow*) with psammoma bodies, whorled cells (*short broad arrow*), probably meningioma, and areas in the center similar to schwannoma. (H & E × 252)

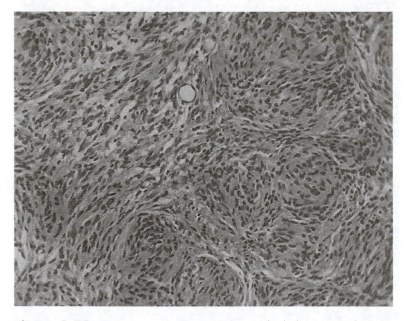

Figure 3–78. Same case as Figure 3–76. Whorled areas (*right*) more resemble meningioma, and elongated cells (*left*) are intermediate in pattern between meningioma and schwannoma. (H & E × 252)

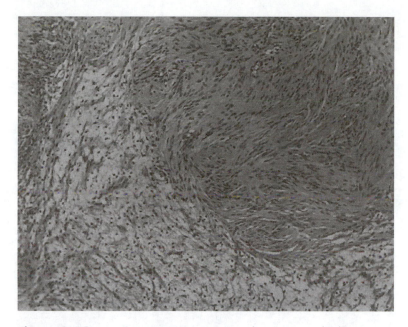

Figure 3–79. Same case as Figure 3–76, showing typical schwannoma at the edge of the tissue (Antoni A, *top right*, Antoni B, *bottom left*). (H & E × 144)

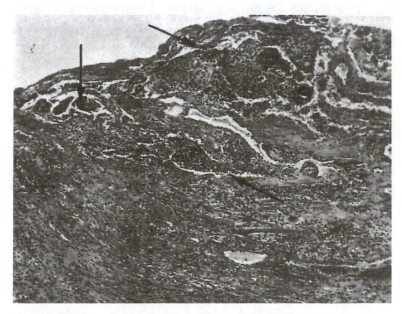

Figure 3–80. Multiple micromeningiomas (or meningeal proliferations) (*arrows*) at the edge of a schwannoma (*bottom*). (H & E × 99)

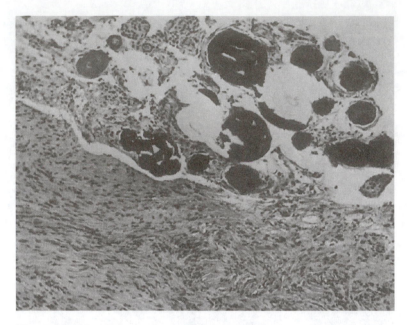

Figure 3–81. Same case as Figure 3–80, different area. "Micromeningioma" with psammoma bodies (*top*) at edge of a schwannoma (*bottom*). (H & E × 144)

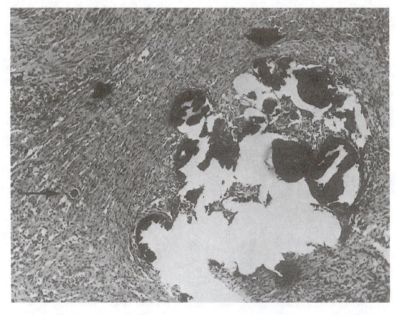

Figure 3–82. Same case as Figures 3–76 through 3–79, different sample of tissue. Meningioma (*broad arrow*) with psammoma bodies is surrounded by schwannoma. (Artifactual fracturing due to calcification.) Ganglion cell (*long arrow*) entrapped by schwannoma. (H & E × 72)

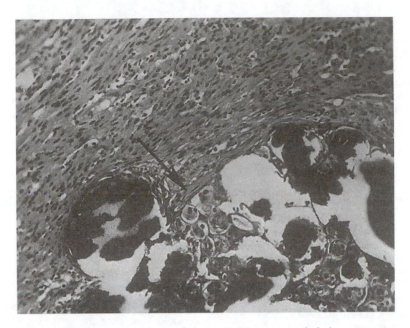

Figure 3–83. Higher power of Figure 3–82. Meningothelial meningioma (*arrow*) with psammoma bodies. Schwannoma at top. (H & E × 180)

can occur in non-NF-2 tumors. We have studied NF-2 tumors restrospectively, including blind studies as well as known NF-2 tumors and special stains for nerve fibers. To date, we are unable to distinguish NF-2 tumors from non-NF-2 tumors by light microscopy. The only distinguishing features are bilateral acoustic schwannomas, multiple, or in combination with meningioma. The combination tumors in patients with NF-2 can be separate, collision, or intermingled tumors.

ACKNOWLEDGMENT

The authors wish to thank Drs. Raymond B. Wuerker and John O. Erickson of the Veteran's Administration Hospital, Long Beach, California, for providing the electron micrographs.

REFERENCES

Ackerman, L. V., & Rosal, J. (1974). *Surgical pathology* (5th ed.) St. Louis: Mosby.

Ash. J.E. (1960). Pathology of the ear. In G. M. Coates & H. P. Schenck (Eds.), *Otolaryngology* (Vol. 1, pp. 1–69). Hagerstown, MD: W.F. Prior

Best, P.V. (1987). Malignant triton tumor in the cerebellopontine angle: Report of a case. *Acta Neuropathological (Berlin), 74*, 92–96.

Burger, P.C., & Scheithauer, B.W. (1994). Tumors of the central nervous system. *Atlas of tumor pathology* (pp. 340–341, 379–381). Washington, DC: Armed Forces Institute of pathology.

Burger, P.C., Scheithauer, B.W., & Vogel, F.S. (1991). *Surgical pathology of the nervous system and its coverings* (3rd ed., pp. 700–709). London: Churchill Livingstone.

Cravioto, H. (1969). The ultrastructure of acoustic nerve tumors. *Acta Neuropathologica, 12*, 116–140.

Cravioto, H., & Lockwood, R. (1968). Long spacing fibrous collagen in human acoustic nerve tumors. *Journal of Ultrastructural Research, 24*, 70–85.

Cravioto, H., & Lockwood, R. (1969). The behavior of acoustic neuroma in tissue culture. *Acta Neuropathologica (Berlin), 12*, 141.

Cushing H. (1932). *Intracranial tumors.* Springfield, Ill: Charles C. Thomas.

Cushing, H. (1963). *Tumors of the nervus acusticus and the syndrome of the cerebellopontile angle.*

New York: Hafner Publishing. (Original work published 1917)

Dastur, D.K., Sinh, G., & Pandya, S.K. (1967). Melanotic tumor of the acoustic nerve. Case report. *Journal of Neurosurgery, 27,* 166–170.

Ducatman, B.S., Scheithauer, B.D., Piepgras, D.G., Reiman, H.M., & Ilstrup, D.M. (1986). Malignant peripheral nerve sheath tumors, *Cancer, 57,* 2006–2021.

Earls, J.P., Robles, H.A., McAdams, H.P., & Rao, K. (1994). General case of the day: Malignant melanotic schwannoma of the eighth cranial nerve. *RadioGraphics, 14,* 1425–1427.

Friedmann, I. (1974). *Pathology of the ear* (pp. 213–223). Oxford: Blackwell Scientific Publications

Gardner, W.J., & Turner, O. (1940). Bilateral acoustic neurofibromas. *Archives of Neurology and Psychiatry, 44,* 76–99.

Gussen. R. (1971). Intramodiolar acoustic neurinoma. *Laryngoscope, 81,* 1979–1984.

Han, D.H., King, D.G., Chi, J.G., Park, S.H., Jung, H.W., & Kim, V.G. (1992). Malignant triton tumor of the acoustic nerve. *Journal of Neurosurgery, 76,* 874–877.

Hardy, M., & Crowe, S.J. (1936). Early asymptomatic acoustic tumor. Report of six cases. *Archives of Surgery, 32,* 292–301

Harkin, J.C., & Reed, R.J. (1969). *Tumors of the peripheral nervous system.* (Fascicles No. 3, 2nd series). Armed Forces Institute of Pathology.

Hirano, A., Dembitzer, H.M., & Zimmerman, H.M. (1972). Fenestrated blood vessels in neurilemmoma. *Laboratory Investigation, 27,* 305.

Hoessly, G.F., & Olivecrona, H. (1955). Report of 280 cases of verified parasagittal meningioma. *Journal of Neurosurgery, 12,* 614.

Information Center for Hearing, Speech and Disorders of Human Communication (1971). *Acoustic neurinoma: Present status and research trends.* Baltimore: The Johns Hopkins Medical Institutions. Distributed by the National Technical Information Service, U.S. Department of Commerce, 5285 Port Royal Road, Springfield, Virginia.)

Kudo, M., Matsumoto, M., & Terao, H. (1983). Malignant nerve sheath tumor of acoustic nerve. *Archives of Pathology and Laboratory Medicine, 107,* 293–297.

Le Blanc, R.A. (1974). Metastasis of bronchogenic carcinoma to acoustic neurinoma. Case report. *Journal of Neurosurgery, 41,* 614–617.

Leonard, J., & Talbot, M. (1970). Asymptomatic acoustic neurilemmoma. *Archives of Otolaryngology, 91,* 117.

Lo, W.W.M., Shelton, C., Waluch, V., Solti-Bohman, L.G., Carberry, J.N., Brackmann, D.E., & Wade, C.T. (1989). Intratemporal vascular tumors: Detection with CT and MRI imaging. *Radiology, 171,* 445–448.

Lumsden, C.E. (1971). The study by tissue culture of tumors of the nervous system. In D.S. Russell & L.J. Rubinstein (Eds.), *Pathology of tumors of the nervous system* (3rd ed.). Baltimore: Williams & Wilkins.

Luse, S.A. (1960). Electron microscopic studies of brain tumors. *Neurology, 10,* 881–905.

Mallory, F.B. (1919). The type cell of the so-called dural endothelioma. *Journal of Medical Research, 41,* 349.

Mangham, C.A., Carberry, J.N., & Brackman, D.E. (1981). Management of intracranial tumors. *Laryngoscope, 91,* 867–876.

McLean, C.A., Laidlaw, J.D., Brownbill, D.S., & Gonzales, M.D. (1990). Recurrence of acoustic neurilemmoma as a malignant spindle cell neoplasm. *Journal of Neurosurgery, 73,* 946–950.

Miller, R.T., Sarikaya H., & Sos, A. (1986). Melanotic schwannoma of the acoustic nerve. *Archives of Pathology and Laboratory Medicine, 10,* 153–154.

Mrak, R.E., Flanigan, S., & Collins, C.L. (1994). Malignant acoustic schwannoma, *Archives of Pathology and Laboratory Medicine, 118,* 557–561.

Murray, M.R. (1942). Comparative data on tissue culture of acoustic neurilemmomas and meningiomas. *Journal of Neuropathology and Experimental Neurology, 1,* 123–124.

Murray, M., & Stout, A.P. (1940). Schwann cell vs. fibroblast as the origin of the specific nerve sheath tumor. *American Journal of Pathology, 16,* 41–60.

Naunton. R., & Petasnick, J. (1970). Acoustic neurinomas with normal internal auditory meatus. *Archives of Otolaryngology, 91,* 437–443.

Pineda, A., & Feder, B.H. (1967). Acoustic neuroma: A misnomer. The *American Surgeon, 33,* 40–43.

Pool, L.J., Pava, A.A., & Greenfield, E.C. (1970). *Acoustic nerve tumors—Early diagnosis and treatment* (2nd ed.). Springfield, IL: Charles C. Thomas.

Revilla, A.G. (1948). Differential diagnosis of tumors at the cerebellopontile recess. *Bulletin of the Johns Hopkins Hospital, 83,* 187.

Rubinstein, L.J. (1972). *Tumors of the central nervous system.* (Fascicle No. 6, 2nd series). Armed Forces Institute of Pathology.

Russell, D.S., & Rubinstein, L.J. (1977). *Pathology of tumors of the nervous system* (4th ed.). Baltimore: Williams & Wilkins.

Schuknecht, H.F. (1974). *Pathology of the ear.* Cambridge, MA: Harvard University Press.

Schuknecht, H.F. Allam, A.F., & Murakami, Y. (1968). Pathology of secondary malignant tumors of the temporal bone. *Annals of Otology, Rhinology, and Laryngology, 77,* 5–22.

Silverberg, S.G. (1983). *Principles and practice of surgical pathology* (Vol. 1, pp. 1508–1509). New York: John Wiley & Sons.

Skinner, H.A. (1929). The origin of acoustic nerve tumors. *British Journal of Surgery, 16,* 440–463.

Sobel, R.A. (1993). Vestibular (acoustic) schwannomas; Histologic features in neurofibromatosis 2 and in unilateral cases. *Journal of Neuropathology and Experimental Neurology, 52,* 106–113.

Stewart, T.J., Liland. J., & Schuknecht, H.F. (1975). Occult schwannomas of the vestibular nerve. *Archives of Otolaryngology, 101,* 91–95.

Stout, A.P. (1935). The peripheral manifestations of the specific nerve sheath tumor (neurilemmoma). *American Journal of Cancer, 24,* 751–796.

Stout, A.P. (1949). *Tumors of the peripheral nervous system.* (Fascicle No. 6, 1st series). Armed Forces Institute of Pathology.

Taylor, C.R., & Cote, R.J. (1994). *Immunomicroscopy: A diagnostic tool for the surgical pathologist* (2nd ed., pp. 354–358). Philadelphia: W.B. Saunders.

Thomsen, J., Klinken, L., & Tos, M. (1984). Calcified acoustic neurinoma. *Journal of Laryngology and Otology, 98,* 727–732.

Tos, M., Drozdziewicz, D., & Thomsen, J. (1992). Medial acoustic neuromas: A new clinical entity. *Archives of Otolaryngology—Head and Neck Surgery, 118,* 127–133.

Walshe, F. (1931). Intracranial tumours; A critical review. *Quarterly Journal of Medicine, 24,* 587–640.

Wanamaker. H.H. (1972). Acoustic neuroma: Primary arising the vestibule. *Laryngoscope, 82,* 1040–1044.

Woolford, T.J., Birzgalis, A.R., & Ramsden, R.T. (1994). An extensive vestibular schwannoma with both intracranial spread and lateral extension to the external auditory canal. *Journal of Laryngology and Otology, 108,* 149–151.

Wu, C., Hwang, C.F., Lin, C-H., & Su, C-Y. (1993). External ear canal schwannoma: An unusual case report. *Journal of Laryngology and Otology, 107,* 829–830.

Zulch, K. (1957). *Brain tumors: Their biology and pathology.* New York: Springer Publishing.

CHAPTER 4

Neurotological Evaluation

Simón I. Angeli, M.D.
Carol A. Jackson, M.D., P.C.

INTRODUCTION

This chapter describes the clinical neuroto-logic manifestations of acoustic neuromas which result from the pressure that these slowly growing tumors exert on the surrounding structures. The cochleovestibular nerve is the most commonly impaired structure, followed by the trigeminal nerve, the facial nerve, labyrinthine vessels, cerebellum and brain, and other adjacent cranial nerves. Larger tumors can interfere with cerebrospinal fluid dynamics and cause hydrocephalus.

Clinical manifestations caused by acoustic neuromas vary greatly. Some tumors grow to a large size without producing symptoms or signs, while much smaller tumors can produce substantial hearing loss, tinnitus, imbalance, and vertigo. Although the classic presentation is asymmetric sensorineural hearing loss with dysequilibrium, symptoms can be insidious or sudden in presentation and can occasionally fluctuate or even "improve" with medical therapies used to treat other inner ear disorders. A high index of suspicion, a complete neurotological and audiological evaluation, and judicious use of adjuvant radiodiagnostic tests can assist in the early diagnosis of an acoustic neuroma.

Harvey Cushing led the way to the diagnosis of acoustic neuromas before reaching premorbid dimension and brilliantly described the chronology of symptoms in his 1917 monograph (Cushing, 1917). By calling attention to the auditory and labyrinthine manifestations that precede other cerebellopontine angle symptoms, he introduced to future generations the diagnostic clues for small acoustic tumors. The goals of treatment of acoustic neuromas have changed from an emphasis on preserving life to preserving neurological function (specifically, cranial nerves VII and VIII). First motor, speech, and swallowing functions were maintained. Later, the facial nerve and, more recently, the cochlear nerve and serviceable hearing can be preserved in many cases. The best functional results occur after removal of small tumors, underscoring the importance of early diagnosis and treatment.

Current advances in microsurgery and neuroimaging have contributed greatly to the increased proportion of small tumors that have been surgically removed in recent years, sometimes in a stage in which symptoms are minimal or absent. Among 1,479 surgically confirmed acoustic neuromas treated at the House Ear Clinic from 1982 through 1992, the percentage of tumors 1.5

cm or less in size has steadily increased from 23% in 1982 to 55%–65% in 1992. Similarly, the percentage of tumors 4 cm or greater in size has decreased from 22% to less than 5%. In this series, the mean patient age was 49 years, there was no sex predilection, and tumors were slightly more frequent on the left than on the right side (59% vs. 41%).

CLINICAL MANIFESTATIONS OF ACOUSTIC NEUROMAS

Auditory symptoms and signs are the first to develop in most acoustic neuroma cases. Table 4–1 delineates these manifestations in 180 consecutive cases treated at the House Ear Clinic during a 15-month period between 1992 and 1993. For early diagnosis of acoustic tumors, every patient with unilateral "inner ear" symptoms should undergo a thorough otologic and neurologic physical examination and audiovestibular testing. Imaging procedures provide the definitive diagnosis when the neurotologic and audiovestibular signs point to an acoustic neuroma.

Hearing Loss

In this series, the complaint of hearing loss was the presenting symptom in 75% of cas-es; 95% of patients had some degree of hearing loss demonstrated on the audiogram. Typically, the sensorineural hearing loss is unilateral and progresses gradually over several years. Patients commonly report difficulty in understanding speech over the telephone, sometimes reporting a recent shift in use of the phone from the side of the tumor to the unaffected side. However, other types of hearing loss can occur. Hearing can fluctuate or even improve. For example, some patients with acoustic neuromas experience acute rotary vertigo, tinnitus, and fluctuating hearing loss typical of Meniere's disease, although this is uncommon .

The prevalence of acoustic neuroma in a recent series of patients with sudden hearing loss from the House Ear Clinic was 2.5%. The severity of hearing loss from acoustic neuroma ranged from mild, when the tumor extends medially, to profound, when the tumor extends to the lateral end of the internal auditory canal. Facial paresthesia, antecedent unilateral tinnitus, or mid-frequency (U-shaped) hearing loss also are signs of an acoustic neuroma. (Saunders, Luxford, Devgan, & Fetterman, in press). Therefore, we caution against ascribing all cases of "idiopathic" sudden hearing loss to either viral infection or vascular accident, even when there is improvement after medical treatment, and recommend a complete

TABLE 4–1. Clinical manifestations of 180 acoustic neuromas diagnosed during the years 1992–1993.

Symptom	Presenting Complaint	Observed on Evaluation
Hearing loss	75%	95%
Tinnitus	9%	86%
Dizziness	9%	57%
Headaches	1%	40%
Facial paresthesia	1%	15%
Facial weakness or spasm	0%	2%
Other	5%	10%

evaluation for acoustic neuroma in cases of unilateral sudden hearing loss.

The tuning fork evaluation will be consistent with the audiometric findings. In the most common presentation of asymmetric sensorineural hearing loss, the Weber test will show lateralization away from the affected ear, and the Rinne test will be positive, with air conduction greater than bone conduction in the affected ear. However, in the frequent scenario of mild asymmetry for hearing loss above 3000 Hz, the tuning fork exam is normal.

Tinnitus

Unilateral tinnitus is frequently an early symptom. Most patients with unilateral or asymmetric hearing loss will have tinnitus on the affected side (86% of cases) but may not complain of tinnitus unless specifically asked. In this series, 9% of patients had tinnitus as the presenting symptom, even in the absence of hearing loss. An acoustic tumor should be diligently sought in cases of unilateral tinnitus of more than 3 months, duration; with durations shorter than this, unilateral tinnitus is highly unlikely to be the sole presenting finding acoustic neuromas or other serious otologic pathology.

Dizziness

Patients with vestibular symptoms due to an acoustic neuroma most often complain of progressive imbalance, positional dizziness, or both. A few patients will experience severe incapacitating rotary vertigo at some stage in their disease, followed by minimal or no unsteadiness (Hitselberger, 1967). Only 9% of patients in this series complained of dizziness at the time of tumor diagnosis, but a history of dizziness was elicited in 57%. The destruction of unilateral peripheral vestibular function by these slowly growing tumors is gradual and fa-

cilitates central vestibular compensation.

The neurotological examination of patients with acoustic tumors often identifies signs of peripheral and central vestibular dysfunction. In small tumors, nystagmus can be found in the horizontal plane beating away from the affected side. Vertical plane nystagmus is a sign of brainstem compression by large tumors. Examination of gait can disclose staggering, called "vestibular ataxia." Deviation toward the lesion sometimes can be demonstrated by asking the patient to walk around a chair, resulting in a fall into the chair when rotating toward the affected side. Walking in tandem, the "straight line walk," which involves placing the heel of one foot directly in front of the toes of the other foot, can be impaired. Romberg's test involves the maintenance of an erect stance while standing with the feet together and the head straight, first with the eyes open and then with the eyes closed. One must determine if balance can be maintained in the absence of vision, which forces reliance on the vestibular system. Patients with acoustic tumors often exhibit a tendency to fall or sway to the affected side when closing the eyes. An abnormal sway or falling is a positive Romberg's sign. To enhance sensitivity, the "sharpened" Romberg's test is performed, in which the patient stands with one foot directly in front of the other, as in the tandem walk test (Figure 4–1). The response is reinforced by having the patient interlock the hands, raise them in front of the chest, and then pull the hands apart.

Dizziness also can be a caused by cerebellar dysfunction. Large acoustic tumors can compress the cerebellum and cause ipsilateral dysfunction. This usually is manifested by difficulty manipulating objects with the hand, past pointing, intention tremor, and a wide based gait. Patients demonstrate difficulty and loss of balance toward the affected side when asked to walk with a narrow base or when standing erect, even with eyes open. Ipsilateral hypotonia and disturbances of posture accompany the

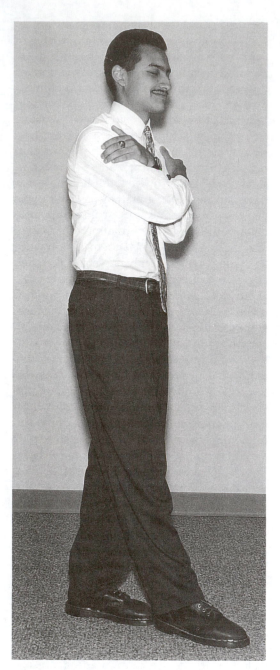

Figure 4–1. The Romberg test is enhanced by placing the feet in the tandem position.

gait disturbance when dysfunction is more severe. Signs of cerebellar dysfunction were present in 7% of patients in our series.

Facial Numbness and Pain

Tumors larger than 2 cm can compress the trigeminal nerve root located superiorly in the cerebellopontine angle (Selesnick, Jackler, & Pitts, 1993). Hypoesthesia of the face can occur if there is involvement of one or more of the three branches of the trigeminal nerve. Absence of the ipsilateral corneal reflex or hypoesthesia was demonstrated in 15% of patients in this series, many of whom were unaware of facial numbness. One patient presented with numbness and tingling in the cheek area. We have seen this complaint more frequently as a presenting symptom of recurrent acoustic neuromas following previous tumor removal if auditory symptoms are absent. Uncommonly, facial pain, reminiscent of "tic douloureaux," can be a feature of large tumors.

The motor division of the trigeminal nerve also should be examined, since some large tumors produce crossbite and atrophy of the temporalis and masseter muscles.

Facial Weakness

The motor division of the facial nerve is surprisingly tolerant of stretch and attenuation and is resistant to compression by acoustic tumor growth. Few cases of overt facial motor dysfunction due to the tumor are seen; in those cases, the tumor is usually large. In our series, none of the patients with previously untreated acoustic neuromas exhibited facial weakness. A more common manifestation of facial nerve dysfunction is quivering of the ipsilateral orbicularis oculi muscle, although afflicted patients usually are not aware of a twitch. On the other hand, marked facial weakness with few auditory signs in the presence of a cerebellopontine angle tumor should raise suspicion of a facial neuroma, a much rarer entity than acoustic neuroma.

The facial nerve is examined by asking the patient to smile, whistle, wrinkle the nose, close the eyes, and elevate the brows.

The House-Brackmann grading scale is used to record any alteration of function (see Chapter 17). Selective dysfunction of individual motor branches also is noted, as well as the presence of mass movement (synkinesis). At the time of tumor diagnosis, 98% of the patients in our series had a House-Brackmann grade I (normal), and 2% of patients had either grades II or III.

The sensory division of the facial nerve is examined best by testing the posterior aspect of the external auditory canal, just within the meatus. Diminished sensation in that region is known as "Hitselberger's sign," which was described first by neurosurgeon William Hitselberger. A wisp of cotton is used for testing, and the sensation is compared to that of the contralateral side. The patient is instructed not to respond to the sensation of sound that is elicited by rubbing the skin of the canal but rather to respond only to the tactile sensation. When present, this sign could correlate highly to the presence of an acoustic neuroma, but this finding is infrequent due to the overlapping sensory innervation in the area (Hitselberger & House, 1966).

Headaches

Although only one patient in our series experienced headaches as the predominant symptom of an acoustic neuroma, 40% of patients with acoustic tumors complained of headaches. The incidence of headache is related to the size of the tumor (Selesnick et al., 1993). Acoustic neuromas produce headaches by causing traction or displacement of intracranial vessels, sinuses, dura, or adjacent cranial nerves. In addition, large tumors can cause hydrocephalus and headaches by interfering with flow or absorption of cerebrospinal fluid. Moreover, dysequilibrium from uncompensated vestibular deafferentation can cause tension headaches and fatigue. In patients with migraine or other vascular headache syndromes unrelated to acoustic neuroma, an increased severity of headaches, frequency of headaches, or both may occur in the perioperative period due to physiologic and emotional stress. A key diagnostic factor that distinguishes migraine headaches from those due to a tumor is that a migraine headache is not alleviated, and is often worsened, by analgesics, including narcotics.

Other Neurological Manifestations

Impaired visual acuity occurs rarely in patients with acoustic tumors. Young patients with neurofibromatosis type 2 occasionally develop cataracts. Patients with large or giant tumors can develop papilledema from hydrocephalus. A fundoscopic examination is an integral part of the neurotologic physical examination of patients with acoustic neuromas. An ophthalmologic consultation should be obtained whenever impaired visual acuity or papilledema is suspected.

Diplopia is rare but may occur from dysfunction of the sixth cranial nerve, due to compression by a large tumor or in the setting of intracranial hypertension. Dysfunction of the lower cranial nerves, IX, X, XI, and XII, is also rare. All patients with acoustic neuromas should be questioned for symptoms and examined for signs of dysphagia, velopharyngeal incompetence, hoarseness, aspiration, shoulder weakness, and tongue weakness.

Due to greater awareness and improved diagnostic techniques, very few patients present today with the devastating neurological consequences common in prior eras due to giant acoustic neuromas in the final premorbid stages. Long tract signs of loss of motor and sensory function in the extremities, respiratory difficulty, and stupor result from brainstem compression and are seldom seen today in untreated patients. However, on rare occasions, an acoustic neuroma will present with sudden neurologic deterioration due to a rapid increase in tumor size from intratumoral hemorrhage. An abrupt onset of hearing loss, facial weakness, facial paresthesia, and somnolence should prompt an emergent evaluation.

The presentation of patients with previously radiated acoustic tumors to the neurotologist for surgical removal has been on the rise in recent years. Most of these patients have medium to large tumors with demonstrated growth postradiation. Hearing loss, facial weakness, and trigeminal nerve dysfunction are the most common neurological signs present in this group. However, lower cranial nerve dysfunction, diplopia, ataxia, and extremity weakness can be present, particularly following the less focused forms of high dosage radiotherapy. These symptoms and signs develop 3 to 6 months following radiation and can progress over several months before stabilizing. Careful documentation of neurotologic impairment is particularly critical in the postradiation patient, because the difficult surgical dissection of the radiated adherent tumor from necrotic adjacent cerebellum, brainstem and temporal lobe increases the risk of postoperative neurological impairment. Multiple observers and videotaping are helpful to document the physical exam when multiple neurological abnormalities are present.

Small acoustic neuromas (≤3 mm in diameter) are now identifiable with enhanced MRI studies. With the ready availability and expanded applications of MRI scanning, the identification of asymptomatic acoustic neuromas is on the rise as an incidental finding in the work-up for headaches, and other neurologic or head and neck disorders. The risks and complications arising from removal of an asymptomatic benign tumor must be balanced against potential future tumor growth and progression of symptoms and signs. Perhaps today's clinician is fortunate to be faced with the dilemma of whether or not to remove tiny, asymptomatic, or minimally symptomatic acoustic neuromas.

Other Considerations

During the initial evaluation of a patient with an acoustic neuroma, associated conditions that could complicate the future management of the patient should be identified. Contralateral hearing should be assessed and considered highly in the recommendation of surgical removal. The patient's life expectancy and general health should be considered in determining the risk of intracranial surgery. Tumor size and symptoms should be taken into consideration. Patients with neurofibromatosis type 2 may have additional cranial and spinal neuromas that should be addressed prior to any intervention. If ipsilateral chronic otitis media is present, it must be adequately resolved prior to microsurgical removal of the tumor.

SUMMARY

Acoustic neuromas produce symptoms and signs by invading or exerting pressure on the cochleovestibular nerve and other structures of the cerebellopontine angle. Despite some variations in clinical presentation, audiovestibular manifestations are the first to develop. They are later followed by neurological changes consequent to involvement of the surrounding structures as the tumor grows. Thus, unilateral tinnitus, progressive hearing loss, and imbalance or positional dizziness usually are symptoms of small-to-medium sized acoustic neuromas. Facial paresthesia, facial weakness, and trigeminal impairment develop with tumor enlargement. Other cranial nerve abnormalities, ataxia, respiratory, and long-tract signs develop with giant tumors. Hydrocephalus, stupor, and vital sign abnormalities of slowed respirations signal the premorbid stage.

Routine audiologic evaluation of acoustic tumors may reveal the characteristic findings of asymmetric sensorineural hearing loss and decreased speech discrimination that is disproportionate to the pure-tone loss. Atypical presentations are not uncommon, and the hearing loss may fluctuate, be minimally asymmetric, or have a sudden onset.

The mainstay of the initial history in the patient with a suspected acoustic neuroma remains a progressive unilateral or asymmetric hearing loss and dysequilibrium. The physical exam includes a lateralizing Weber, positive Romberg test, a search for facial weakness, a reduced corneal reflex, and facial hypoesthesia. The atypical presentation poses a challenge to the clinician. Sophisticated diagnostic tests identify tumors in patients with other patterns of hearing loss, vertigo, and cranial nerve dysfunction. The discovery of an asymptomatic small tumor is becoming more commonplace. Therefore, the clinician must rule out the possibility of acoustic neuroma in patients who present for neurotologic care with unexplained audiovestibular complaints and perform a thorough history and physical exam, as described here, searching for the atypical or infrequent presentations, as well as the classic abnormalities of acoustic neuromas.

REFERENCES

Cushing, H. (1917). *Tumors of the nervus acusticus and the syndrome of cerebellopontile angle*; Philadelphia: W.B. Saunders Co.

Hitselberger, W.E. (1967). Tumors of the cerebellopontine angle in relation to vertigo. *Archives of Otolaryngology—Head and Neck Surgery, 85*, 95–97.

Hitselberger, W.E., & House, W.F. (1966). Acoustic neuroma diagnosis: External auditory canal hypesthesia as an early sign. *Archives of Otolaryngology—Head and Neck Surgery, 83*, 50–53.

Saunders, J.E., Luxford, W.M., Devgan, K.K., & Fetterman, B.L. (in press). Sudden hearing loss in acoustic neuroma patients. *Archives of Otolaryngology—Head and Neck Surgery.*

Selesnick, S.H., Jackler, R.K., & Pitts, L.W. (1993). The changing presentation of acoustic tumors in the MRI era. *Laryngoscope, 103*, 431–435.

CHAPTER 5

Audiologic Testing

Debara L. Tucci, M.D.

Cushing was the first to note, in 1917, that unilateral hearing loss is an early symptom in patients diagnosed with acoustic neuroma, a fact reiterated in many subsequent publications (Selesnick & Jackler, 1992). The development of sophisticated techniques of audiological assessment has permitted the earlier diagnosis of acoustic neuroma in patients with unilateral auditory symptoms. The goal of a comprehensive assessment battery is to identify these tumors at an early stage, when complete resection can be accomplished with minimal morbidity and mortality.

PATIENT PRESENTATION

Recent reviews report the incidence of asymmetric sensorineural hearing loss in patients with documented acoustic tumors as 85% (Chandrasekhar, Brackmann, & Devgan, 1995; Selesnick & Jackler, 1992; Welling, Glasscock, Woods, & Jackson, 1990). The next most common symptoms reported were tinnitus (80%), dizziness (57%), headache (20%), and paresthesias (17%) (Chandrasekhar et al., 1995). Hearing loss is by far the most important presenting complaint, documented in 65% of patients (Chandrasekhar et al., 1995; Selesnick &

Jackler, 1992). The incidence of hearing loss increases with tumor size and is reported as 77% in patients with tumors smaller than 1 cm, 88% in patients with tumors 1 to 3 cm, and 95% in patients with tumors larger than 3 cm (Selesnick & Jackler, 1992). In most cases, the hearing loss is unilateral and gradual in onset over an average of 3 to 4 years. However, many investigators have reported atypical presentations, including normal hearing, symmetrical hearing loss, and sudden onset hearing loss.

It is now well recognized that sudden hearing loss is not an uncommon presentation for patients with acoustic neuromas. While only 1–2% of patients with sudden sensorineural hearing loss will have an eighth nerve tumor, as many as 26% of acoustic tumor patients have been documented to have an abrupt decrement in hearing at some time prior to diagnosis (Selesnick & Jackler, 1993). A large series reported by Pensak, Glasscock, Josey, Jackson, and Gulys (1985) identified 15% of patients with cerebellopontile angle tumors as having a past history of sudden hearing loss. It is not uncommon for the hearing loss to improve or resolve completely with steroid therapy (Welling et al., 1990). Pensak et al. (1985) and others stress that every patient with a unilateral sensorineural hearing loss, no matter how long it has been present and no matter what the apparent etiology may be, should be evaluated to rule out an acoustic tumor (Shaia & Sheehy, 1976). Recent series report a significant incidence of normal hearing (4%–7%) or symmetrical hearing loss (7%) in acoustic tumor patients (Selesnick & Jackler 1993; Welling et al., 1990). These patients may present with isolated symptoms such as unilateral tinnitus or, rarely, vertigo.

The incidence of normal hearing in documented acoustic neuroma cases has increased as gadolineum-enhanced magnetic resonance imaging (MRIg) comes into more widespread use. MRIg was first introduced in 1987, and has become the "gold standard" for diagnosis of acoustic neuroma with the capability of detecting tumors as small as 3 mm in diameter. Prior to the introduction of MRIg, tests of audiological and vestibular function served as the most sensitive indicators of possible eighth cranial nerve pathology. Due to the expense involved in obtaining an MRI, audiological testing continues to serve a role in the cost effective assessment of patients determined to be at risk for the diagnosis of acoustic neuroma. This chapter will summarize some of the historically important tests of audiological function used to assess patients with unilateral or asymmetrical hearing loss, examine currently utilized assessment strategies, and discuss suggested protocols for the work-up of patients with suspected acoustic neuroma.

BEHAVIORAL ASSESSMENT: HISTORICALLY IMPORTANT TESTS OF RETROCOCHLEAR PATHOLOGY

Early assessments of auditory function defined several characteristics of retrocochlear pathology, including: (1) abnormal neural adaptation (or tone decay), (2) absence of loudness recruitment, (3) poor speech recognition ability relative to pure tone thresholds, and (4) an abnormal performance-intensity function on phonetically balanced

(PI-PB) word recognition tests. These early tests were based on behavioral assessments of auditory abilities, and have, for the most part, been replaced with more objective and more accurate electrophysiological methods of assessment, as described below. However, a discussion of these tests provides historical context as well as a useful understanding of auditory capabilities in these patients. While abnormal results on some of these tests, particularly the tone decay and PI-PB function tests, are reportedly accurately predictive of an acoustic neuroma in as many as 70%–75% of patients (Turner, Shepard, & Frazer, 1984), it must be noted that most reports are based on assessment of patients prior to the availability of MRI and, hence, are based on the diagnosis of tumors larger than those that we are able to detect reliably with current methods.

Tests of Neural Adaptation

It was first noted in the 1950s that neural adaptation is abnormal in acoustic neuroma patients. This concept was first utilized in site-of-lesion testing in the context of Bekesy automated audiometry. Bekesy audiograms included separate threshold tracings across frequency for continuous and pulsed signals. The combination of test findings and proposed associated pathologies was described in a classification scheme by Jerger (1960). The Type IV audiogram, thought to be consistent with retrocochlear pathology, consists of a continuous tone threshold tracing that falls below that of the pulsed tone by at least 20 dB. Thus, thresholds were better for pulsed than for continuous tones in patients with retrocochlear pathology, a finding attributed to their inability to maintain perception of a tone presented near threshold. Later refinements in Bekesy audiometry improved the detection rate for retrocochlear lesions. However, the test was limited by the fact that special instrumentation was required for administration.

Tone decay measurements, on the other hand, can be made with conventional audiometric equipment. Tone decay refers to the inability of a subject to maintain perception of a tone presented at either a barely audible or a suprathreshold level. Abnormal tone decay has been identified in patients with a variety of pathologies involving the eighth cranial nerve, including acoustic neuroma, and typically is not observed in patients with a hearing loss of cochlear origin. In the modification of the test as described by Carhart (1957), the subject is instructed to indicate either a change in tonality or a change in audibility of a signal presented at 5 dB above the established threshold at the test frequency. An adaptation of the test, proposed by Jerger and Jerger (1975), called the suprathreshold adaptation test (STAT), is based on the authors' observation that symptoms of abnormal tone decay appear first at high sound intensities. Neural adaptation may also be tested in the context of acoustic reflex decay, as discussed below.

Tests of Loudness Recruitment

Recruitment is defined as the abnormal growth of loudness for signals presented at suprathreshold intensities and is one hallmark of a cochlear hearing loss. Two procedures, the alternate binaural loudness balance (ABLB) and the short increment sensitivity index (SISI) have been utilized to differentiate cochlear from retrocochlear disorders.

Fowler (1936) first proposed the ABLB as a test for otosclerosis, prior to the introduction of bone conduction audiometry. The ABLB requires the subject to match in loudness two tones of the same frequency presented alternately to the two ears. Application of this test to the differential diagnosis of hearing loss was suggested by Dix, Hallpike, and Hood (1948), who reported that, while loudness recruitment was reliably present in 30 patients with Ménière's disease, it was absent in 14 of 20 patients with acoustic neuroma.

Bekesy (1947), noting that subjects with cochlear hearing loss had narrower continuous tone tracings than those with conductive hearing loss, suggested that the excursion width measured with his threshold tracking procedure was a method of monaural assessment of loudness recruitment. Further developments included the advent of direct assessment of intensity difference limens (Luscher & Zwislocki, 1948) and the subsequently related development of the SISI test. The SISI test was developed by Jerger and colleagues (1959) as a simple test of loudness recruitment and requires only that the subject report when a steady tone presented 20 dB above threshold periodically increases in intensity. Individuals with retrocochlear pathology often are unable to detect small changes in intensity, perhaps because of excessive tone decay. The high-level SISI test, thought to be more sensitive to retrocochlear pathology, was introduced by Thompson (1963). Test results in patients with eighth nerve tumors are noted to be affected by the size of the tumor and, presumably, by the amount of cochlear involvement (such as by interruption of cochlear blood supply). Although all tests of loudness recruitment are sensitive to cochlear pathology, they lack sensitivity for identification of retrocochlear lesions and are some of the least reliable tests for differential diagnosis (Brunt, 1994). Our ability to distinguish between a cochlear and retrocochlear pattern of hearing loss is complicated further by the fact that patients with a documented acoustic neuroma may demonstrate a cochlear pattern of hearing loss. This is thought to be secondary to anoxic injury as the tumor compresses the coch-lear blood supply (Flood & Brightwell, 1984).

Speech Recognition Assessment

In general, patients with acoustic neuromas exhibit poor speech discrimination for the degree of hearing loss, relative to patients with cochlear pathology. However, there is considerable overlap in speech recognition scores in these two groups of patients (Johnson, 1968).

Speech Recognition Performance-Intensity Function

Determination of a performance-intensity function has been shown to enhance the diagnostic significance of speech recognition testing by identifying those patients who exhibit a significant decrease in performance as presentation intensity is increased. Jerger and Jerger (1971) proposed the performance intensity function for phonetically balanced words (PI-PB function), or "rollover" test, as a means of identifying patients at risk for acoustic neuroma. The rollover ratio is defined as: (PB max − PB min) / PB max, where PB max is the best and PB min is the worst score as measured up to a maximum intensity of 110 dB sound pressure level (SPL).

ELECTROPHYSIOLOGIC TESTS FOR ASSESSMENT OF RETROCOCHLEAR PATHOLOGY

Acoustic Reflex Testing

Anderson, Bart, and Wedenberg (1969) were the first to apply acoustic reflex measurements to the evaluation of patients with suspected eighth nerve tumors. Acoustic reflex thresholds higher than the 90th percentile are considered elevated, and this finding, or that of absent reflexes, in the absence of conductive pathology, should raise suspicion of the presence of retrocochlear pathology (see Figure 5–1). Abnormal acoustic reflex decay is also a relatively strong indicator of retrocochlear pathology. Reflex decay is determined by presenting a stimu-

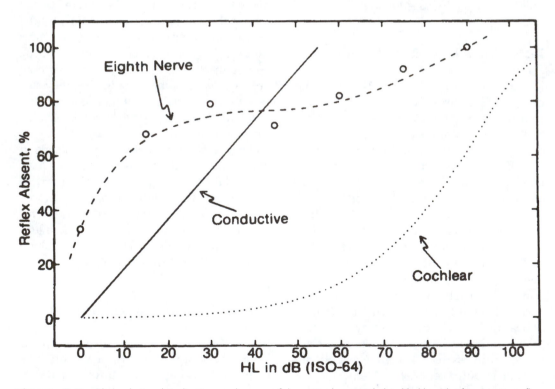

Figure 5–1. The relationship between degree of hearing loss and the likelihood of acoustic reflex absence in patients with conductive, cochlear, and eighth nerve pathology. From "The acoustic reflex in VIIIth nerve disorders," by K. F. Jerger, E. Harford, J. Clemis, B. Alford, 1994, Figure 2. *Archives of Otolaryngology 99*, pp. 409–413. Reprinted with permission.

lus test tone at 10 dB above the reflex threshold at 500 and 1000 Hz. Abnormal reflex decay is present if the amplitude of the reflex declines by more than half its original magnitude in less than 10 seconds. Turner, Shepard, and Frazer (1984) reviewed 23 studies involving 1,333 ears with acoustic neuromas and reported that the combined use of acoustic reflex thresholds and reflex decay correctly predicted retrocochlear pathology in 84% of patients. However, as noted above, these tests may be less sensitive than originally reported in detecting the small tumors which may be identified using newer radiographic imaging techniques.

Auditory Brainstem Evoked Response Testing (ABR)

ABR is the most sensitive auditory test available for identification of patients with acoustic neuromas. Selters and Brackmann (1977) first focused attention on the use of ABR testing for diagnosis of acoustic neuromas. They reported abnormal ABR results in 94% of 46 patients with confirmed tumors and advocated that the ABR be added to the battery of tests used to screen patients for retrocochlear pathology.

The ABR is a far-field recording of neuroelectric activity of the eighth cranial nerve and brainstem auditory pathways that occurs over the first 10 to 15 ms after delivery of an eliciting stimulus to the subject's ear. In a normal population, the ABR is characterized by five to seven peaks (designated by convention with Roman numerals) that represent synchronous neural discharge from sources along the auditory pathway. Although the neural generators of the ABR are known only partially at this time, it is generally accepted that waves I and II arise from the distal and proximal portions of the eighth nerve, respectively, and that the later waveforms are generated by multiple, overlapping neural sources within the auditory brainstem (Ruth & Lambert, 1991).

Neurodiagnostic testing using the ABR focuses on several characteristics of the response: (1) interwave latencies (I–III, I–V, III–V), (2) the interaural latency difference of wave V, (3) absolute latencies, (4) the presence or absence of waveform components, (5) amplitude ratios (V/I), and (6) overall waveform morphology (see Figure 5–2). The most widely used and diagnostically reliable parameters are the measures of interwave latency and the interaural latency difference of wave V. Latency is thought to be prolonged in patients with acoustic neuroma because of compression of the eighth nerve by the tumor mass, resulting in disruption of synchronous neural firing in response to the auditory stimulus (Ruth & Lambert, 1991; Selters & Brackmann, 1977). In cases of cochlear, rather than retrocochlear, hearing impairment, all wave peaks are thought to be equally prolonged, depending on the extent of the patient's peripheral hearing loss. Thus, for these patients, the interwave intervals remain constant, and are not prolonged. However, prolongation of the I–V interval is considered indicative of retrocochlear impairment. Assessment of the I–V interwave latency measurement is complicated when, as is often the case with high frequency hearing loss, wave I is absent. In this situation, wave V is compared between the ears. Since wave V can be delayed in the presence of cochlear hearing loss, a correction factor is generally applied to account for this discrepancy between the ears due to the hearing loss. Selters and Brackmann (1977) suggested that a 0.1 ms latency correction factor be applied for every 10 dB of hearing loss exceeding 50 dB HL at 4000 Hz. In the case that a response cannot be generated to the typical click stimulus in a patient with a severe-to-profound high frequency hearing loss, it may be possible to measure responses to lower frequency tone pips for assessment of interaural latency differences (Telian & Kileny, 1989).

Interpretation of Abnormal Findings

Clinicians differ in their criteria for abnormal absolute latency and interaural latency

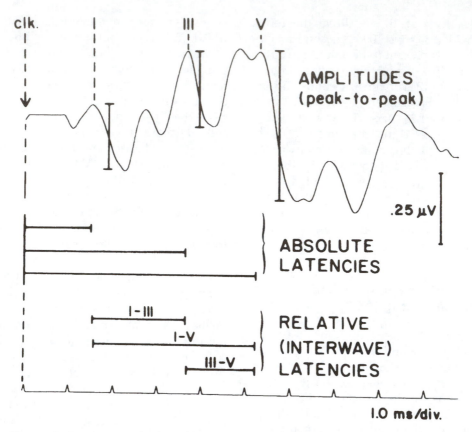

Figure 5–2. Basic amplitude and latency measurements of the ABR. The onset of the eliciting stimulus (click) is indicated by "Clk." From "The short latency auditory evoked potentials." A tutorial paper by the Audiologic Evaluation Working Group on Auditory Evoked Potential Measurements, 1988. Rockville, MD: ASHA. Reprinted with permission.

differences, and these criteria must be noted when interpreting data from studies that attempt to assess the predictive value of ABR in screening for acoustic neuroma.

Of all audiologic tests in the "retrocochlear" screening battery, ABR is the most valuable, because it has the highest sensitivity and specificity for identification of an acoustic neuroma. Sensitivity and specificity of the ABR are determined by ABR assessment in a population of patients who have been studied with MRIg and, therefore, are known either to have an acoustic neuroma or to be free of this pathology. In this case, MRIg is regarded as the gold standard test for identification of acoustic neuroma. Sensitivity is defined in this case as the ratio of true-positive ABR (abnormal ABR and presence of an acoustic neuroma) to all subjects with known pathology. Specificity is defined as the ratio of true-negatives (normal ABR in the absence of acoustic neuroma) to all subjects with no evidence of pathology. The predictive value of a test (the ratio of true-positive results to all positive results) will be affected by the sensitivity and specificity as well as the prevalence of the disease in the population tested (Bance, Hyde, & Malizia 1994; Weiss, Kisiel, & Bhatia, 1990). Most large series which have documented the reliability of ABR in screening for acoustic neuromas have been performed within large neuro-otologic practices, and most have focused on the incidence of abnormal ABR in patients with a known acoustic neuroma. Few studies have documented ABR sensitivity and specificity in general otology or general otolaryngology practices, and those that have report a less frequent finding of acoustic neuroma in patients with an abnormal ABR (Hendrix, DeDio, & Sclafani, 1990; Weiss, et al., 1990). It should be noted that the ABR may be abnormal in patients with retrocochlear pathology other than an acoustic neuroma, such as multiple sclerosis (Hendrix et al., 1990).

Most large series have reported an ABR sensitivity of 92%–98% and specificity of 80%–90% (Chandrasekhar et al., 1995; Selesnick & Jackler, 1992; Selters & Brackmann, 1977; Welling et al., 1990). The incidence of false-negative ABR appears to be greatest in small intracanalicular tumors, particularly those involving the superior vestibular nerve (Telian et al., 1989; Wilson, Hodgson, Gustafson, Hogue, & Mills, 1992).

VESTIBULAR ASSESSMENT

Electronystagmography (ENG) was used often in the past as one of a battery of tests designed to identify patients with suspected acoustic neuroma. Prior to the advent of modern diagnostic methods, the ENG could be expected to demonstrate a unilaterally reduced caloric response in more than 95% of patients. However, with the advent of more sophisticated methods of diagnosis and the ability to diagnose smaller tumors, the frequency of an abnormal vestibular response has dropped to about 70% (Linthicum, 1983; Welling et al., 1990). At least in part, poor sensitivity is due to the fact that the bithermal caloric portion of the ENG tests only the function of the horizontal semicircular canal and its innervation, the superior vestibular nerve. Hence, tumors originating from the inferior vestibular nerve may not be associated with ENG abnormal-ities, particularly if they are small. ENG abnormalities other than weakness of the response to caloric testing may include failure of fixation suppression, bilateral slowing of optokinetic nystagmus, saccadic pursuit, and occasional bilateral horizontal gaze nystagmus (Selesnick & Jackler, 1992).

ENG may provide information useful in planning postsurgical treatment for patients with a known acoustic neuroma. Patients with little demonstrated loss of vestibular function prior to surgery may be expected to experience more severe vestibular dysfunction after surgery than patients who have already experienced a significant loss of function over time. Presumably, patients with poor preoperative vestibular function have had the opportunity to compensate for this gradual unilateral vestibular loss. Another potential use of the information provided by ENG is in predicting the outcome of hearing preservation surgery. Hearing is more likely to be preserved in patients with small tumors of the superior vestibular nerve than in patients with tumors of the inferior vestibular nerve, which are more likely to involve the cochlear nerve at an early stage of tumor growth. Hence, the presence of a unilateral vestibular weakness, indicating a probable tumor of the superior vestibular nerve, may help to predict successful hearing preservation (McFarland, Linthicum, & Waldorf, 1989).

AN EFFICIENT APPROACH TO THE DIAGNOSIS OF AN ACOUSTIC NEUROMA

Identification of the Patient "At Risk" for Acoustic Neuroma

The primary presenting symptoms that should raise a suspicion of this diagnosis include asymmetric sensorineural hearing loss (sudden, slowly progressive, or long-standing), unilateral tinnitus, poor speech recognition ability relative to pure tone thresholds, and vertigo or imbalance. The degree of hearing asymmetry that should prompt further evaluation is unclear. While Welling and colleagues (1990) suggest that a 15 dB difference at any frequency from 500 to 4000 Hz should be considered significant, Mangham (1991) suggests that as little as a 5 dB difference in averaged thresholds at 1000, 2000, 4000, and 8000 Hz should lead to further evaluation. Hendrix et al. (1990) pursue further testing of patients who demonstrate a threshold difference of 10 dB at any two consecutive frequencies or at least a 15 dB difference at any frequency between 250 and 4000 Hz. Bu-Saba, Bebeiz, Salman, Thornton, and West (1994) list the following indications for ABR testing: (1) an unexplained interaural difference in pure-tone thresholds of ≥10 dB at two frequencies or 15 dB at one frequency, (2) an unexplained difference in speech discrimination scores between ears, or scores judged to be unusually poor for the patient's hearing loss (not otherwise specified), (3) unexplained unilateral or asymmetric tinnitus, (4) unexplained unilateral or bilateral aural pressure, (5) any unexplained equilibrium disturbance. Obviously, the more strict the diagnostic strategy, the more patients with the disease will be identified. However, implementation of too strict a strategy may lead to inappropriately high costs for the detection of each tumor.

Figure 5–3 shows audiologic, ABR, and MRIg findings for a patient who was initially screened with an ABR because of unilateral symptoms of left ear hearing loss, fullness, and tinnitus. This patient underwent resection of her tumor via a suboccipital approach, with successful preservation of residual hearing.

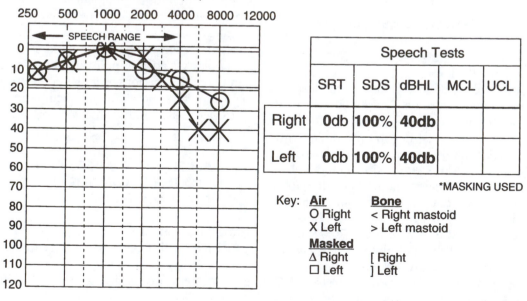

a

Figure 5–3. Preoperative audiologic **(a)**, ABR **(b)**, MRIg **(c)**, and postoperative audiologic **(d)** findings in a 54-year-old woman who presented with symptoms of left ear fluctuating hearing loss, fullness, tinnitus, and episodic vertigo. An ENG revealed a 64% left unilateral weakness.

Preoperative ABR

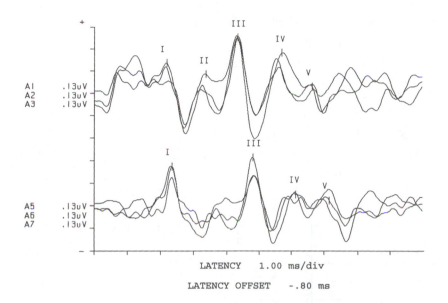

A1 .13uV
A2 .13uV
A3 .13uV

A5 .13uV
A6 .13uV
A7 .13uV

LATENCY   1.00 ms/div

LATENCY OFFSET   -.80 ms

	LATENCIES (ms)									
	I	II	III	IV	V	VI	VII	I'	III'	V'
A1	1.38	2.55	3.53	4.89	5.83					
A7	1.54		4.00	5.32	6.34					

b

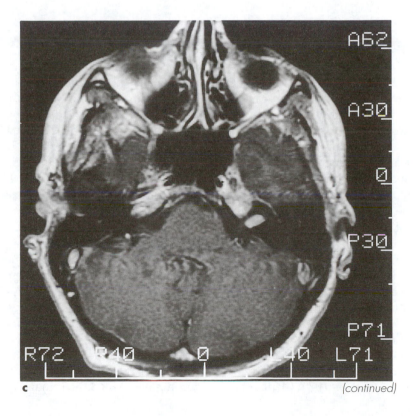

A62

A30

0

P30

P71

R72   R40   0   L40   L71

c

(continued)

Figure 5–3. *(continued)*

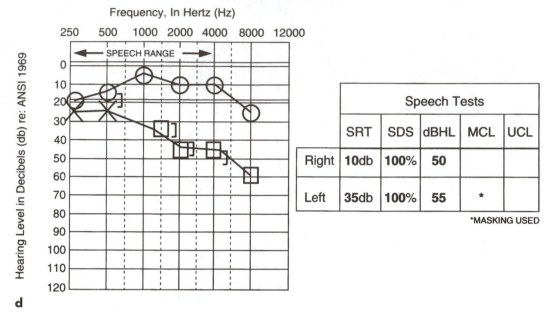

d

Cost-Effective Patient Evaluation

The issue of the most cost-effective strategy for evaluation of patients thought to be at risk for an acoustic neuroma is a controversial one, and no clearly superior strategy has been described. Multiple factors affect cost-benefit analyses, including test sensitivity and specificity, test costs, acceptable cost per incremental case diagnosed, accepted value of a missed tumor, and the prevalence of the disease in the population tested (Bance et al., 1994; Dobie, 1992). Prevalence of the disease is difficult to determine and is a major variable in studies dealing with cost analysis. While the prevalence of acoustic neuroma in unselected temporal bones has been reported as 0.8% (Bance et al., 1994) and 1.7% (Welling et al., 1990), the reported prevalence of identified tumors, calculated from the yearly incidence, is much lower, or 0.07% (Bance et al.,

1994). Although it is certainly desirable to identify tumors at a stage at which they are small in size, it is difficult to assess the value of a missed tumor in this number of asymptomatic individuals. Reports from large otologic practices often specify a prevalence of 1% (Mangham, 1991). However, the prevalence of this disease in a general otolaryngology practice is likely to be much lower (Dobie, 1992). Thus, the applicability of decision-cost analyses performed in otologic practices with a relatively high prevalence of acoustic neuroma patients to the development of optimal strategies in a more general practice may be questioned.

Despite the controversy, the great majority of authors who have written about cost-effective diagnostic strategies have recommended some combination of ABR and MRIg for evaluation of patients deemed at risk for acoustic neuroma. Most authors recommend ABR as an initial screening test, followed by MRIg if the ABR is abnormal (Bance et al., 1994; Bu-Saba et al., 1994; Hendrix et al., 1990). If hearing is too poor for an ABR to be obtained, an MRIg is obtained as the initial screening test.

Recent attention has focused on the decreased sensitivity of ABR in detecting the small acoustic neuroma (Chandrasekhar et al., 1995; Telian et al., 1989; Wilson et al., 1992), prompting some investigators (Chadrasekhar et al., 1995; Welling et al., 1990) to propose that that the ABR be bypassed in favor of the MRIg as the initial screening test. This strategy has the advantage of identifying small tumors at a stage when resection results in minimal morbidity and mortality but increases the cost of each tumor identified. Some authors have advocated the use of a less costly abbreviated MRI to rule out the presence of an acoustic neuroma. However, this approach has the disadvantage of failing to diagnose other potential causes of retrocochlear pathology, such as multiple sclerosis.

Whatever evaluation strategy is utilized, vigilant patient follow-up is of critical importance. Patients with significant hearing asymmetry and a normal ABR should undergo a repeat ABR in 6–12 months, particularly if the hearing loss progresses or the patient develops other symptoms suspicious for acoustic neuroma. Although MRIg is regarded as the gold standard for diagnosis of acoustic neuroma, some consideration should be given to a follow-up study in patients with an abnormal ABR, progression of symptoms, or both (Hendrix et al., 1990).

REFERENCES

Anderson, H., Barr, B., & Wedenberg, E. (1969). Intra-aural reflexes in retrocochlear lesions. In C. A. Hamberger & J. Wersall (Eds.), *Nobel Symposium: Vol. 10, Disorders of the Skull Base Region* (pp 48–54). Stockholm: Almquist and Wikell.

Bance, M.L., Hyde, M.L., & Malizia, K. (1994). Decision and cost analysis in acoustic neuroma diagnosis. *Journal of Otolaryngology, 23,* 109–120.

Bekesy, G.V. (1947). A new audiometer. *Acta Oto-Laryngologica, 45,* 411–422.

Brunt, M. (1994). Tests of cochlear function. In J. Katz (Ed.), *Handbook of clinical audiology* (4th ed.). Baltimore: Williams and Wilkins.

Bu-Saba, N.Y., Rebeiz, E.E., Salman, S.D., Thornton, A.R., & West, C. (1994). Significance of false-positive auditory brainstem response: A clinical study. *American Journal of Otology, 15,* 233–236.

Carhart, R. (1957). Clinical determination of abnormal auditory adaptation. *Archives of Otolaryngology—Head and Neck Surgery, 65,* 32–39.

Chandrasekhar, S., Brackmann, D.E., & Devgan, K.K. (1995). Utility of auditory brainstem audiometry in diagnosis of acoustic neuromas. *American Journal of Otology, 16,* 63–67.

Cushing, H. (1917). *Tumors of the nervus acusticus and the syndrome of the cerebellopontile angle.* Philadelphia: W. B. Saunders Company.

Dix, M.R., Hallpike, C.S., & Hood, J.D. (1948). Observations upon the loudness recruitment phenomenon, with especial reference to the differential diagnosis of the internal ear and VIIIth nerve. *Proceedings of the Royal Society of Medicine, 41,* 516–526.

Dobie, R.A. (1992). Hearing threshold differences and risk of acoustic tumor. [Letter to the Editor]. *Archives of Otolaryngology—Head and Neck Surgery, 107,* 493.

Flood, L.M., & Brightwell, A.P. (1984). Cochlear deafness in the presentation of a large acoustic neuroma. *Journal of Laryngology and Otology, 98,* 87–92.

Fowler, E.P. (1936). Method for early detection of otosclerosis. *Archives of Otolaryngology, 24,* 731–741.

Hendrix, R.A., DeDio, R.M., & Sclafani, A.P. (1990). The use of diagnostic testing in asymmetric sensorineural hearing loss. *Archives of Otolaryngology—Head and Neck Surgery, 103,* 593–598.

Jerger, J. (1960). Bekesy audiometry in analysis of auditory disorders. *Journal of Speech and Hearing Research, 3,* 275–287.

Jerger, J.J., Shedd, L., & Harford, E. (1959). On the detection of extremely small changes in sound intensity. *Archives of Otolaryngology—Head and Neck Surgery, 69,* 200–211.

Jerger, J., & Jerger, S. (1971). Diagnostic significance of PB word functions. *Archives of Otolaryngology—Head and Neck Surgery, 93,* 573–580.

Jerger, J., & Jerger, S. (1975). A simplified tone decay test. *Archives of Otolaryngology—Head and Neck Surgery, 101*, 403–407.

Johnson, E.W. (1968). Auditory findings in 200 cases of acoustic neurinomas. *Archives of Otolaryngology—Head and Neck Surgery, 88*, 598–603.

Linthicum, F.H. (1983). Electronystagmography findings in patients with acoustic tumors. *Seminars in Hearing, 4*, 47–53.

Luscher, E., & Zwislocki, J. (1948). A simple method of monaural determination of the recruitment phenomenon. *Practica Oto-Rhino-Laryngologica, 10*, 521–522.

Mangham, C. (1991). Hearing threshold difference between ears and risk of acoustic tumor. *Archives of Otolaryngology—Head and Neck Surgery, 105*, 814–817.

McFarland, W.H., Linthicum, F.H., & Waldorf, R.A. (1989). Auditory and vestibular tests. *Seminars in Hearing, 10*, 313–326.

Pensak, M.L., Glasscock, M.E., Josey, A.F., Jackson, C.G., & Gulya, A.J. (1985). Sudden hearing loss and cerebellopontine angle tumors. *Laryngoscope, 95*, 1188–1193.

Ruth, R.A., & Lambert, P.R. (1991). Auditory evoked potentials. *Otolaryngologic Clinics of North America, 24*, 349–370.

Selesnick, S.H., & Jackler, R.K. (1992). Clinical manifestations and audiologic diagnosis of acoustic neuromas. *Otolaryngology Clinics of North America, 25*, 521–551.

Selesnick, S.H., & Jackler, R.K. (1993). Atypical hearing loss in acoustic neuroma patients. *Laryngoscope, 103*, 437–441.

Selters, W.A., & Brackmann, D.E. (1977). Acoustic tumor detection with brain stem electric response audiometry. *Archives of Otolaryngology—Head and Neck Surgery, 103*, 181–187.

Shaia, F., & Sheehy, J. (1976). Sudden sensorineural hearing impairment: A report of 1,220 cases. *Laryngoscope, 86*, 389–398.

Telian, S.A., & Kileny, P.R. (1989). Usefulness of 1000 Hz tone-burst-evoked responses in the diagnosis of acoustic neuroma. *Archives of Otolaryngology—Head and Neck Surgery, 101*, 466–471.

Telian, S.A., Kileny, P.R., Niparko, J.K., Kemink, J.L, & Graham, M.D. (1989). Normal auditory brainstem response in patients with acoustic neuroma. *Laryngoscope, 99*, 10–14.

Thompson, G.A. (1963). Modified SISI technique for selected cases with suspected acoustic neurinoma. *Journal of Speech and Hearing Disorders, 28*, 299–302.

Turner, R.G., Shepard, N.T., & Frazer G.J. (1984). Clinical performance of audiological and related diagnostic tests. *Ear and Hearing, 5*, 187–194.

Weiss, M.H., Kisiel, D.L., & Bhatia, P. (1990). Predictive value of brainstem evoked response in the diagnosis of acoustic neuroma. *Archives of Otolaryngology—Head and Neck Surgery, 103*, 583–585.

Welling, D.B. , Glasscock, M.E., Woods, C.I., & Jackson, C.G. (1990). Acoustic neuroma: A cost-effective approach. *Archives of Otolaryngology—Head and Neck Surgery, 103*, 364–370.

Wilson, D.F., Hodgson, R.S., Gustafson, M.F., Hogue, S., & Mills, L. (1992). The sensitivity of auditory brainstem response testing in small acoustic neuromas. *Laryngoscope, 102*, 961–964.

CHAPTER 6

Radiologic Findings in Acoustic Tumors

Charles A. Syms, III, M.D.
Antonio De la Cruz, M.D.
William W.M. Lo, M.D.

HISTORY

The investigation into neurotologic symptoms to detect acoustic tumors has progressed through plain films, tomography, air contrast and then oil-based contrast cisternography, angiography, computed tomography (CT) with and without cisternal air or contrast and, most recently, magnetic resonance imaging (MRI) with and without paramagnetic contrast agents. Each successive imaging modality has provided increased sensitivity for detecting acoustic tumors and decreased potential for adverse reactions.

The introduction of paramagnetic contrast agents into clinical imaging in the late 1980s gave radiologists and clinicians the most sensitive tool to detect and precisely outline vestibular schwannomas. At last, a noninvasive "gold" standard, replacing craniotomy, was available to which other diagnostic strategies could be compared. Contrast enhancement on MRI, however, is not specific for tumors (Arriaga, Carrier, & Houston, 1995; Barbara, Saliola, & Filipo,

1993; Donnelly, Cass, & Ryan, 1944; vonGlass et al, 1981). Rarely, inflammatory lesions may simulate neoplasms, especially small areas of enhancement in the lateral aspect of the internal auditory canal. Further, the cost of this modality as the initial part of a screening paradigm for acoustic tumors is prohibitive. Phelps (1994) introduced T2 fast spin echo (FSE), and Casselman and colleagues (1993) started three dimensional Fourier transformation-constructive interference in steady state sequence (3DFT-CISS) magnetic resonance imaging for the investigation of otologic and neurotologic diseases. By maximizing the contrast between cerebrospinal fluid (CSF) and soft tissue and bone, these techniques outline acoustic tumors, nerves, and vessels in the cerebellopontine angle (CPA) and internal auditory canal (IAC), without paramagnetic contrast. While the sensitivity of these approaches is yet to be determined, these techniques promise to be the most cost effective methods for screening acoustic tumors by decreasing imaging time, obviating paramagnetic contrast and the need for a radiologist to inject it.

IMAGING PROTOCOL

A comprehensive study of the internal auditory canal, cerebellopontine angle, and brain is the best imaging scheme. As done in most facilities, this includes T1-weighted images (T1WI) in contiguous or overlapping 2–4 mm sections through the IAC before and after intravenous contrast is given. T2-weighted images (T2WI) then are obtained in 5–8 mm sections throughout the brain. Our current, full survey protocol is depicted in Table 6–1. When reviewing films of patients with neurotologic com-

TABLE 6–1. Sample MRI protocol for comprehensive study of CPA/IAC.

I. Axial survey of brain: PDWI and T2WI

    Repetition time (TR): 2500 ms
    Echo Delay time (TE): 22.90 ms
    Section thickness: 6 mm
    Interslice gap: 1.2 mm
    Field of view (FOV): 200 mm
    Image matrix: 200 × 256
    Acquisition NO (Acq): 1
    Acquisition time (TA: 8:24 min or 4:34 min, half Fourier)
    Saturation pulse applied

II. Axial posterior fossa detail: T1WI precontrast

    TR/TE: 580/15
    3-mm sections, 0.3 mm gap
    FOV: 170 cm
    Image matrix: 256 × 256
    Acq: 2
    TA: 5:00 min
    Saturation pulse applied

III. Axial posterior fossa detail: T1WI postcontrast

    Repeat sequence II.

IV. Choice of one of four

    A. For vestibulocochlear/IAC detail, repeat III at interleaving levels
    B. For localization of lesion, repeat III in coronal plane
    C. For NF-2, do coronal whole brain
        TR/TE: 580/15
        6-mm sections, 1.2-mm gap
        FOV: 200 mm
        Image matrix: 200 × 256
        Acq: 2
        TA: 3:55 min
    D. For nonspecific posterior fossa signs and symptoms, do sagittal whole brain with same parameters as in (C), except for FOV 230 mm

Note: CPA = cerebellopontine angle; IAC = internal auditory canal. Magnetic resonance imaging (MRI) was conducted with a superconducting magnet operating at 1.5 T (Helicon, Seimens, Islin, NJ). Gd-DTPA (Magnevist-Berlex Laboratories, Wayne, NJ) was administered intravenously.

Source: From Imaging of the Cerebellopontine Angle by W.M. Lo, 1994, p.366. *Neurotology* (Chap. 21), by R.K. Jackler and D.E. Brackmann (Eds.), St. Louis: Mosby-Year Book. Copyright 1994 by Mosby-Year Book. Reprinted with permission.

plaints obtained from outside institutions, it is important to review the slice thickness, since a small tumor may be missed. The facial and acoustic nerves must be seen for a study to be considered "adequate." False negative examinations in patients who are given gadolinium are rare and, more often, the result of an inadequate imaging protocol, rather than failure of the gadolinium to show the tumor. At our institution, we had a case in which a small intracanalicular tumor was missed when the proper imaging protocol was not followed.

In patients with an asymmetric or unilateral hearing loss, speech understanding that is worse than expected for the degree of hearing loss, unilateral tinnitus, dizziness, or other suspicious symptoms or signs, we obtain an "IAC examination". The sole goal of the imaging is to "rule out" an acoustic tumor. The ideal tests would be the FSE or the 3DFT-CISS examinations, although they are not yet widely available. If any questions remain after examining the images, or if these imaging techniques are not available, then a T1 with gadolinium (T1Gd) study is appropriate (Figure 6–1A, B, and C). We prefer this protocol to a screening survey with postcontrast T1 images through the internal auditory canal. In the future, the anticipated cost of these examinations may obviate current electrophysiologic screening methods. The advantages of the FSE and 3DFT-CISS techniques are: (a) the ability to differentiate lipomas and hemangiomas, since a T1 unenhanced image would be obtained; (b) less time consumed, since the FSE takes only 5 min and the T1 Gad images take approximately 15 min; (c) most importantly, lower cost, since a physician does not need to inject any substance and no contrast agent needs to be purchased.

Both FSE and 3DFT-CISS show cerebrospinal fluid in the internal auditory canal and cerebellopontine angle in excellent detail. These images are not unlike iophendylate or metrizamide computerized meatography. When comparing these two techniques, the relative merits and disadvantages are beyond the scope of this chapter. One possible advantage with the present use of T1Gd is showing the internal auditory canal free of masses. In neuritis, the nerve enhances with gadolinium, and differentiation from a mass is difficult, if not impossible (Figure 6–2 A and B). Currently, these patients either are explored or followed with serial imaging. The FSE and 3DFT-CISS techniques would allow the demonstration of CSF occupying the entire internal auditory canal without filling defects, if neuritis is the underlying pathology. Casselman et al. (1994) recently have described such a case, and this possibly could eliminate the false positive T1Gd examinations.

CHARACTERISTICS OF ACOUSTIC NEUROMAS

The intracanalicular tumor is smaller than 1 cm in length and has a convex medial border (Figure 6–3). In the earliest stages, the tumor appears rounded (Figure 6–1A). After it fills the internal auditory canal, it appears more sausage-shaped (Figure 6–4A and B). The tumor tends to widen the internal auditory canal and assume an "ice cream on cone" shape when it expands into the CPA (Figure 6–5A and B). A cisternal tumor tends to be spherical and centered on the porous acousticus (Figure 6–6A and B) (Lo, 1994). A large cisternal tumor may assume an ovoid appearance (Figure 6–7A and B). Most acoustic tumors show an acute angle at the posterior bone-tumor interface, whereas meningiomas tend to have an obtuse angle (Valavanis, Schubiger, Hayak, & Pouliadis, 1981). On T1WI, the tumor is isotense or mildly hypointense when compared with the brain and hyperintense when compared with CSF (Figure 6–4A). Viewing T2WI reveals the tumor to be almost isointense with brain and hypo- to isointense with CSF (Figure 6–4B).

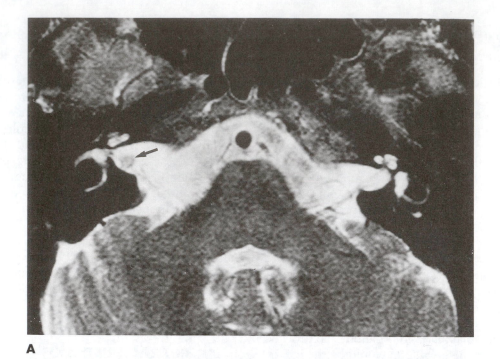

A

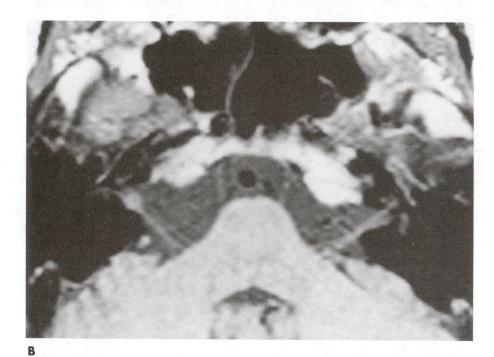

B

Figure 6–1. Intracanalicular acoustic schwannoma. **A.** Fast spin echo technique shows a small tumor (arrow) in the right internal auditory canal (IAC), between gray matter and cerebrospinal fluid (CSF) in intensity. **B.** T1WI shows the tumor isointense to brain. **C.** Gd-T1WI shows marked contrast enhancement in tumor.

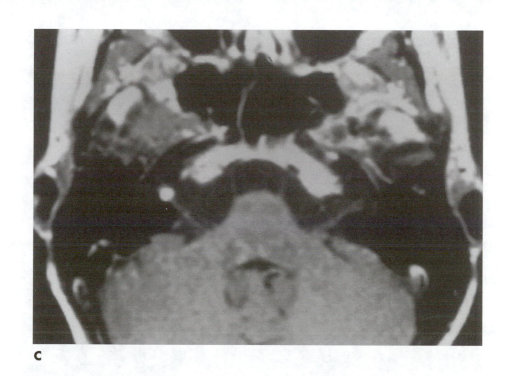

C

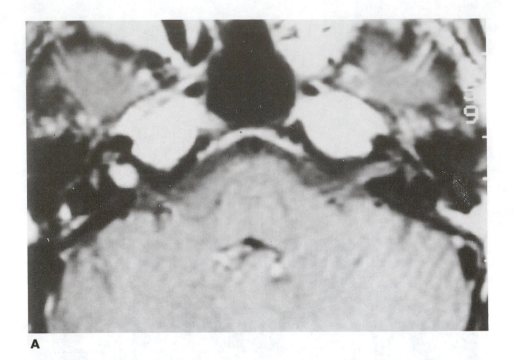

A

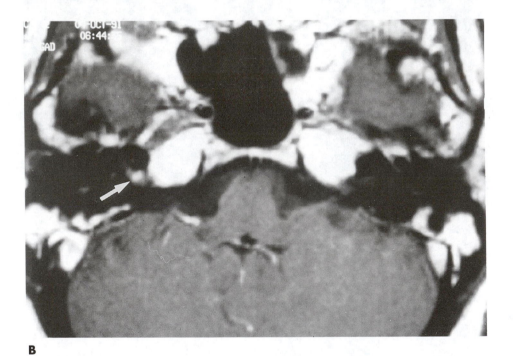

B

Figure 6–2. Vestibulocochlear neuritis. **A.** Gd-T1WI shows marked globular enhancement filling the distal right IAC. Note similarity to Figures 6–1C, 6–3, and 6–4B. **B.** Gd-T1WI 3 months later shows near complete resolution of enhancement *(arrow)*.

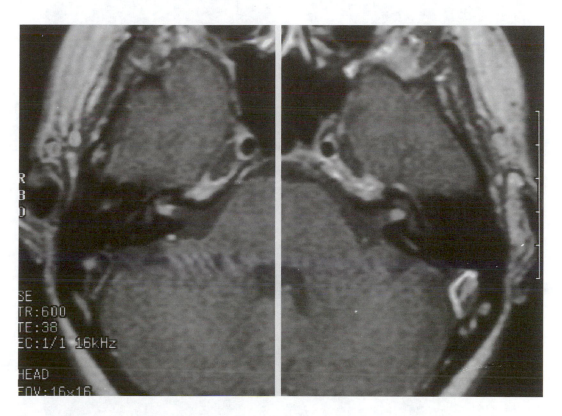

Figure 6–3. Synchronous bilateral intracanalicular lesions. Gd-T1WI shows the typical convex medial border of a left acoustic schwannoma. The concave medial border of the hemangioma on the right would be atypical for a schwannoma.

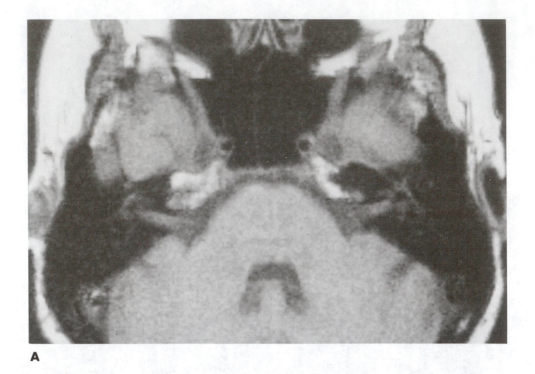

A

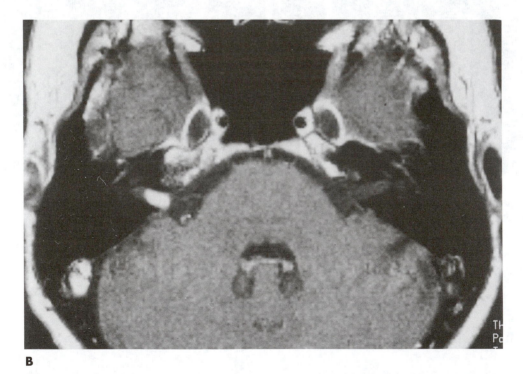

B

Figure 6–4. Intracanalicular acoustic neuroma. **A.** T1WI and **B.** Gd-T1WI show a typical sausage-shaped, markedly enhancing intracanalicular acoustic schwannoma.

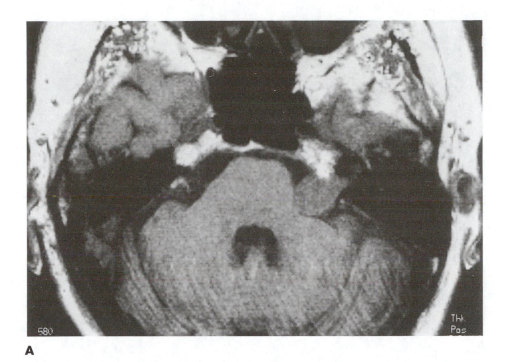

A

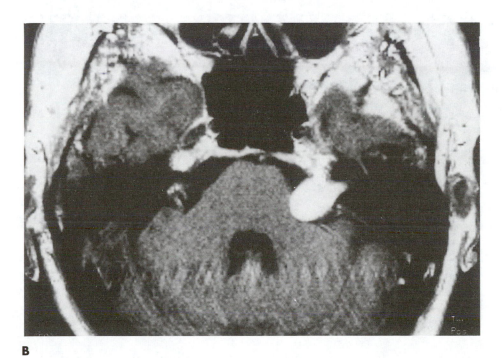

B

Figure 6–5. Acoustic neuroma with an "ice cream on cone" appearance. **A.** T1WI shows a smoothly marginated tumor partly in the IAC and partly "mushrooming" out of the IAC into the cerebellopontine angle (CPA), mildly hypointense to gray matter. **B.** Gd-T1WI shows a marked homogenous enhancement that is typical of schwannomas.

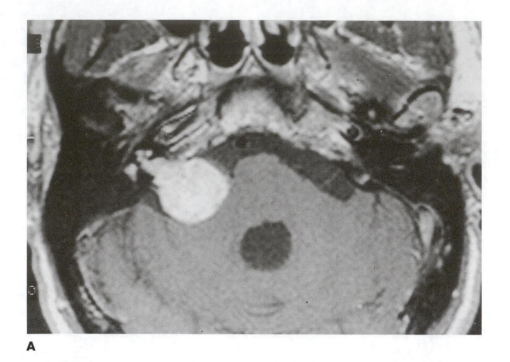

A

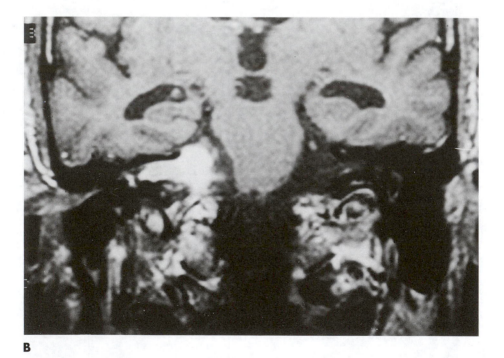

B

Figure 6–6. Large acoustic schwannoma in the CPA and IAC, extending into the labyrinth. **A.** Gd-T1WI. **B.** Gd-T1WI, coronal plane. Arrows indicate tumor extension from the IAC into the vestibule and cochlea, a relatively rare finding for an acoustic schwannoma.

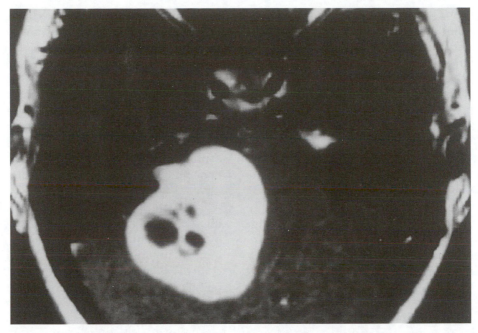

A

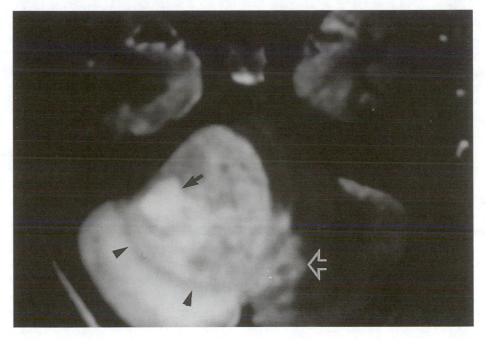

B

Figure 6–7. Large ovoid acoustic neuroma with multiple intratumor cysts. **A.** Gd-T1WI shows hypointense cysts within the markedly enhancing solid component of the tumor. **B.** T2WI shows markedly hyperintense cysts *(arrow)* within the slightly inhomogeneous hyperintense tumor (arrowhead). Hyperintensity in the adjacent cerebellum *(open arrow)* suggests edema.

Displaced vessels along the tumor edge or within the tumor usually are apparent, if present, and should be identified if surgery is planned. Intratumor cysts (Figure 6–7A and B) should be recognized, since they recently have been correlated with a more difficult dissection and worse postoperative facial nerve outcome (Charabi, Klinken, Tos, & Thorisen, 1994). An arachnoid cyst or cysts (Figure 6–8A and B) may accompany the schwannoma or, rarely, predominate the mass. Dural tails (Figure 6–9A and B), although more commonly seen in meningiomas, can occur rarely with acoustic tumors. Intratumor hemorrhage or, infrequently, subarachnoid hemorrhage, may occur, but are seldom detected by imaging.

DIFFERENTIAL DIAGNOSIS

The differential diagnosis of intracanalicular lesions is shown in Table 6–2. Ninety percent of the time, the mass will be a vestibular schwannoma (Lo, 1994). Facial schwannomas in the IAC or CPA may be indistinguishable from vestibular schwannomas by imaging. This is an important caveat, since these tumors call for different management strategies. Although uncommon, we counsel all patients undergoing surgical removal of an acoustic neuroma because of the small possibility that it may be a facial neuroma, and we discuss the alternative management schemes. Hemangiomas (Figures 6–3, 6–10A and B) and vascular malformations may show the typical "honeycomb" changes of the adjacent bone on CT images, but they are similar to acoustic tumors on MRI. Although rare, lipomas (Figure 6–11A, B, and C) can be diagnosed with proper imaging. They appear markedly hyperintense on T1WI and hypointense on T2WI. Confirmation of the diagnosis can be made with fat suppression techniques. Metastatic lesions can be suspected by a short duration of symptoms, facial nerve manifestations, progression of symptom intensity, and a known history of malignant disease. The key to suspecting any of these lesions be-

fore surgery includes facial nerve symptoms. Intracanalicular vestibular schwannomas infrequently show signs of facial nerve involvement (Neely & Neblett, 1983). Vestibulocochlear neuritis (Figure 6–2A and B) may be present with an MRI finding of a small area of enhancement, particularly in the lateral internal auditory canal (Han et al., 1991). If the FSE or 3DFT-CISS techniques are not available to confirm the absence of a mass, then observation and repeat imaging would be the recommended approach.

Small areas of enhancement outside the internal auditory canal also may be caused by intravestibular schwanommas (Figure 6–12). With improved MRI resolution, especially FSE or 3DFT-CISS techniques, this pathologic process no longer will be the diagnostic dilemma that it was in the past.

The incidence of the mass lesions that occur in the cerebellopontine angle differs from that of intracanalicular tumors. The difficulty is in distinguishing vestibular schwannomas from meningiomas. Meningiomas are a distant second to schwannomas in frequency of occurrence in the cerebellopontine angle. They typically are sessile and hemispherical (Figure 6–13A, B, and C) in their configuration. They usually are placed eccentrically around the porous acousticus (Lo, 1994). Their appearance on T2WI is variable but, since vestibular schwannomas tend to be isointense with brain, if the mass is hypointense with brain on T2WI, then it most likely is a meningioma (Gentry et al, 1987). A dural tail frequently is present.

Congenital cholesteatomas or epidermoids are third in incidence among cerebellopontine angle masses. In most cases, MRI imaging reveals the mass to be iso- or mildly-hyperintense to CSF on T1WI, but isotense to CSF on T2WI, and they are nonenhancing (Figure 6–14A, B, C). They are variable in shape and show a finely irregular, "cauliflower" surface. Schwannomas originating from other cranial nerves are rare and are distinguished from acoustic tumors primarily by their location (Lo, 1994) (Figure 6–15A–E). Vascular lesions, both ve-

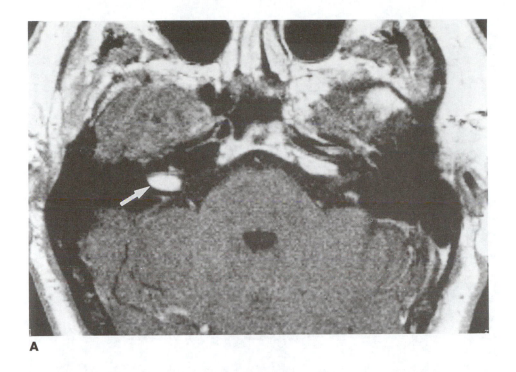

A

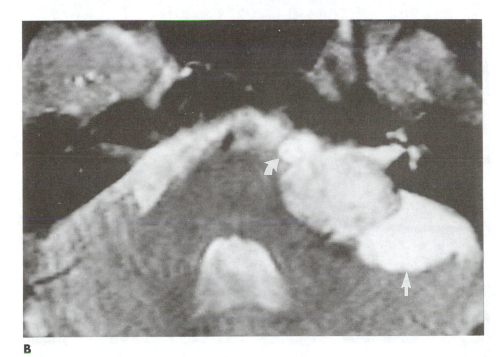

B

Figure 6–8. Large acoustic neuroma with adjacent arachnoid cysts. **A,** T1WI and **B,** T2WI show arachnoid cyst (*arrow*) and cystic component of tumor (*curved arrow*), approximating CSF in intensity, overlying a schwannoma.

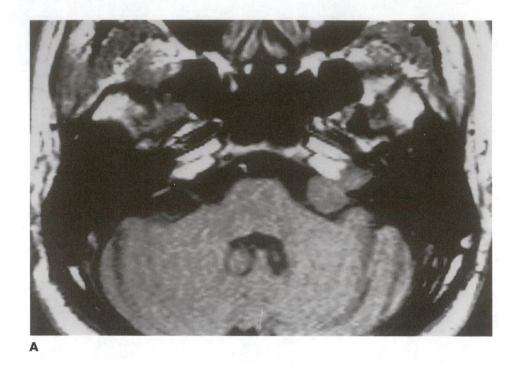

A

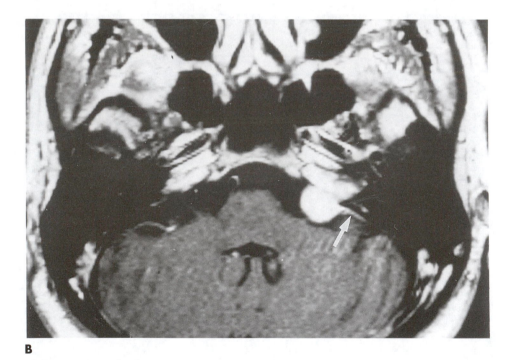

B

Figure 6–9. Acoustic neuroma with a dural "tail." **A,** T1WI and **B,** Gd-T1WI show a reactive dural thickening (*arrow*) adjacent to the tumor.

TABLE 6–2. Intracanalicular lesions

Neoplastic	Nonneoplastic
Vestibular Schwannoma	AICA (Anterior inferior cerebellar artery) loop
Facial Schwannoma	AICA aneurysm
Hemangioma	Meningitis
Meningioma	Neuritis
Lipoma	Hamartoma
Metastasis	
Lymphoma	
Melanoma	
Glioma	
Osteoma	

Source: From Imaging of the Cerebellopontine Angle by W.M. Lo, 1994, p.368. Neurotology, by R.K. Jackler and D.E. Brackmann (Eds.), St. Louis: Mosby-Year Book. Copyright 1994 by Mosby-Year Book. Reprinted with permission.

nous and arterial, may be confused with a tumor (Figure 6–16A, B, and C). Better magnetic resonance imaging resolution and magnetic resonance angiography allow the patient to avoid invasive angiography to resolve this diagnostic problem.

POSTOPERATIVE IMAGING

We usually recommend a follow-up enhanced MRI within 3 to 5 years of surgery if the removal is considered to be complete. Residual tumor readily can be identified if it is large enough but may be difficult to differentiate from enhancing dura or scar tissue. Fat suppression techniques help decrease the interference from the free adipose graft that is used for closure. Serial imaging studies may be necessary to distinguish postsurgical enhancement from residual tumor.

IMAGING IN SPECIAL CIRCUMSTANCES

Patients who cannot undergo an MRI because of pacemakers, aneurysm clips, cochlear implants, or claustrophobia that is resistant to se-

dation may be imaged with CT. This would detect all cisternal and some intracanalicular tumors. Small intracanalicular tumors will require the addition of gas cisternography for better contrast and sensitivity.

We do not recommend irradiation for the treatment of benign lesions, including vestibular schwannomas. If a patient has undergone stereotactic irradiation, annual enhanced-MRI evaluations are recommended to observe tumor growth, communicating hydrocephalus, adjacent brain parenchymal changes (Figure 6–17A, B and C), osteoradionecrosis and, later, secondary malignancies. Since lesions in this area can be silent for extended periods of time, the need for continued annual follow-up cannot be overemphasized.

When bilateral acoustic tumors are detected in a patient (Figure 6–18), further diagnostic imaging and examination are needed. All of our patients with bilateral acoustic tumors undergo ophthalmologic evaluations to look for posterior capsular cataracts. Patients with neurofibromatosis type 2 (NF-2) are at high risk to develop other CNS tumors, such as meningiomas, astrocytomas, spinal ependymomas and, especially, other schwannomas (Figure 6–19). Upon making

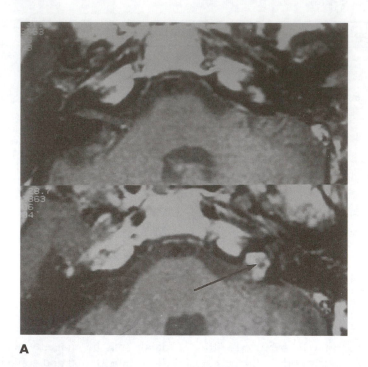

A

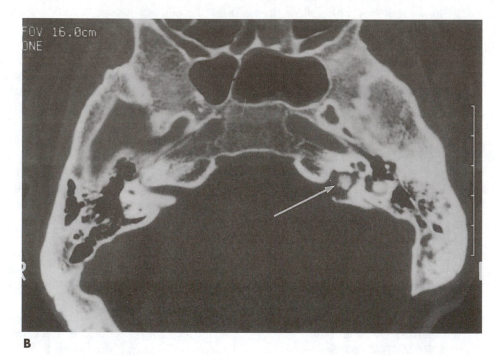

B

Figure 6–10. Intracanalicular hemangioma. **A.** Gd-T1WI shows a central hypointensity (*arrow*) in the enhancing tumor, corresponding to the intratumoral lamellar bone (*arrow*) in the high resolution CT, shown in **B.** (CT Courtesy of Gary A. Press, M.D., San Diego, CA.)

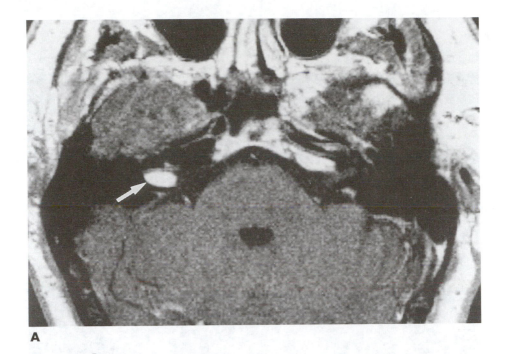

A

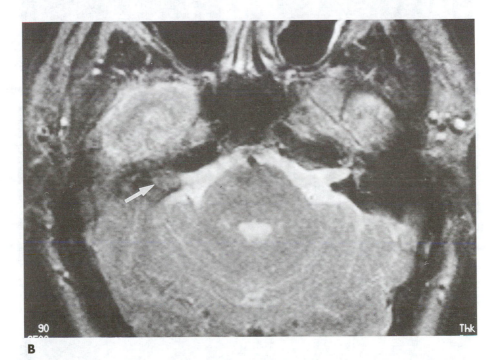

B

Figure 6–11. Intracanalicular lipoma. **A.** T1WI shows hyperintensity of the tumor (*arrow*) without gadolinium. **B.** T2WI shows hypointensity of tumor (*arrow*). **C.** Fat suppression MRI showing hypointensity of the tumor (*arrow*) confirms a fatty lesion and differentiates it from a melanotic melanoma, which may show intensities paralleling those of fat on standard spin-echo sequences.

(continued)

Figure 6–11. *(continued)*

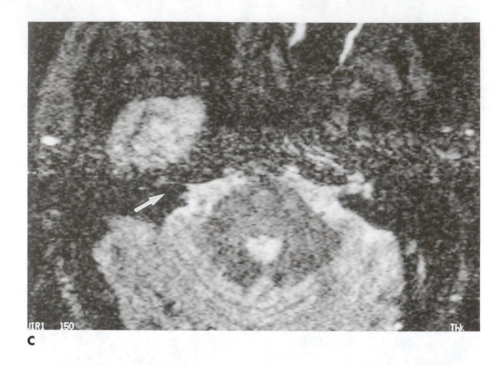

C

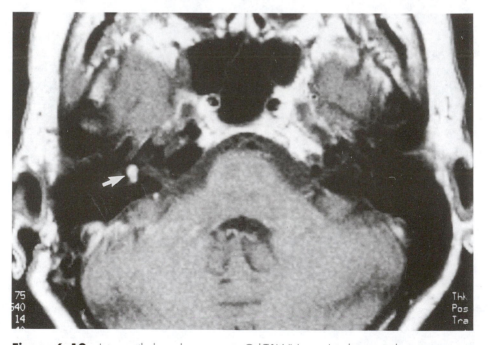

Figure 6–12. Intravestibular schwannoma. Gd-T1WI (arrow) indicates enhancing tumor.

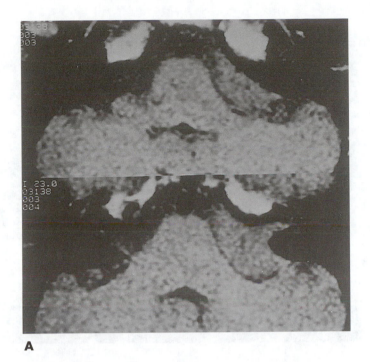

A

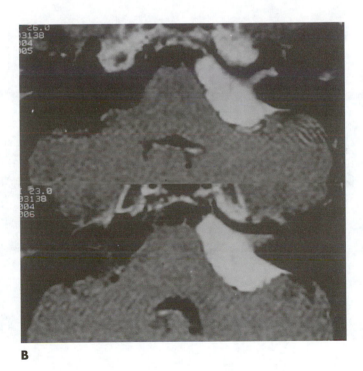

B

Figure 6–13. CPA meningioma. **A.** T1WI shows a mildly hypointense, and **B,** Gd-T1WI shows a markedly enhancing extraaxial mass in the left CPA cistern. The mass extends into the IAC but differs from an acoustic schwannoma because it is hemispherical with its broad base against the dural surface, rather than round. A dural "tail" extends from the tumor laterally. **C.** Gd-T1WI, coronal plane, shows tumor lying against the inferior surface of the tentorium *(arrow)*.

(continued)

Figure 6–13. *(continued)*

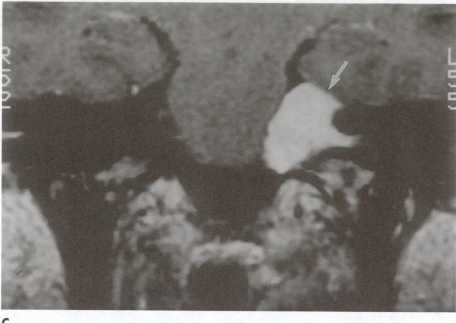

C

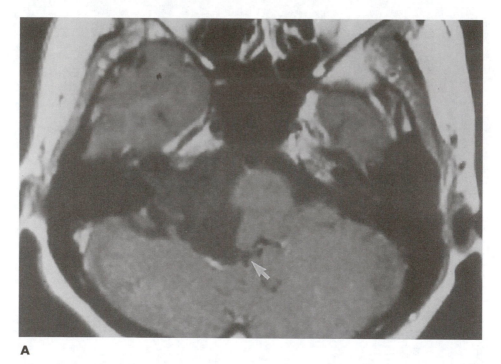

A

Figure 6–14. CPA cholesteatoma. **A.** T1WI shows an irregular, nonenhancing extraaxial mass mildly hyperintense to CSF, widening the right porous acousticus, displacing the pons and cerebellum, and insinuating into the lateral recess (*arrow*) of the fourth ventricle. **B.** T2WI shows isointensity of the mass to CSF. There is fine surface irregularity and mild internal inhomogeneity that distinguish an intradural cholesteatoma from an arachnoid cyst. **C.** Gd-T1WI, coronal plane, shows a small component of the tumor (*arrow*) herniating through the tentorial incisura into the middle cranial fossa.

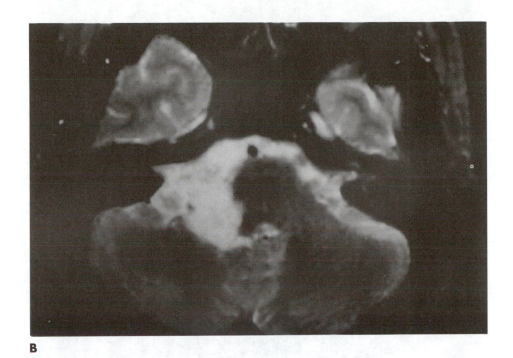

B

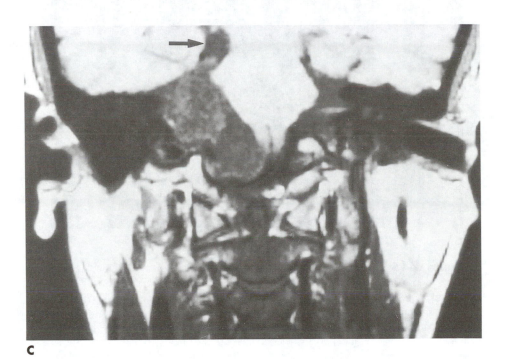

C

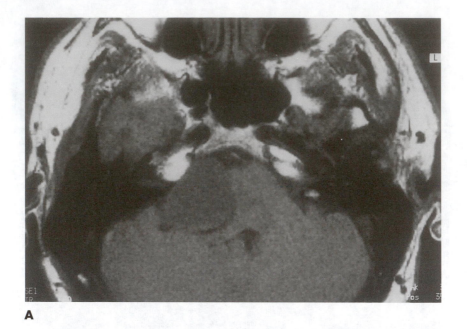

A

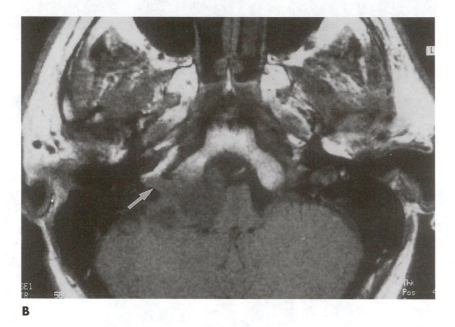

B

Figure 6–15. Glossopharyngeal schwannoma. **A.** T1WI shows a smooth, nearly rounded extraaxial mass mildly hypointense to brain in the right CPA overlying a normal IAC, simulating a CPA acoustic schwannoma. **B.** T1WI, 6 mm inferior to **A,** shows a stem of the mass extending into the pars nervosa (*arrow*) of the right jugular foramen. **C.** T2WI shows marked hyperintensity of a large cystic component of the tumor, a common finding in schwannomas. **D,** Gd-T1WI, coronal plane, shows an enhancing rim around the cystic component of the tumor in the right CPA outside of the normal IAC (*arrow*). E. Gd-T1WI, coronal plane, 3 mm posterior to **D,** shows an enhancing solid stem of the tumor (*arrow*) extending into the pars nervosa over the jugular tubercle (*curved arrow*).

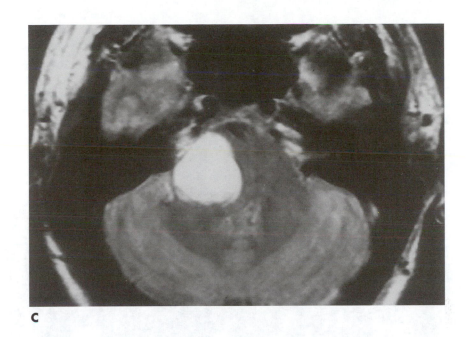

C

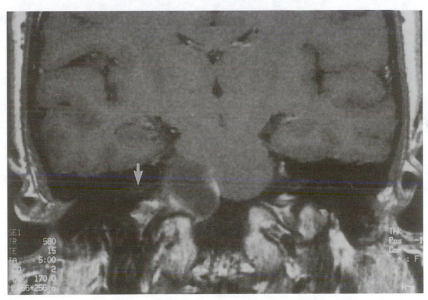

D

(continued)

Figure 6–15. *(continued)*

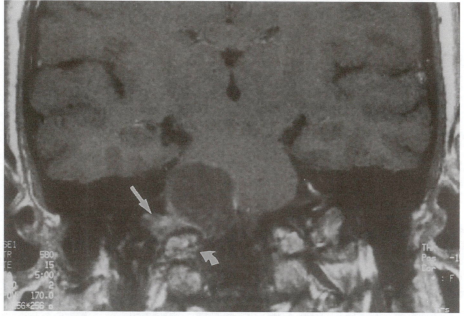

E

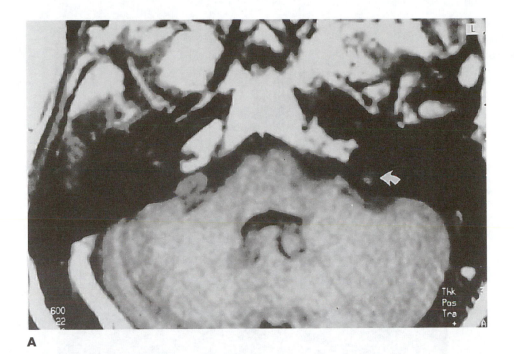

A

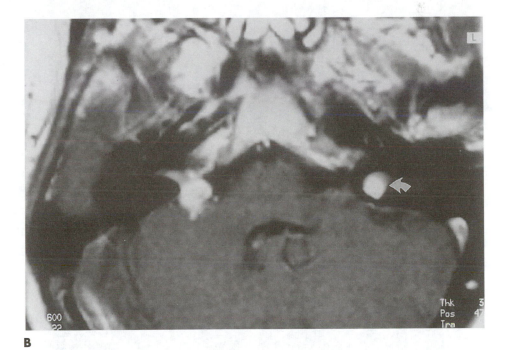

B

Figure 6–16. Real and pseudotumors. **A.** T1WI and **B.** Gd-T1WI show a mushroom-shaped enhancing right CPA acoustic schwannoma extending into the IAC and a rounded enhancing "lesion" in the left jugular fossa *(curved arrows)* from slowly flowing blood, forming a pseudotumor. **C.** Gd-T1WI, coronal plane, shows a right IAC/CPA acoustic schwannoma *(arrow)* and bilateral jugular enhancements *(curved arrows)* immediately medial to the descending facial nerve canals *(arrowheads)*. Jugular pseudotumors are occasional pitfalls on MRI.

(continued)

Figure 6–16. *(continued)*

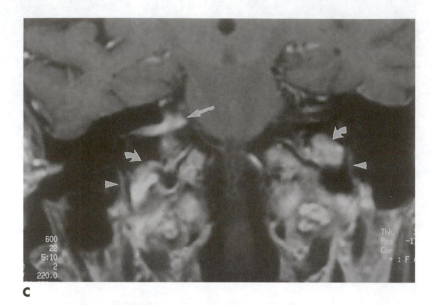

C

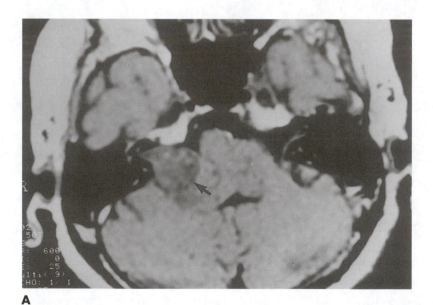

A

Figure 6–17. Acoustic neuroma 1 year after stereotactic radiation ("gamma knife"). **A.** T1WI shows tumor (*arrow*) in the right IAC/CPA slightly indenting the pons. **B.** T1WI shows enhancement in the tumor (*arrow*) and inhomogeneous enhancement in the adjacent pons (*arrowheads*), indicating breakdown in blood-brain barrier. **C.** T2WI shows hypervascularity (*arrows*) in the pons, consistent with edema.

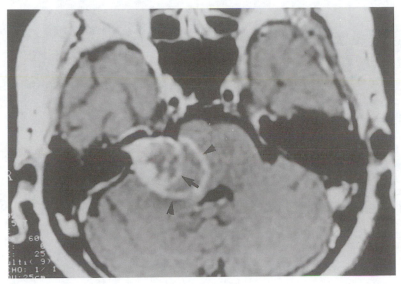

B

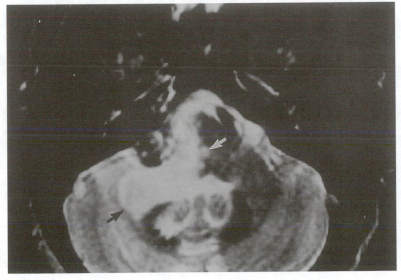

C

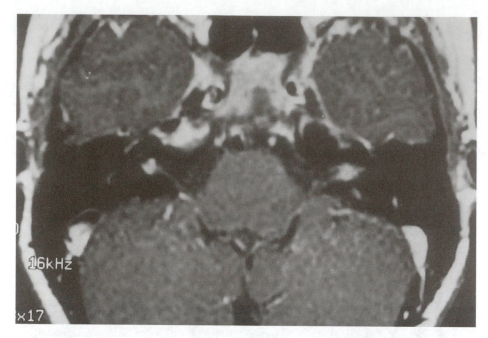

Figure 6–18. Neurofibromatosis type 2. Gd-T1WI shows small, bilateral intracanalicular schwannomas in a 10-year-old boy.

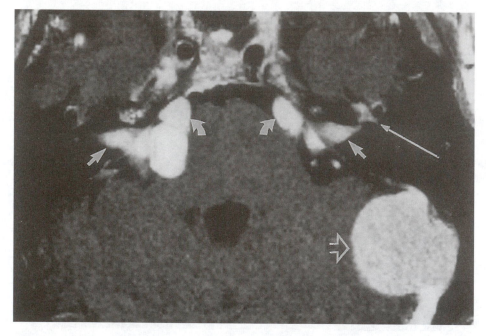

Figure 6–19. Neurofibromatosis type 2. Gd-T1WI shows bilateral IAC/CPA acoustic schwannomas (*arrows*), bilateral trigeminal schwannomas (*curved arrows*), a left facial schwannoma in the geniculate ganglion region (*long arrow*), and a left posterior fossa meningioma (*open arrow*).

the diagnosis of NF2, the entire neural axis should be imaged before any neurotologic intervention is initiated.

CONCLUSION

Magnetic resonance imaging with paramagnetic contrast has simplified greatly the definitive diagnosis of vestibular schwannomas. Usually, there is little controversy over the diagnosis. The FSE and 3dFT-CISS techniques are exciting, recent developments in the goals to develop a more cost-effective screening strategy and decrease the incidence of false positive images.

Acknowledgments. The authors would like to thank Butch Welch for his aid in preparation of the figures and Karen I. Berliner for her editorial assistance.

The views expressed in this chapter are those of the authors and do not necessarily reflect the official policy of the Department of Defense or the United States Air Force.

REFERENCES

Arriaga, M.A., Carrier, D., & Houston, G.D. (1995). False positive magnetic resonance imaging of small internal auditory canal tumors: A clinical, radiologic, and pathologic correlation study. *Archives of Otolaryngology—Head and Neck Surgery, 113,* 61–70.

Barbara, M., Saliola, S., & Filipo, R. (1993). False-positive MRI in a patient with otoneurological pathology. *Journal of Laryngology and Otology, 107,* 465–467.

Casselman, J.W., Kuhweide, Deimling, M., Ampe, W., Meeus, L. & Steyaert, L. (1993). Pathology of the Membranous Labryinth: Comparison of T1- and T2-weighted and gadolium-enhanced spin-echo and 3DFT-CISS imaging. *American Journal of Neuroradiology, 14,* 47–57

Casselman, J.W., Kuhweide, R., Deimling, M., Ampe, W., & Devlies, F. (1994). Magnetic resonance examination of the inner ear and cerebellopontine angle in patients with vertigo and/or abnormal findings at vestibular testing. *Acta Otolaryngologica (Stockholm) 513,* (Suppl.), 15–27.

Charabi, S., Klinken, L., Tos, M., & Thomsen, J. (1994). Histopathology and growth pattern of cystic acoustic neuromas. *Laryngoscope, 104,* 1348–1352.

Donnelly, M.J., Cass, A.D., & Ryan, L. (1994). False positive MRI in the diagnosis of small intracanalicular vestibular schwannomas. *Journal of Laryngology and Otology, 108,* 986–988.

Gentry, L.R., Jacoby, C.G., Turski, P.A., Houston, L.W., Strother, C.M., & Sackett, J.F. (1987). Cerebellopontine angle-petromastoid mass lesions: Comparative study of diagnosis with MR imaging and CT. *Radiology, 162,* 513–520.

Han, M.H., Jabour, B.A., Andrews, J.C., Canalis, R.F., Chen, F-H., Anzai, Y., Becker, D.P., Lufkin, R.B., & Hanafee, W.N. (1991). Nonneoplastic enhancing lesions mimicking intracanalicular acoustic neuroma on gadolinium-enhanced MR images. *Radiology, 179,* 795–796.

Lo, W.W.M. (1994). Imaging of the cerebellopontine angle. In R.K. Jackler & D.E. Brackmann (Eds.), *Neurotology.* St. Louis. Mosby-Year Book.

Neely, J.G., & Neblett, C.R. (1983). Differential facial nerve function in tumors of the internal auditory meatus. *Annals of Otology, Rhinology, and Laryngology, 92,* 39–41.

Phelps, P.D. (1994). Fast spin echo in otology. *Journal of Laryngology and Otology, 108,* 383–394.

Valavanis, A., Schubiger, O., Hayek, J., & Pouliadis, G. (1981). CT of meningiomas on the posterior surface of the petrous bone. *Neuroradiology, 22.* 111–121.

vonGlass, W., Haid, C., Cidlinsky, K., Stenglein, C., & Christ, P. (1981). False-positive MR imaging in the diagnosis of acoustic neuromas. *Archives of Otolaryngology—Head and Neck Surgery, 104,* 863-867.

CHAPTER 7

Surgical Decision-Making in Acoustic Tumor Surgery

William M. Luxford, M.D.

A recent consensus conference on acoustic tumors determined that treatment of acoustic tumor patients should be individualized and provided by an experienced, well-integrated multidisciplinary team (National Institutes of Health Consensus Development Conference, 1994). Therapeutic options include surgery, stereotactic irradiation, and observation. The ideal treatment, as decided at the consensus conference, is total surgical excision of the tumor in a single stage, with preservation of neurologic function. In the group of patients for whom conservative approaches may be indicated, including long-term observation, the risk of neurologic deterioration needs to be discussed. Sufficient verbal and written materials need to be provided so that patients and families have realistic expectations of treatment outcomes.

SURGICAL OPTIONS

There are three major surgical approaches for removal of acoustic tumors: the translabyrinthine approach (Chapter 9), the mid-dle fossa approach (Chapter 11), and the retrosigmoid/suboccipital approach (Chapter 12). Each of these approaches has advantages and disadvantages. The overall objectives of acoustic tumor surgery are tumor removal to prevent mortality, total removal to prevent recurrence, preservation of facial nerve function and, when possible, preservation of hearing. The first three objectives are possible with any of the three major surgical approaches. The use of the operating microscope and facial nerve monitoring have decreased the mortality and morbidity of acoustic tumor surgery markedly. Facial nerve function following acoustic tumor surgery at established referral centers is comparable when examining translabyrinthine versus middle fossa removal and translabyrinthine versus retrosigmoid/suboccipital removal of similar tumors.

Hearing preservation is possible with either the middle fossa or retrosigmoid/suboccipital approach, but it is not possible with the translabyrinthine approach. There is a wide range of audiometric criteria for hearing preservation surgery. The ideal candidate for hearing preservation has a speech reception threshold (SRT) of 30 dB HL and a word recognition score (WRS) of at least 70%. The chances for hearing preservation would appear to be improved in patients who have hypoactive calorics on electronystagmography (ENG) testing and auditory brainstem response interaural wave V latency differences of less than 0.4 ms (Shelton, 1992). The choice of surgical approach depends on several factors, including the patient's preoperative hearing, the size and location of the tumor, and the experience of the surgical team (Jackler & Pitts, 1992).

The Translabyrinthine Approach

The translabyrinthine approach provides a direct route to the cerebellopontine angle and requires minimum extradural cerebellar retraction, thereby decreasing the incidence of postoperative ataxia (Brackmann & Green, 1992). Dissection of the lateral end of the internal auditory canal ensures complete tumor removal from that area and allows definitive identification of the facial nerve in the temporal bone. If the facial nerve is lost during acoustic tumor removal, the translabyrinthine approach offers the best opportunity for immediate repair by end-to-end anastomosis or insertion of a nerve graft.

The obvious disadvantage of the translabyrinthine approach is the sacrifice of any residual hearing in the operated ear. In most patients undergoing translabyrinthine removal, useful hearing either already has been lost or the size and location of the tumor make it very unlikely that useful hearing will remain postoperatively.

The use of the translabyrinthine approach is not limited by either tumor size or location (Briggs, Luxford, Atkins, & Hitselberger, 1994). Tumors that are small or large and that are located in the lateral or medial internal auditory canal, the cerebellopontine angle, or both can be removed through the translabyrinthine approach.

The Middle Fossa Approach

The advantage of the middle fossa approach is that it provides complete exposure of the contents of the internal auditory canal, allowing removal of laterally placed tumors without the need for blind dissection (House & Shelton, 1992). This exposure ensures total removal and is well suited for the removal of very small acoustic tumors. The inner ear structures are preserved, allowing for the possibility of hearing preservation. Positive identification of the facial nerve is possible at the lateral end of the internal auditory canal, facilitating tumor dissection from the facial nerve.

The first disadvantage of this approach is that the surgeon must work past the facial nerve to remove the tumor. This subjects the facial nerve to more manipulation than does the translabyrinthine approach for a similarly sized tumor, particularly if the tumor arises from the inferior vestibular nerve. Fortunately, at an experienced referral center that employs microsurgery techniques and intraoperative facial nerve monitoring, this increased manipulation of the nerve during the middle fossa approach has not led to a decrease in long-term facial nerve function when compared to results obtained following the translabyrinthine approach (Arriaga, Luxford, & Berliner, 1994). A second problem that sometimes is encountered with the middle fossa approach is postoperative unsteadiness that results from partial preservation of vestibular function. Careful dissection of the remaining vestibular nerve fibers reduces the incidence of postoperative unsteadiness, but it also increases the risk of further hearing loss. The middle fossa approach provides limited access to the posterior fossa to control any bleeding that may occur there. Patients older than 60 years do not tolerate the middle fossa approach as well as younger patients because of the fragility of the dura and retraction of the temporal lobe.

The middle fossa approach is used primarily for patients with small acoustic tumors that extend less than 5 mm into the cerebellopontine angle and good preoperative hearing. Because the approach allows good visualization of both the medial and lateral ends of the internal auditory canal, it does not matter where in the canal the tumor is located. Tumors that extend farther than 5 mm into the cerebellopontine angle have been removed by the middle fossa approach with good preservation of facial nerve function and hearing. However, tumors that extend 2 cm or more into the cerebellopontine angle probably are best removed by either the translabyrinthine or retrosigmoid/suboccipital approach.

The Retrosigmoid/Suboccipital Approach

With the retrosigmoid/suboccipital approach, preservation of hearing is possible in selected cases of moderate size tumors within the cerebellopontine angle (Cohen, 1992). The disadvantage of this approach is that the most lateral portion of the internal auditory canal is not visible. Exposure of this area requires drilling through the labyrinth and results in total loss of hearing. Therefore, when attempting to preserve hearing, removal of tumor in the lateral internal auditory canal may not be complete. Growth of the residual tumor will require a revision surgical procedure. This approach also requires more cerebellar retraction than the translabyrinthine approach. There also is a higher incidence of cerebrospinal fluid (CSF) leakage and postoperative headaches. The headaches are believed to be due to bone dust resulting from drilling the posterior aspect of the internal auditory canal. In the translabyrinthine and middle fossa approaches, bone removal is extradural; in the retrosigmoid/suboccipital approach, the bone removal is intradural.

The retrosigmoid/suboccipital approach is useful for patients who have moderate size tumors (≤2 cm) in the cerebellopontine angle that have little extension into the in-

ternal auditory canal. It is difficult to ensure complete tumor removal and preserve hearing for patients whose tumors extend into the lateral internal auditory canal. It also is difficult to preserve hearing in patients whose tumors extend more than 2 cm into the cerebellopontine angle. For patients with these larger tumors, for whom hearing preservation is unlikely, some surgical teams opt for the translabyrinthine approach because it has less morbidity. Hearing preservation is dependent on preserving not only the cochlear nerve, but also the blood supply to the inner ear. Maintaining circulation is the more difficult task, because the cochlear blood supply often is affected by the tumor, either within the cerebellopontine angle or the internal auditory canal.

STEREOTACTIC IRRADIATION

Stereotactic radiosurgery (Chapter 21) is an alternative treatment for carefully selected patients with acoustic tumors (Flickinger, Lunsford, Linskey, Duma, & Korziolka, 1993). Indications for treatment include patients who are medically unable to undergo surgery, elderly patients, the presence of bilateral acoustic tumors or contralateral deafness, recurrent tumor despite surgical resection, and patients who refuse microsurgery. Radiosurgery is contraindicated in patients with symptomatic brainstem or cerebellar compression from large acoustic tumors. Patients whose tumors are at least 3 cm in size are not considered candidates for radiosurgery. Previous posterior fossa radiotherapy is a relative contraindication.

Stereotactic radiosurgery does not eliminate the tumor, but it appears to arrest tumor growth through cell death and necrosis. The goal of radiosurgery is not tumor shrinkage but, rather, "tumor control," meaning absence of tumor growth. Prolonged imaging follow-up is required to ensure that apparently inactivated tumors do not begin to grow again.

OBSERVATION

Candidates for observation include patients with bilateral acoustic tumors who already have been treated unilaterally and who have either small- or medium-sized tumors and good or serviceable hearing in the contralateral ear, patients with unilateral acoustic tumors in the only hearing ear, elderly patients in poor health with small acoustic tumors, and patients who decline to undergo surgical treatment (Nedzelskui, Schessel, Pfleiderer, Kassel, & Rowed, 1992). Patients who choose to undergo observation must be followed closely with serial magnetic resonance imaging (MRI) scans at 6-month intervals for 3 years. If there is not significant change in tumor size, patients then can be followed annually. Surgery is suggested for those patients who show a rate of tumor growth that is equal to or exceeding 0.2 cm per year. The rate of tumor growth appears to be influenced by duration of symptoms and the neuroradiologic architecture of the tumor (Charabi et al., 1995). In the Charabi et al. study, tumors in patients with a short duration of symptoms grew faster than did tumors in patients with a long prediagnostic duration of symptoms. Patients with cystic tumors and bilateral acoustic tumors had a faster rate of growth when compared to unilateral noncystic tumors. Most patients who are candidates for hearing preservation surgery should not be observed. Observation also is not suggested for patients with significant brainstem compression or hydrocephalus.

TREATMENT OPTIONS FOR SELECTED PATIENT GROUPS

Advances in diagnostic and imaging techniques have allowed the accurate diagnosis of tumors when they are smaller and produce fewer symptoms. Besides the tumor size and location, patient characteristics can influence the kind and timing of therapy.

Patients with Bilateral Acoustic Tumors

Bilateral acoustic tumors occur in the autosomal dominant disorder, neurofibromatosis type 2 (NF-2) (Chapter 20). Treatment options to be considered are: (a) hearing preservation surgery with total tumor removal, (b) observation without surgical intervention, (c) middle fossa canal and internal auditory canal decompression without tumor removal, (d) retrosigmoid craniotomy with partial tumor removal, (e) nonhearing preservation with translabyrinthine total tumor removal, and (f) auditory brainstem implant (ABI) or cochlear implantation (Briggs, Brackmann, Baser, & Hitselberger, 1994).

Hearing Preservation Surgery— Total Tumor Removal

Since the introduction of gadolinium-enhanced magnetic resonance imaging, many patients with NF-2 have been diagnosed while they still have good hearing. In a patient with bilateral small tumors, total tumor removal with attempted hearing preservation on the side with the larger tumor or greater hearing impairment, or both, is advised. Of the two hearing preservation approaches, the middle fossa and retrosigmoid/suboccipital approaches, the middle fossa approach is used more often. If hearing is successfully preserved at a serviceable level, removal of the contralateral tumor after 6 months is recommended. The delay is necessary to show that hearing is stable in the initially operated ear. If the initial tumor removal resulted in loss of hearing, the contralateral tumor is observed, and hearing preservation surgery is not attempted.

In choosing the tumor to be treated, the relative chances of hearing preservation must be assessed carefully. For patients with NF-2, any preserved hearing is potentially useful, so audiologic criteria that are less conservative than the 50/50 rule (50% speech reception threshold and 50% WRS) may be used when hearing preservation is considered.

Observation without Surgical Intervention

Observation without surgical intervention is recommended either when a small tumor is present in an only hearing ear or when hearing is bilateral, but the tumors are probably too large for hearing preservation. There must be no risk to the patient from tumor size (e.g., brainstem compression or hydrocephalus). Regular follow-up at 6-month intervals for 2 years and annually thereafter is essential and should include repeated MRIs to document tumor size or development of hydrocephalus. Surgical intervention is necessary if further hearing loss occurs or when the tumor reaches sufficient size (approximately 3 cm) to produce symptoms of increased intracranial pressure and involvement of other cranial nerves.

Retrosigmoid Craniotomy— Partial Tumor Removal

Partial tumor removal usually is not recommended, because even partial tumor removal in patients with NF-2 usually results in hearing loss. Partial tumor removal may be considered when a patient has good unilateral hearing and a tumor that is symptomatic because of its largeness. In this circumstance, debulking of the tumor via retrosigmoid craniotomy may be performed. A cuff of tumor capsule is left in an attempt to protect the seventh and eighth nerves and the cochlear blood supply. Unfortunately useful hearing is not often preserved and, when it is, rapid regrowth of the tumor often occurs.

Nonhearing Preservation— Translabyrinthine Total Tumor Removal

When hearing preservation is no longer an issue, total tumor removal with preservation of the facial nerves is the goal. The translabyrinthine approach is used for tumors of any size in an ear without useful hearing or for large tumors that produce symptomatic brainstem compression, even if there is residual hearing. For NF-2, perhaps the greatest advantage of the translabyrinthine approach is that it allows direct access to the lateral recess of the fourth ventricle for placement of an auditory brainstem implant electrode array (Brackmann et al., 1993).

Stereotactic Radiation Therapy

Opinions differ on the use of stereotactic radiosurgery in patients with NF-2. In general, stereotactic radiosurgery is not recommended.

Education, Counseling, Screening, and Rehabilitation

Education of patients and screening of family members to identify other affected or at-risk individuals is essential. Genetic counseling should be available and part of the family screening. DNA analysis and gadolinium-enhanced MRI provide the most definitive diagnosis. Rehabilitation of all patients with NF-2 should begin in anticipation of eventual profound or total hearing loss. Instruction in speechreading, signing, and use of telephone typewriter devices should be undertaken.

Patients with a Unilateral Acoustic Tumor in the Only Hearing Ear

Microsurgical techniques and facial nerve monitoring have improved the mortality and morbidity of acoustic tumor removal. It is difficult to predict preservation of hearing following microsurgery or stereotactic radiosurgery with any certainty. Because of this uncertainty, patients with unilateral tumors in their only hearing ear usually are observed. In patients with rapidly deteriorating hearing in their only hearing ear, middle fossa decompression of the internal auditory canal is offered (Gadre, Kwartler,

Brackmann, House, & Hitselberger, 1990). The decompression procedure appears to relieve the pressure exerted by the tumor on the seventh and eighth nerves. The relief of this pressure may enhance blood supply to the nerve and end organ. The decompression procedure, although not curative, appears to slow down the rapid hearing loss. This provides additional time for patients to learn speechreading or manual communication skills before all hearing is finally lost. Once hearing has been lost, total tumor removal is achieved through the translabyrinthine approach. In these cases, a cochlear implant may be appropriate for the nontumor ear.

Patients with Small Acoustic Tumors

Gadolinium-enhanced MRI allows the detection of small tumors in patients with very early symptoms. Some of these intracanalicular tumors present with minimal hearing loss and no other associated symptoms. Although gadolinium-enhanced MRI has very high sensitivity for an acoustic tumor, it unfortunately has a low specificity; that is, a negative gadolinium-enhanced MRI essentially eliminates the possibility of an internal auditory canal tumor. However, enhancement in the internal auditory canal may be caused by a variety of processes other than an acoustic tumor. It is important to have corroborating information (e.g., unilateral hearing loss, abnormal ABR, and reduced vestibular response on caloric testing) suggesting that an acoustic tumor is present within the internal auditory canal (Arriaga, Carrier, & Houston, 1995; Chandrasekhar, Brackmann, & Devgan, 1995).

Patients who have enhancement on an MRI scan with gadolinium without corroborating information should be observed; they should have repeat gadolinium-enhanced MRI scans performed at 6-month intervals. If follow-up testing is consistent with an acoustic tumor and the repeated scans show persistent enhancement or enlargement of the lesion in the internal auditory canal, a middle fossa approach should be used for removal of the tumor.

Observation with serial imaging also should be used for the elderly patient with small internal auditory canal lesions. Young patients with corroborating evidence of an acoustic tumor and positive gadolinium-enhanced MRI scans should undergo middle fossa removal of the tumor. The probability of hearing preservation following surgery is higher in patients with smaller tumors. Therefore, patients with symptoms, screening studies, and enhanced MRI findings consistent with an acoustic tumor and preservable hearing should undergo early middle fossa surgical resection of their small acoustic tumor (Shelton & Hitselberger, 1991). A few groups advocate stereotactic radiosurgery for these patients.

Acoustic Tumors in Elderly Patients

Questions regarding surgical risk, tumor growth rate, and life expectancy have led to discussions concerning the best and safest treatment modality in elderly patients with acoustic tumors. The growth rate of acoustic tumors has been found to vary. The estimated average growth rate is 2 mm per year, but some tumors never show any signs of growth over time, whereas others show accelerating growth, perhaps due to hemorrhage or cyst formation within the tumor.

Microsurgery is accepted as the primary treatment for acoustic tumors in the general population. In the elderly patient who has hearing loss, whose tumor is 2 cm or larger, and who is medically stable, the translabyrinthine approach is used for surgical removal of the acoustic tumor (Ramsay & Luxford, 1993). Stereotactic radiosurgery is considered in elderly patients who are at increased surgical risk because of medical problems and who have tumors less than 3 cm in size. A recent study showed that, in experienced hands, translabyrinthine removal of tumors of all sizes is safe, regardless of the age of the patient (Ramsay & Luxford, 1993). Observation is considered in the elderly patient who has a small tumor and who is asymptomatic.

Tumor removal should be considered sooner, rather than later, because surgery becomes more difficult, and the rate of complications rises with increasing tumor size. Increased life expectancy, as well as the unpredictable growth rate of acoustic tumors, make surgery warranted even in patients of advanced age. Microsurgery has the advantage of achieving total ablation of the disease in most cases. Partial tumor removal is accepted only if the tumor is adherent to the facial nerve or if changes in vital signs are observed during surgery.

Acoustic Tumors in the Pregnant Patient

Acoustic tumors are statistically more common in women, and the larger, more vascular tumors are twice as common in women. Although case reports of known acoustic tumors in pregnant patients are few, they generally show that the signs and symptoms of these tumors can dramatically worsen during the last 3 or 4 months of pregnancy (Doyle & Luxford, 1994). Techniques of general anesthesia and monitoring have advanced to the point where nonelective surgery can be performed safely in pregnant mothers with some limitations. Surgery is performed best during the second trimester to minimize risk to both fetus and mother. Removal during the second trimester allows the patient to avoid the increasing signs and symptoms of accelerated tumor growth that may occur in the last trimester. As with other patients, the smaller the tumor, the easier it is to remove. Stereo-

tactic radiosurgery and observation are not treatment options that are suitable for the pregnant patient with an acoustic tumor.

COMMENT

With the recent advances in diagnostic and imaging techniques, more patients are being diagnosed with acoustic tumors. Options for therapy include surgery, stereotactic irradiation, and observation. The size and location of the tumor(s) and patient characteristics influence the choices of the type and timing of therapy.

REFERENCES

Arriaga, M.A., Carrier, D., & Houston, G.D. (1995). False-positive magnetic resonance imaging of small internal auditory canal tumors: A clinical, radiologic, and pathologic correlation study. *Archives of Otolaryngol-ogy—Head and Neck Surgery, 113,* 61–70.

Arriaga, M.A., Luxford, W.M., & Berliner, K.I. (1994). Facial nerve function following middle fossa and translabyrinthine acoustic tumor surgery: A comparison. *American Journal of Otology, 15,* 620–624.

Brackmann, D.E., & Green, J.D. (1992). Translabyrinthine approach for acoustic tumor removal. *Otolaryngology Clinics of North America, 25,* 311–329.

Brackmann, D.E., Hitselberger, W.E., Nelson, R.A., Moore, J., Waring, M.D., Portillo, F., Shannon, R.V., & Telischi, F.F. (1993). Auditory brainstem implant: I. Issues in surgical implantation. *Archives of Otolaryngology—Head and Neck Surgery, 108,* 624–633.

Briggs, R.J.S., Brackmann, D.E., Baser, M.E., & Hitselberger, W.E. (1994). Comprehensive management of bilateral acoustic neuromas. *Archives of Otolaryngology—Head and Neck Surgery, 120,* 1307–1314.

Briggs, R.J.S., Luxford, W.M., Atkins, J.S., Jr., & Hitselberger, W.E. (1994). Translabyrinthine removal of large acoustic neuromas. *Neurosurgery, 34,* 785–791.

Chandrasekhar, S.S., Brackmann, D.E., & Devgan K.K. (1995). Utility of auditory brainstem response audiometry in diagnosis of acoustic neuromas. *American Journal of Otology, 16,* 63–67.

Charabi, S., Thomsen, J., Mantoni, M., Charabi, B., Jorgensen, B., Borgesen, S.E., Gyldensted, C., & Tos, M. (1995) Acoustic neuroma (vestibular schwannoma): Growth and surgical and nonsurgical consequences of the wait-and-see policy. *Archives of Otolaryngology—Head and Neck Surgery, 113,* 5–14.

Cohen, N.L. (1992). Retrosigmoid approach for acoustic tumor removal. *Otolaryngology Clinics of North America, 25,* 295–310.

Doyle, K.J., & Luxford, W.M. (1994). Acoustic neuroma in pregnancy. *Archives of Otolaryngology—Head and Neck Surgery, 15,* 111–113.

Flickinger, J.C., Lunsford, L.D., Linskey, M.E., Duma, C.M., & Kondziolka, D. (1993). Gamma knife radiosurgery for acoustic tumors: Multivariate analysis of four year results. *Radio therapy and Oncology, 27,* 91–98.

Gadre, A.K., Kwartler, J.A., Brackmann, D.E., House, W.F., & Hitselberger, W.E. (1990). Middle fossa decompression of the internal auditory canal in acoustic neuroma surgery:

A therapeutic alternative. *Laryngoscope, 100,* 948–952.

House, W.F., & Shelton, C. (1992). Middle fossa approach for acoustic tumor removal. *Otolaryngology Clinics of North America, 25,* 347–359.

Jackler, R.K., & Pitts, L.H. (1992). Selection of surgical approach to acoustic neuroma. *Otolaryngology Clinics of North America, 25,* 361–387.

National Institutes of Health Consensus Development Conference. (1994). Statement of acoustic neuroma. *Archives of Neurology, 51,* 201–207.

Nedzelski, J.M., Schessel, D.A., Pfleiderer, A., Kassel, E.E., & Rowed, D.W. (1992). Conservative management of acoustic neuromas. *Otolaryngology Clinics of North America, 25,* 691–705.

Ramsay, H.A., & Luxford, W.M. (1993). Treatment of acoustic tumors in elderly patients: Is surgery warranted? *Journal of Laryngology and Otology, 107,* 295–297.

Shelton, C. (1992). Hearing preservation in acoustic tumor surgery. *Otolaryngology Clinics of North America, 25,* 609–621.

Shelton, C., & Hitselberger, W.E. (1991). The treatment of small acoustic tumors: Now or later? *Laryngoscope, 101,* 925–928.

CHAPTER 8

Anesthesia in Acoustic Tumor Surgery

Karen Jo Doyle, M.D., Ph.D.
Brett R. Broderson, M.D.

This chapter outlines anesthetic management in acoustic neuroma surgery. It is organized into sections on preoperative assessment, intraoperative management, and postoperative care. We will cover monitoring, pharmacologic agents, and anesthetic procedures used in neuroanesthesia so that we may enable the reader to anticipate problems inherent to acoustic neuroma surgery.

PREOPERATIVE MANAGEMENT

Preoperative Assessment

The preanesthesia interview and examination of the patient usually take place on the day before surgery. Ideally, the written history and physical examination are available to the anesthesiologist, as well as any laboratory and radiologic studies (Broderson & Barky, 1979). Recording the patient's history includes cardiac, pulmonary, renal, gastrointestinal, hepatic, endocrine, and hemotologic status. A medication history is taken, including drug allergies, and the patient's physician and anesthesiologist decide which

medications should be continued perioperatively. Previous anesthetic records are reviewed for problems and complications. Based on the examination, further tests, such as those of pulmonary function, arterial blood gases, coagulation, blood chemistries, and liver function may be ordered by the anesthesiologist.

After the anesthetic history and examination, the anesthesiologist describes the steps involved in the induction, maintenance, and conclusion of general anesthesia for the patient. The risks of general anesthesia are described, and the patient's questions are answered.

Blood transfusions are unusual in acoustic neuroma surgery, except for the largest tumors. Autologous blood donations may be made by patients from several weeks to a few days before surgery.

Premedication

The typical anesthetic premedications used today include the benzodiazapine, midazolam, and the narcotic, fentanyl. Midazolam

143

has a short half-life, anxiolytic and amnestic properties, and can reduce the doses of anesthetics required for induction without prolonging recovery time after anesthesia (De Lucia & White, 1992). Midazolam and fentanyl both can cause respiratory depression and should be used at the smallest effective doses. Judicious use of intravenous premedication will alleviate patient anxiety and pain without producing unwanted respiratory, hypodynamic, or cerebral effects.

INTRAOPERATIVE MANAGEMENT

Monitors

Monitors used frequently in acoustic neuroma surgery include (a) a blood pressure cuff, (b) an electrocardiogram, (c) an esophageal stethoscope, (d) a core temperature probe, (e) a urinary catheter, (f) a pulse oximeter, (g) a mass spectrometer, (h) a peripheral nerve stimulator, (i) a nasogastric tube, (j) an arterial line, and (k) facial or auditory nerve monitors. An intravenous line is started in the preoperative area. After the patient is moved to the operating table, the blood pressure cuff, electrocardiogram, pulse oximeter, and precordial stethoscope are placed before induction of anesthesia. After induction, the other monitors are placed, and an additional large-bore intravenous line may be established. Central venous pressure monitoring may be employed for patients with cardiovascular disease. Electrophysiologic monitoring of the seventh cranial nerve now is used routinely in acoustic tumor surgery, as are intraoperative recordings of the eighth cranial nerve and auditory brainstem responses in hearing preservation procedures. The anesthesiologist ensures that the monitors are safely and securely placed and will not interfere with safe anesthetic procedure.

During the operation, the anesthesiologist periodically enters the heart rate, blood pressure, electrocardiogram interpretation, temperature, oxygen saturation, and urine output into the anesthetic record. Ventilator settings, drugs and fluids administered, and peripheral nerve responses are recorded, as well. When required for decision-making, intraoperative measures of hemoglobin count, blood chemistries, and arterial blood gases may be obtained.

Induction

After pre-oxygenation with 100% oxygen for several minutes, induction is performed for most patients using intravenous agents. Muscle relaxant then is given for laryngoscopy and endotracheal intubation, procedures that are conducted after observation of reduced or absent twitch to tetanic peripheral nerve stimulation. For patients with anticipated airway problems, this induction sequence is modified, using awake intubation with local anesthesia and direct or fiberoptic laryngoscopy. The chest is auscultated to verify proper endotracheal tube placement. Next, cranial nerve monitors are placed and the eyes are taped to prevent corneal injury.

Positioning

The middle fossa, suboccipital, and translabyrinthine procedures all may be performed with the patient supine and the head turned. With head-turning beyond 30°, there can be increases in intracranial pressure (Hung, Brien, & Hope, 1992). It is sometimes necessary to place the patient in the lateral position with the head in a Mayfield clamp. Today, the prone and sitting positions are rarely used in neurotologic surgery. The dangers of the sitting position include venous air embolism, cervical spinal cord ischemia, and hypotension (Albin, 1992). Acoustic tumors can be accessed readily without using the sitting position (Hitselberger & House, 1980).

Carefully positioning the patient is important. The table is turned 180°, with the patient's draped head away from the anesthesiologist; therefore, all monitors must be taped securely to prevent inadvertent disconnection. The patient is securely belted to the operating table with additional wrappings of sheets and adhesive tape to prevent slippage during rotation of the table. All pressure points are padded, including the elbows, heels, and sacrum. Anti-embolism stockings or sequential compression devices are placed to prevent venous thrombosis, especially if a lengthy operating time is anticipated.

Drugs Used in Anesthetic Maintenance

In this section, we will review some of the more commonly used inhaled and intravenous pharmacologic agents employed in the maintenance of anesthesia, as well as some of the intravenous neuromuscular blocking agents.

Inhaled Agents

Isoflurane is the most often used of the volatile inhaled anesthetics in neuroanesthesia (Gonzales, 1993). It produces less marked cerebral vasodilation than the other volatile agents, thereby minimizing increases in intracranial pressure and cerebral blood flow. Other advantages of its use include the possible depression of cerebral metabolism, with resultant cerebral protection during oxygen deprivation, and induced hypotension, to decrease surgical bleeding and treat hypertension. Nitrous oxide, which is usually given in combination with a narcotic, probably has minimal effects on cerebral blood flow, intracranial pressure, and cerebral metabolism (Messick, Newberg, Nugent, & Faust, 1985). The advantage of using nitrous oxide is that it is insoluble and washes out rapidly when compared with the volatile agents. The disadvantages include its high concentration requirements and, therefore, less protection from hypoxemia;

the necessity of combining it with other anesthetics to produce adequate anesthesia level; and its role in the formation of tension pneumocephalus (Artru, 1982).

Intravenous Agents

The narcotics fentanyl, meperidine, morphine, and sufentanil are used frequently in neuroanesthesia. The advantages of their use include the reduction of intracranial pressure and reversibility with naloxone. Both meperidine and morphine release histamine and are associated with tachycardia and hypotension, while fentanyl and the other, newer narcotics do not release histamine (Moss & Rosow, 1983). Propofol is an intravenous agent that can be used in induction or maintenance of anesthesia. Recovery from maintenance anesthesia is very rapid with propofol, and it has antiemetic properties. In addition, it decreases cerebral blood flow, intracranial pressure, and cerebral metabolism (Eng, Lam, Mayberg, Mathison & Lee, 1992; Muzzi, Losasso, Weglinski, and Milde, 1992). The main disadvantages of its use are pain at the injection site and possible precipitous drops in arterial blood pressure on induction. It is packaged as an emulsion without antibacterial preservatives and must be handled aseptically to prevent septicemia.

Neuromuscular Blocking Agents

The neuromuscular blocking agents are used for laryngoscopy and endotracheal intubation in acoustic tumor surgery. Succinylcholine, the short-acting, depolarizing agent, can produce increases in arterial pressure and intracranial blood pressure (Messick et al., 1985). The well-known muscle fasciculations produced by succinylcholine may be avoided by pretreatment with D-tubocurare. The nondepolarizing agents, vecuronium, atracurium, mivacurium, and nocuronium all are relatively short-acting and have negligible effects on cerebral blood flow and intracranial pressure. Because facial nerve electromyographic monitoring is carried out routinely in acoustic tumor surgery, the use of neuromuscular blocking agents generally is avoided after anesthetic induction.

Fluid Management

The anesthesiologist manages intravenous fluids during acoustic tumor surgery to correct hypovolemia and avoid overhydration. Because most patients initially are hypovolemic when entering the operating room, isotonic solutions are given at induction to prevent the hypotension that frequently occurs with inhaled or intravenous induction agents. To prevent cerebral ischemia, the anesthesiologist replaces fluid losses detected by changes in pulse, blood pressure, blood loss, and urine output. Simultaneously, overhydration is avoided to prevent cerebral edema, increased intracranial pressure, congestive heart failure, and pulmonary edema. Glucose-containing solutions are avoided on the basis of animal studies showing their use may result in greater neurologic injury when given prior to episodes of cerebral ischemia. The mechanism of neurologic injury is thought to be lactic acidosis (Newberg, 1985).

The osmotic diuretic, mannitol, and the loop diuretic, furosemide, often are administered in acoustic neuroma surgery to reduce brain swelling. Because mannitol initially may produce increased intravascular volume and, thus, a transient increase in intracranial pressure, furosemide is administered first to offset this effect (Wilkinson & Rosenfeld, 1983). After diuretic administration, the anesthesiologist closely monitors pulse, blood pressure, and urine output. Deficits in potassium, chloride, and sodium are detected by serum measurements.

Ventilator Management

During anesthetic maintenance, mechanical ventilation is employed, and the anesthesiologist monitors endtidal oxygen and car-

bon dioxide using the mass spectrometer. In neurosurgical procedures, hyperventilation is a tool for decreasing cerebral blood flow and, therefore, brain swelling, with carbon dioxide pressure maintained at 25–30 mm Hg. If cerebral ischemia becomes a concern, hypocarbia may produce cerebral vasospasm, and should be avoided to maintain cerebral perfusion (Domino, 1987).

POSTOPERATIVE MANAGEMENT

Emergence from Anesthesia

Anesthetic agents must be titrated appropriately to permit smooth emergence from anesthesia and prevent complications. The volatile anesthetics must be stopped in advance, and their endtidal concentrations must be observed with the mass spectrometer. Nitrous oxide must be discontinued before dural closure to prevent tension pneumocephalus. Because of its rapid offset, propofol infusion may be continued until minutes before desired emergence. Narcotics must be used lightly at the end of anesthesia to prevent respiratory depression. Naloxone may be used to reverse narcotic effects, but its temporary influence must be considered. The peripheral nerve stimulator should be used to verify reversal of nondepolarizing muscle relaxants.

When the patient is breathing spontaneously and the surgical dressing has been applied, 100% oxygen then is administered to prepare for extubation. The endotracheal tube cuff is deflated, then removed. Coughing on the endotracheal tube may result in increased intracranial pressure or bleeding; this may be prevented with intravenous lidocaine (Donegan & Bedford, 1980). After extubation, 100% oxygen via face mask is applied for transport to the intensive care unit.

Postoperative Nausea

After removal of the vestibular nerves or labyrinth in acoustic neuroma surgery, postoperative nausea and vomiting are common. The stomach is emptied via a nasogastric tube, which is usually left in place, with intermittent suction provided overnight. Several medications, including droperidol, metoclopramide, or ondansetron may be administered to control postoperative emesis.

SPECIAL PROBLEMS IN ACOUSTIC NEUROMA SURGERY

In this section, we will present three problems encountered in anesthesia for acoustic neuroma surgery: tension pneumocephalus, venous air embolism, and vital sign changes with cranial nerve retraction. We will discuss anesthetic strategies used to solve these uncommon, yet potentially devastating, problems.

Tension Pneumocephalus

Tension pneumocephalus occurs when subdural intracranial gas produces mass effect and neurologic deficit. It has been reported most commonly following posterior fossa surgery performed in the sitting position, but it also has occurred following the translabyrinthine removal of acoustic neuromas using the lateral position (Toung, Donham, Lehner, Alano, & Campbell, 1983). Nitrous oxide has been implicated in the genesis of tension pneumocephalus by diffusion into and expansion of an entrapped volume of intracranial air, thereby raising intracranial pressure (Artru, 1982). Discontinuing nitrous oxide prior to dural closure may prevent tension pneumocephalus. Close neurologic monitoring postoperatively will enable early detection of tension pneumocephalus, and the diagnosis is made by computed tomographic scan. Tension pneumocephalus is treated by reopening the surgical wound or by burr-hole craniotomy to evacuate the entrapped air.

Venous Air Embolism

Venous air embolism occurs when air enters the circulation through openings in the dural sinuses or diploic veins. When air enters the pulmonary circulation, it may increase dead space, impair gas exchange, and produce hypercarbia or hypoxia. In the right side of the heart, air can result in decreased ventricular outflow, venous return, and cardiac output, producing arrhythmias, hypotension, and cyanosis (Albin, 1992). In the left side of the heart, air may produce cerebral embolism with resultant brain infarction if an intracardiac defect exists or if the air diffuses into the systemic circulation (Marquez, Sladen, Gendell, Boehnke, and Mendelow, 1981). In the sitting position, craniotomy carries a 20% to 60% risk of venous air embolism, while the risk in the lateral position is significantly less (Albin, Carroll, & Maroon, 1978). Intravascular air can expand in the presence of nitrous oxide, but it does not appear to increase the incidence of venous air embolism (Losasso, Muzzi, Black, & Cucchiara, 1989). Small amounts of air are detectable intraoperatively by a precordial Doppler ultrasound transducer or transesophageal echocardiography (Cucchiara, Nugent, Seward, & Messick, 1984). Transesophageal echocardiography has been conducted following induction of anesthesia for patients undergoing neurosurgery in the sitting position, to detect intracardiac defect prior to beginning surgery, thereby identifying patients at risk for cerebral air embolism (Losasso, Muzzi, & Weglinski, 1992). Signs of the presence of air embolism include decreased end-tidal carbon dioxide, increased arterial blood gas carbon dioxide, and decreased oxygen saturation (Russell & Graybeal, 1989). Nitrous oxide should be discontinued after venous air embolism has been detected to avoid expansion of the embolism. Treatment includes placing the patient on the left side with the head down. Air then is aspirated through a central venous catheter or pulmonary artery catheter. Blood pressure should be maintained with volume expansion, vasopressors or both.

Vital sign changes with cranial nerve retraction

During removal of an acoustic tumor, surgical manipulation of the cranial nerves or brainstem may produce apnea, hypotension, hypertension, bradycardia, or cardiac arrhythmias (Lall & Jain, 1969). With large posterior fossa tumors, dissection in the floor of the fourth ventricle may produce sinus arrhythmia (Drummond & Todd, 1984). Manipulation of the trigeminal nerve may cause abrupt hypertension, bradycardia, or ventricular arrhythmias (Domino, 1987). Sectioning the upper vagus rootlets for glossopharyngeal neuralgia has produced acute hypotension and right bundle branch block (Nagashima, Sakaguchi, Kamisasa, & Kawanuma, 1976). The anesthesiologist must be aware of these potential changes, and alert the surgeon to them when they occur. Likewise, the surgeon should notify the anesthesiologist when tumor is dissected from cranial nerves or brainstem. With termination of surgical manipulation, vital sign changes usually resolve but may persist and require treatment.

REFERENCES

Albin, M.S. (1992). Neuroanesthesia. In J.R. Youmans (Ed.), *Neurological surgery* (pp. 903–921). Philadelphia: W.B. Saunders Company.

Albin, M.S., Carroll, R.G., & Maroon, J.C. (1978). Clinical considerations concerning detection of venous air embolism. *Neurosurgery, 3,* 380–384.

Artru, A.A. (1982). Nitrous oxide plays a direct role in the development of tension pneumocephalus intraoperatively. *Anesthesiology, 57,* 59–61.

Broderson, B.R., & Barky, N. (1979). Acoustic tumor surgery: Anesthetic considerations. In W.F. House & C.M. Luetje (Eds.), *Acoustic tumors* (pp. 3–14). Baltimore: University Park Press

Cucchiara, R.F., Nugent, M., Seward, J.B., & Messick, J.M. (1984). Air embolism in upright neurosurgical patients: Detection and localization by two-dimensional transesophageal echocardiography. *Anesthesiology, 60,* 353–355.

De Lucia, J.A., & White, P.F. (1992). Effect of midazolam on induction and recovery characteristics of propofol. *Anesthesia and Analgesia, 74,* S63.

Domino, K.B. (1987). Anesthesia for cranial base tumor operations. In L.N. Sekhar & V.L. Schramm (Eds.). *Tumors of the cranial base: Diagnosis and treatment* (pp. 107–121). Mount Kisco, NY: Futura Publishing.

Donegan, M.F., & Bedford, R.F. (1980). Intravenously administered lidocaine prevents intracranial hypertension during endotracheal suctioning. *Anesthesiology, 52,* 516–518.

Drummond, J.C., & Todd, M.M. (1984). Acute sinus arrhythmia during surgery in the fourth ventricle: An indicator of brain-stem irritation. *Anesthesiology, 60,* 232–235.

Eng, C., Lam, A., Mayberg, T., Mathison, T., & Lee, C. (1992). The influence of propofol with and without nitrous oxide on cerebral blood flow velocity and CO_2 reactivity in man. *Anesthesia and Analgesia, 74,* S87.

Gonzales, R.M. (1993). Special anesthetic considerations in cranial base tumor surgery. In L.N. Sekhar & I.P. Janecka (Ed.), *Surgery of cranial base tumors (pp. 69–81).* New York: Raven Press.

Hitselberger, W.E., & House, W.F. (1980). A warning regarding the sitting position for acoustic tumor surgery. *Archives of Otolaryngology–Head and Neck Surgery, 106,* 69.

Hung, O.R., Brien, S., & Hope, C.E. (1992). The effect of head position on the intracranial pressure in patients with intracranial tumors. *Anesthesiology, 77,* A197.

Lall, N.G., & Jain, A.P. (1969). Circulatory and respiratory disturbances during posterior cranial fossa surgery. *British Journal of Anaesthesiology, 41,* 447–449.

Losasso, T.J., Muzzi, D.A., Black, S., & Cucchiara, and R.F. (1989). The "risk" of nitrous oxide in sitting neurosurgical patients: A prospective, randomized study. *Anesthesiology, 71,* A1137.

Losasso, T.J,. Muzzi, D.A., & Weglinski, M.R. (1992). The risk of paradoxical air embolism in sitting neurosurgical patients with and without a demonstrable right-to-left shunt. *Anesthesiology, 77,* A198.

Marquez, J., Sladen, A., Gendell, H., Boehnke, M., & Mendelow, H. (1981). Paradoxical cerebral air embolism without an intracardiac septal defect. *Journal of Neurosurgery, 55,* 997–1000.

Messick, J.M., Newberg, L.A., Nugent, M., & Faust, R.J. (1985). Principles of neuroanesthesia for the nonneurosurgical patient with CNS pathophysiology. *Anesthesia and Analgesia, 64,* 143–174.

Moss, J., & Rosow, C.E. (1983). Histamine release by narcotics and muscle relaxants in humans. *Anesthesiology, 59,* 330–339.

Muzzi, D., Losasso, T,. Weglinski, M., & Milde, L. (1992). The effect of propofol on cerebrospinal fluid pressure in patients with supratentorial mass lesions. *Anesthesiology, 77,* A216.

Nagashima, C., Sakaguchi, A., Kamisasa, A., & Kawanuma, S. (1976). Cardiovascular complications on upper vagal rootlet section for glossopharyngeal neuralgia. *Journal of Neurosurgery, 44,* 248–253.

Newberg, L.A. (1985). Use of intravenous glucose solutions in surgical patients. *Anesthesia and Analgesia, 64,* 559.

Russell, G.B., & Graybeal, J. M. (1989). Sensitivity of venous air embolism detection by continuous monitors of oxygenation and ventilation. *Anesthesiology, 71,* A133.

Toung, T., Donham, R.T., Lehner, A., Alano, J., & Campbell, J. (1983). Tension pneumocephalus after posterior fossa craniotomy: Report of four additional cases and review of postoperative pneumocephalus. *Neurosurgery, 12,* 164–168.

Wilkinson, H.A., & Rosenfeld, S. (1983). Furosemide and mannitol in the treatment of acute experimental intracranial hypertension. *Neurosurgery, 12,* 405–410.

CHAPTER 9

Translabyrinthine Approach

William F. House, M.D.

In the first edition of *Acoustic Tumors: Diagnosis and Management*, the translabyrinthine surgical approach was presented in Chapter 3. The first part of that chapter was a history of surgical management of acoustic neuromas from 1961 to 1977. In this new edition, the surgical description of the translabyrinthine approach has been left unchanged,[1] while the history section has been updated by Drs. Glasscock, Bohrer, and Steenerson and included as Chapter 2.

SURGICAL TECHNIQUE

The translabyrinthine approach in its present form developed and evolved over a period of 20 years. It was made possible by the operating microscope and modern otologic surgical technique. The operation encompasses two major aspects: exposure of the tumor through the temporal bone and acoustic tumor removal. Obviously, there has never been a surgical technique developed that cannot be improved, and it is our hope that further improvements will continue.

For this technique, the patient lies on the table on his back with his head turned to the side. We usually arrange for the patient's head to be at the foot of the table. This gives the surgeon, seated at the side of the table, room for his legs and the anesthesiologist, at the head of the table, easy access to controls under the patient's feet (Figure 9–1). In our experience, electrically driven tables have proven inadequate, since small adjustments necessary for microsurgery are difficult or impossible. We prefer that the surgeon be seated, allowing greater stability and relaxation during exacting microsurgical techniques.

Temporal Bone Exposure

Before the incision, the surgeon must again confirm that the proper ear has been prepped and draped.

The postauricular incision (Figure 9–2) is curved, extending from the ear down to the mastoid tip. It is about 2 cm back of the postauricular fold. Curving the incision avoids a great deal of foreshortening when

[1]Reprinted from *Acoustic Tumors: Volume 2. Management* (pp. 42–87), by W.F. House and C.M. Luetje (Eds.), 1979, Baltimore: University Park Press. Copyright 1985 by the House Ear Institute. Reprinted with permission.

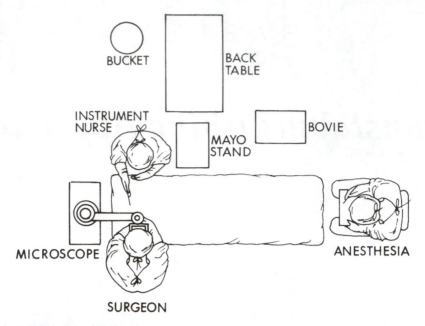

Figure 9–1. Translabyrinthine approach, room arrangement. Note positions of surgeon, anesthesiologist, and nurse.

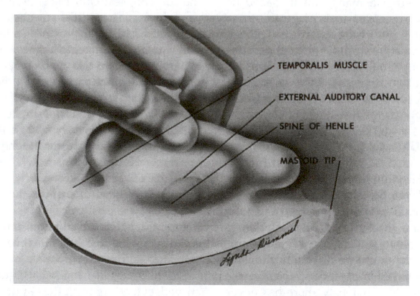

Figure 9–2. Skin incision 2 cm behind the postauricular sulcus.

the retractor is placed to push the external ear forward. The curve also helps to keep the incision posterior to the access to the areas over the sigmoid sinus and sinodural angle. Most of the surgical view of the cerebellopontine angle occurs along the plane of the posterior fossa dura. For this reason, posterior access is important. If an error is to be made, it should be in the direction of putting the incision more posterior.

To make the incision, I use a cutting current, which puts the dermal vessels in spasm, since the electric current passes through these vessels as a path of least resistance. The current does not spread out along the surface of the skin because it is less conductive than the subdermal tissues. Thus, there is little burning of the skin edges as long as the cutting cautery is kept moving at a reasonable speed to prevent buildup of heat. At first, half of the incision was made with a cold knife and half with a hot knife. Because there was no difference in the appearance of the healing of the wound in the postoperative period, we now use only the electrocautery knife for postauricular incisions.

The incision extends down to the temporalis muscle fascia and the bone inferior to the linea temporalis. Bleeding points are cauterized, and a plane is developed over the temporalis muscle above the external auditory canal. It is important not to develop this plane more than necessary, since it minimizes postoperative hematoma above the operative area. The Lempert periosteal elevator is used to free the postauricular tissues from the underlying bone cortex posterior to the sinodural angle and forward as far as the spine of Henley and the external auditory canal. Postauricular retractors are placed to elevate the external ear forward and elevate the temporalis muscle superiorly. A suction on the posterior blade of the retractor will remove excess irrigation fluid and blood from the wound (Figure 9–3). Without a suction, they will run over the wound and onto the drapes. We use plastic drapes taped to the patient's head. If they come loose, the irrigating solution and blood can run directly down onto the patient's head and hair. Soaking the drapes with irrigating solution, a potential source of contamination, should be avoided.

After adequate exposure of the cortex, the bone removal is carried out with irrigation suction and cutting burr. The bone removal should be started forward at the region of the external auditory canal. The strokes of the cutting burr are anterior to posterior, which allow the operator more control of the burr than strokes toward him. Bone then is removed down along the posterior aspect of the external canal and along the middle fossa plate so that a fan-shaped cortex removal is developed. The apex of the fan is at the posterior and superior portion of the external auditory canal. As soon as the cortex has been removed, mastoid air cells will be visualized. Bone removal is extended and deepened. Take care to saucerize—not to undercut—the cortex and to keep the external opening as large as possible. The middle fossa plate soon is identified, and the sigmoid sinus is visualized. Bone is removed liberally back along the sinodural angle and over the sigmoid sinus posterior to the sigmoid.

In large tumors with elevated intracranial pressure, the bony removal posterior to the sigmoid sinus is carried out liberally. In some cases, the bone is removed with a rongeur as far as an inch or an inch and a half posterior to the sigmoid sinus and inferior down under the cerebellar hemisphere. This gives more decompression of the posterior fossa and a little room for stretching of the dura to relieve pressure. Care must be taken, however, not to injure the dura. This would allow the cerebellum to be forced into the dural tear and cause the small portion that exudes out to become infarcted. Removal of bone over the sigmoid must be performed carefully. If the cutting burr crashes into the sigmoid, serious bleeding can ensue that would require Surgicel pack. Also, emissary veins that protrude from the posterior aspect of the sigmoid must be approached with caution. They can be identified through the bone as it is being removed, since the irrigation suction, which keeps the bone clean, allows visualization of structures developed during the bone removal.

As soon as the cortex is removed and the sigmoid sinus is well outlined, the operating microscope is brought into place. It allows more accurate bone removal and development of all the structures of the temporal bone. A thin layer of bone is left over the sigmoid sinus and around the

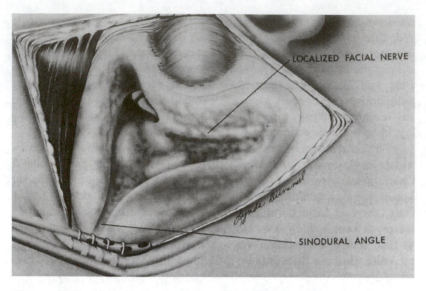

LOCALIZED FACIAL NERVE

SINODURAL ANGLE

Figure 9–3. Mastoidectomy completed. Facial nerve localized and sigmoid sinus skeletonized.

emissary veins, and the mastoidectomy is completed down to the level of the horizontal canal (Figure 9–3). It is important that the antrum be opened and that the horizontal (lateral) canal be visualized accurately. The lateral canal is the basic landmark in temporal bone surgery. Once the position of this canal is known, the depth and three-dimensional relationships of the facial nerve and posterior and superior semicircular canals can be visualized.

The ability to visualize three-dimensional relationships of all the structures in the temporal bone as the angle of the microscope changes for different views comes only after many hours of diligent temporal bone dissection. Temporal bone microsurgery depends upon thorough knowledge of anatomy and the ability to visualize the structures just under the cutting burr or diamond stone. One should always be watching for the next structure to be encountered in the surgical approach.

In the translabyrinthine approach, the facial nerve is an important landmark whose position must be established early in the surgical dissection. The facial nerve usually is located in the mastoid portion following

skeletonization of the posterior semicircular canal (see Figure 9–5). The mastoidectomy part of the translabyrinthine operation is considered complete when the posterior canal, horizontal canal, middle and posterior fossa plates, and the sigmoid sinus are skeletonized. The position of the facial nerve then is known accurately. At this point, the labyrinthectomy begins.

Labyrinthectomy involves drilling down the superior petrosal sinus, which is the junction of the middle posterior fossa plates, gradually deepening and enlarging this area to include the labyrinth and, finally, identifying the internal auditory canal and jugular bulb. Therefore, with a round cutting burr, the dissection is carried down along the superior petrosal sinus and gradually enlarged. The next structure encountered is the posterior semicircular canal, which is opened and followed along its course (Figure 9–4). When approaching the ampulla of this canal, care must be taken, of course, to watch for the facial nerve, which is just lateral to the ampulla of the posterior canal. The lateral canal is now opened and removed. The surgeon begins watching for the superior canal as he progresses forward

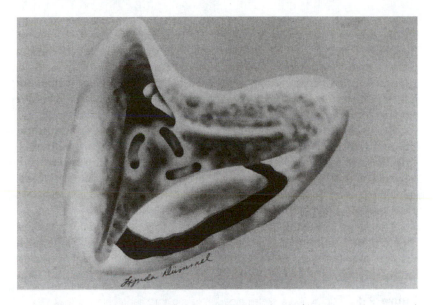

Figure 9–4. Semicircular canals opened. Bill's island of bone over the sigmoid sinus is created.

along the middle fossa plate. When these structures have been opened and removed with a diamond stone, the facial nerve is now skeletonized (Figure 9–5).

The final skeletonization of the facial nerve is performed at this point, since there is room to use the side, rather than the end, of the diamond stone. The end is slower and more dangerous, as it obscures visualization of the cutting surface. At this point, it is best to skeletonize the mastoid portion of the facial nerve around the genu and the tympanic portion of the facial nerve just past the area of the ampulla of the superior canal (see Figure 9–7). The superior and lateral canal ampullae usually lie just below the facial nerve. This portion of the dissection is important, because the facial nerve is the anterior limiting structure of this section. Adequate skeletonization allows for visualization of the vestibule and also of the lateral end of the internal auditory canal.

Now that the position of the facial nerve is established accurately, the vestibule is opened widely, and the dissection is carried more inferiorly. It is important to remember that the jugular bulb can come up into the

mastoid as high as the ampulla of the posterior canal. Therefore, when removing the ampulla of the canal or drilling anywhere inferior to the posterior semicircular canal, always be alert for the jugular bulb. In removing this area inferior to the posterior semicircular canal, the first structures encountered are the retrofacial air cells. They are removed until the top of the jugular bulb is visualized (see Figure 9–7).

Removing this area usually includes removing the vestibular aqueduct and the endolymphatic sac with a cutting burr. When the approximate location of the jugular bulb is well established, the dissection is deepened so that the bone is removed between the internal auditory canal and the posterior fossa dura. This removal completes the skeletonization of the sigmoid sinus.

The sinus overhang into the cavity now obscures vision, making work around the internal auditory canal difficult. Therefore, the bone is removed over the sinus so that it can be collapsed and retracted against the underlying dura and cerebellum. This is accomplished with a large diamond stone and liberal irrigation. Care must be taken to

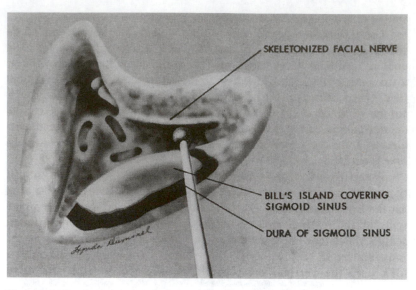

SKELETONIZED FACIAL NERVE

BILL'S ISLAND COVERING SIGMOID SINUS

DURA OF SIGMOID SINUS

Figure 9–5. Facial nerve skeletonized in its mastoid segment.

avoid a tear in the sinus. An island of bone is left over the sinus (named Bill's island by Dr. Antonio De la Cruz) to protect the surface from the trauma of retraction and the wearing of the rotating burr shank (Figures 9–5 and 9–6). Retracting the sigmoid sinus allows dissection to be carried around and into the internal auditory meatus.

The vestibule is opened more widely, and the lateral end of the internal auditory canal is identified. The first structure to look for is the superior vestibular nerve canal, keying off the ampullated end of the superior semicircular canal. It is best to dissect in this area with a diamond stone. Great caution must be exercised. If the diamond stone is brought into the vestibule, it can come up under the facial nerve as it traverses the superior lateral aspect of the vestibule, and it can damage the facial nerve (Figures 9–7 and 9–8). Therefore, the entire length of the superior vestibular nerve is outlined.

Then, the dissection is carried medially to begin outlining more of the internal auditory canal. The lateral part of the canal is exposed so that the transverse crest is visible and the superior and inferior compartments of the internal auditory canal are identified. It is important to identify the lat-

eral-most extent of the internal auditory canal at this point. Failure to remove bone here will not allow later identification of Bill's bar, the vertical crest extending superiorly from the crista falciformus. Thus, identification of the seventh nerve will be compromised somewhat. Usually, the foramen singulare, with the contained nerve to the posterior canal ampulla, is identified. When it is removed, the inferior compartment is opened well at the lateral end of the internal auditory canal.

It is now important to expose completely the posterior one-half to two-thirds of the internal auditory canal and to remove all the bone here. Accordingly, the dissection again is carried inferiorly. The inferior portion of the internal auditory canal is exposed and the jugular bulb is skeletonized carefully with a diamond stone. Dissection is carried down to the posterior fossa dura. In removing the final bone between the porus acusticus and the jugular bulb, care is taken to watch for the cochlear aqueduct. When a diamond stone is used, this aqueduct usually appears as a white spot, since the soft tissues of the duct are pushed back into the duct. If a needle is inserted in this opening, spinal fluid will gush out, unless,

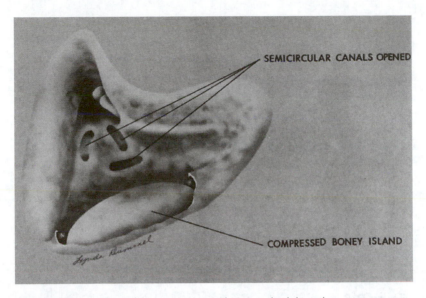

Figure 9–6. Sigmoid sinus compressed to start the labyrinthectomy.

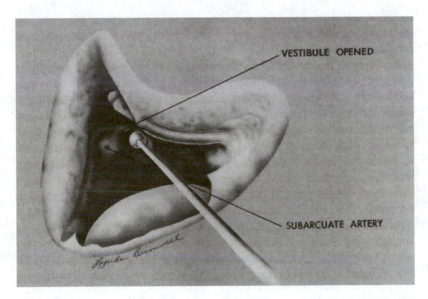

Figure 9–7. Lateral and posterior semicircular canals removed, vestibule opened, and facial nerve skeletonized in its tympanic segment.

of course, the tumor is so large that it has obliterated this duct.

Locating the exact position of the cochlear aqueduct is important, because the ninth nerve and the cochlear aqueduct exit the cranial cavity at about the same spot, the cochlear aqueduct being just slightly supe-

rior to the ninth nerve. If the dissection of bone is carried forward, the ninth nerve is injured in its canal as it comes out of the cranial cavity and proceeds across the medial and superior aspect of the jugular bulb. Inferiorly, the bone removal is complete when the jugular bulb is skeletonized, the

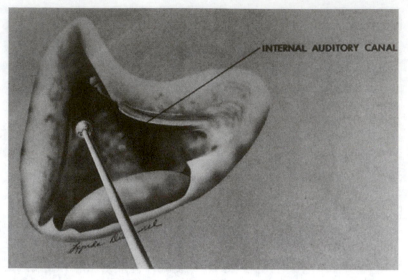

Figure 9–8. Internal auditory canal skeletonized. Note direction of rotation of burr.

cochlear aqueduct has been identified, and the inferior part of the internal auditory canal bone is removed from the porus acusticus to the lateral aspect of the canal.

A word of caution: If the jugular bulb is opened accidently with the diamond stone or burr, the bleeding must be controlled quickly with a large Surgicel (oxidized cellulose) pack. No part of the pack should extend into the lumen of the jugular bulb. If the bleeding is allowed to continue while large suctions are being mobilized and used to check the size of the hole, a pint of blood can be lost. Fortunately, with the patient lying on the table, the venous pressure is above atmospheric pressure, so air embolism is not a problem. Rapid loss of blood from a hole in the jugular bulb apparently lowers the intracranial pressure and triggers a hypotensive reaction (opposite of hypertension-elevation of intracranial pressure). Despite rapid blood replacement, the shock may continue for some time and be more profound than can be explained by the one-pint blood loss.

Assuming that the blood loss has been stopped promptly by a large pack, how then do we control the bleeding from the bulb and still have access to continue the surgery? Attempting to place small plugs of Surgicel can be hazardous, because they can loosen and disappear into the lumen of the bulb. From here, obviously, the Surgicel would proceed through the right heart and into the lung, where a serious infarction could result. To prevent this possibility, tie the jugular vein in the neck before attempting to deal with the jugular bulb tear, if the tear is significantly large.

Tying the jugular vein is accomplished by extending the postauricular incision down along the border of the sternomastoid muscle about 1.5 in. The muscle is detached partially from the mastoid tip and retracted posteriorly. The lateral process of C-1 is palpated just below the mastoid tip. The posterior border of the digastric muscle is pushed forward off of the lateral process of C-1. The jugular vein, on the anterior aspect of the lateral process of C-1, can be located at this point. Care should be taken to locate the accessory nerve, which usually runs posteriorly over C-1 or just below it. In two thirds of the cases, the nerve passes lateral to the vein; in the rest of the cases, it passes medial to the vein. By locating this nerve and carefully dissecting it off of the vein, it will not be included in the tie around the vein. Once the jugular vein has been tied, it is safe to pack a small piece of Surgicel into the opening in the jugular bulb to stop the bleeding. In one case, however, the opening became larger as attempts were made to pack into the tear. A large wad of Surgicel was placed in the jugular bulb, and the bleeding was controlled. However, swelling of the Surgicel later caused pressure on the ninth, tenth, and eleventh nerve complex (in this case, the jugular ganglion area), and the patient developed vocal cord paralysis. This complication can be avoided by using smaller amounts of Surgicel or a combination of Surgicel and Avitene (microfibrillar collagen).

Attention now is directed to the superior aspect of the internal auditory canal. The superior vestibular nerve canal already having been identified, the bone is removed superior to the internal auditory canal, and the facial nerve canal is sought. When the entrance of the facial nerve canal into the internal auditory canal is identified, a small point of bone, the landmark to the separation between the superior vestibular nerve and the facial nerve, will be found (Figures 9–9 and 9–10). This point of bone was named Bill's bar by the late Dr. Frank Ellis of Sydney, Australia. (My constant emphasis on identification of this important landmark during his dissections was the occasion for giving this piece of bone its name.) Bill's bar is the vertical crest extending superiorly from the crista falciformis, dividing the superior compartment of the lateral part of the internal auditory canal (see Figure 9–12).

Once Bill's bar has been located, the exact position of the facial nerve where it is not involved with tumor can be determined. On the rare occasion when the tumor extends along the facial canal, it is necessary to follow the facial nerve from the tympanic portion around the geniculate ganglion to identify the facial nerve at a point where it is not involved with tumor. This problem occurs only in very invasive tumors that break out into the vestibule, the inner ear and, occasionally, as far as the middle ear.

It is important now for the surgeon to adequately remove the bone between the middle fossa dura and the superior aspect of the internal auditory canal. This is a confined and difficult area in which to work because of possible damage to the facial nerve. The facial nerve lies just inside the dura of the internal auditory canal. The diamond stone must remove all of this bone straight medially from Bill's bar to the porus acusticus, thus exposing at least the posterior half of the internal auditory canal throughout its entire length from the lateral end to the porus acusticus.

At this point, it is important to control the direction of rotation of the cutting diamond stone. The sharp edge of the bone just above the internal auditory canal can catch the diamond stone and flip it directly into the internal auditory canal, injuring the facial nerve. To avoid this possibility, the burr is rotated so that the diamond fragments cut from the middle fossa dura to the internal auditory canal (Figure 9–8). This direction makes the burr tend to move toward the middle fossa dura, rather than toward the facial nerve. In a left ear, this requires clockwise rotation; in a right ear, it requires counterclockwise rotation. Exposure then is completed.

ACOUSTIC TUMOR REMOVAL

Entrance to the cerebellopontine angle through the temporal bone begins with the incision of the posterior fossa dura. The incision is designed to protect the surface of the cerebellum by keeping a flap of dura over it and to avoid opening the dura more than necessary for tumor exposure. In the event that elevated intracranial pressure occurs, the opening should allow no cerebellum to extrude into the wound. The incision is started just above the jugular bulb, carried around the porus acusticus, and extended just inferior to the superior petrosal sinus (Figure 9–10). The incision is made

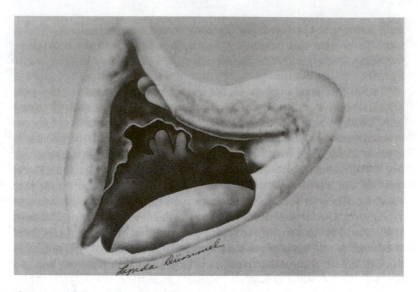

Figure 9–9. Superior and inferior vestibular nerves identified in the internal auditory canal. Note transverse crest in between.

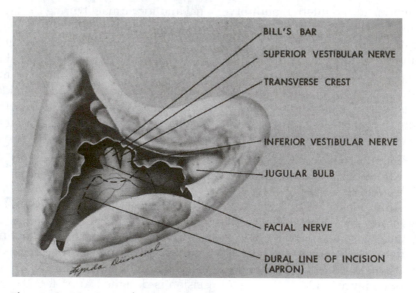

BILL'S BAR

SUPERIOR VESTIBULAR NERVE

TRANSVERSE CREST

INFERIOR VESTIBULAR NERVE

JUGULAR BULB

FACIAL NERVE

DURAL LINE OF INCISION
(APRON)

Figure 9–10. Dura of posterior fossa exposed.

with Bellucci scissors. Care must be taken to prevent the blade of the scissors from deeply penetrating the posterior fossa, which could damage the petrosal vein (vein of Dandy). This vein, providing important drainage of the cerebellar hemisphere, usually extends around the posterior aspect of the tumor and drains into the superior petrosal sinus just above the internal auditory canal. The dura usually adheres to the surface of the tumor all the way around the porus acusticus. Obviously, when opening the dura, care must be taken not to damage nerves across the surface of the tumor, such as the facial nerve, which occasionally comes up posteriorly across the superior aspect of the tumor.

It is important to delineate the posterior surface of the tumor and the junction of the tumor with the cerebellum. This is done by extending the inferior incision along the jugular bulb posteriorly along the sigmoid sinus. The superior incision, which is just inferior to the superior petrosal sinus, is extended back toward the sigmoid sinus. As the apron flap of dura is pulled backward, the posterior aspect of the tumor can be visualized (Figure 9–11). The beginning of the cerebellum which, in large tumors, is compressed, also will be visualized. Rarely is a tumor so large that it extends back posterior to the sigmoid sinus. Therefore, in most cases, this junction of cerebellum and posterior tumor can be identified simply by extending the incision far enough back.

In rare cases in which the patient has a far forward sigmoid sinus, it is advisable to liberally remove the bone behind the sigmoid sinus, especially if the CT scan has shown a large tumor with an extension back toward the sigmoid sinus. This particular point can be fairly well evaluated on the CT scan. If this combination of far forward sigmoid sinus and large tumor is encountered, it may be advisable to open the dura posterior to the sigmoid sinus. Rarely do we actually ligate the sigmoid sinus; we prefer to push it posteriorly and anteriorly and work around it. Ligation of the sinus, although not a major obstacle, does take time and, for this reason, we rarely use the transsigmoid approach today.

On the posterior aspect of the tumor is a cyst, which is a thickening of arachnoid filled with cerebrospinal fluid with an increased protein content. It is called a "herald cyst" because, in the suboccipital approach, it is the first thing observed before exposing the tumor, thus "heralding" the tumor. The reason for the existence of this cyst is not known. Apparently, however, a fold of arachnoid is closed off as the tumor grows out through the porus acusticus. The cyst is opened. The exact layer between the arachnoid and the posterior and inferior surface of the tumor is developed. If the proper plane is not established during this development, increased bleeding occurs. Because major blood vessels around the tu-

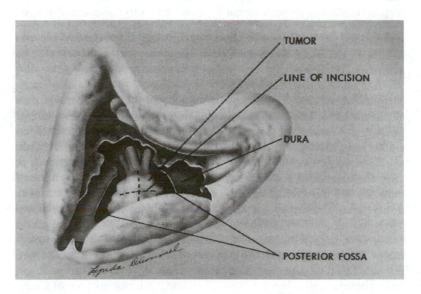

Figure 9–11. Tumor exposed by incising the dura covering the internal auditory canal and posterior fossa.

mor are outside its arachnoid sheath, proper development of the plane between the arachnoid and the surface of the tumor capsule will prevent bleeding. The apron of dura now is pushed down between the tumor surface and the surface of the cerebellum in the plane developed when the arachnoid has been stripped away from the tumor.

Let me emphasize the necessity of developing the plane between the surrounding arachnoid sheath of the tumor and the tumor capsule itself. When the tumor starts in the region of the vestibular nerve, it apparently lies within the arachnoid sheath that surrounds the entire seventh and eighth nerve bundle. The arachnoid sheath is pushed ahead and expanded as the tumor grows out into the cerebellopontine angle. As growth occurs, the anterior-inferior cerebellar artery, whose lateral branch usually loops up into the internal auditory canal, is pushed out of the internal auditory canal and usually is pushed to the inferior aspect of the tumor. The internal auditory arteries, which are branches off this vessel, are enlarged to supply the tumor and elongated over the surface of the tumor. These arteries are the only vessels that cross the plane between the arachnoid sheath and the tumor capsule. Therefore, by staying exactly in the plane between the arachnoid sheath and the capsule, one can ensure that the only vessels that need be cauterized or clipped are the smaller vessels, which sometimes can be numerous around the periphery of a tumor that extends into the cerebellopontine angle. In most cases, the small vessels can be separated off the surface of the tumor. Bipolar cautery will control bleeding from these vessels without causing retrograde thrombosis to the main lateral branch of the anterior-inferior cerebellar artery.

Careful dissection of the capsular surface has been made possible by the operating microscope. Previously, it was not possible to observe the minute details of circulation to these tumors. Therefore, the large veins around the tumor and the larger vessels surrounding the tumor usually were opened during surgery, causing considerable bleeding that further obscured the dissection. This type of bleeding prompted Cushing to call the cerebellopontine angle "the bloody angle." By virtually eliminating this massive bleeding, microsurgical techniques have made possible a controlled, systematic dissection of the tumor capsule. This has been the major factor in lowering the mortality of acoustic tumors. Only rarely with microsurgical techniques is the anterior-inferior cerebellar artery or its main branches thrombosed, cauterized, or clipped. The syndrome of the anterior-inferior cerebellar artery is discussed in Chapter 19.

In describing tumor removal through the translabyrinthine approach, we indicated that the apron of dura was pushed down between the tumor surface and the surface of the cerebellum. In close proximity to the posterior surface of the tumor is a vein that drains the cerebellar hemisphere. The vein runs across the posterior aspect of the tumor to empty into the superior petrosal sinus just above the internal auditory canal. This vein is called the petrosal vein, or the vein of Dandy. In most cases, it is possible to keep the dural flap over this vein so that it is compressed against the cerebellum and not subject to the trauma of tumor removal. This is one of the principal advantages of a U-shaped dural flap.

If the petrosal vein is damaged, clip or cauterize it. If it is torn off close to the superior petrosal sinus, pack it with Surgicel up under the tentorium. In some cases, an opening can be made in the superior petrosal sinus and the sinus can be filled with Surgicel, completely closing off the opening of the petrosal vein to control annoying bleeding. In very large tumors, the posterior lobe of the tumor may extend under the vein, making work around the vein difficult. In this case, elective clipping or cautery of the vein is preferred to isolating the vein by pushing it off the back of the tumor.

The posterior surface of the tumor now is inspected carefully. If no nerve bundles transverse it, an opening is made into the tumor, and the intracapsular removal of the tumor is begun (Figures 9–11 and 9–12). It is important to avoid excessive movement of the tumor, and it is especially important not to push the tumor forward when developing the plane around the posterior aspect of the tumor. If the tumor is pushed forward, it will further stretch the facial nerve, which could cause considerable damage to this structure. Pushing and pulling on the tumor also can lead to increased spasm of the surrounding blood vessels, particularly the anterior-inferior cerebellar artery, causing brainstem ischemia and vital sign changes.

In the intracapsular enucleation of larger tumors, we have found the Urban dissector to be of great value. It is a suction tube with an inner rotating tube that sucks the tumor into the opening of the tube, where the inner rotating cannula clips it off (Figure 9–13). The Urban dissector allows the surgeon to gut the interior of the acoustic tumor without pushing and pulling it, as would be necessary with techniques utilizing cup forceps or various types of punches. If an Urban dissector is not available, it is important to place a suction in the tumor when it is being removed with a cup forceps. The suction tip will stabilize the interior of the tumor while portions of the tumor are being removed, thus avoiding major traction.

Practice with the Urban dissector allows the surgeon to develop a "feel" for the time when the interior has been totally removed and the capsule is only a few millimeters thick. Fortunately, the Urban dissector is less effective in removing capsule than in removing the softer interior of the tumor, thus affording protection against penetrating the surface of the tumor to surrounding nerves or vessels. Obviously, care should be taken to avoid this complication. Occasionally, considerable bleeding occurs from the interior of the tumor. It can be controlled by packing or simply by further development of the capsule with progressive removal of feeder vessels coming in through the surface of the tumor.

Once the tumor is extensively gutted (Figure 9–14), selective removal and development of the tumor capsule are carried

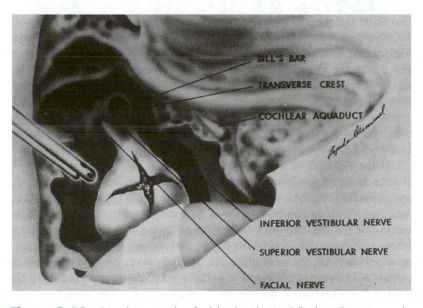

Figure 9–12. Facial nerve identified by localizing Bill's bar. Tumor capsule incised.

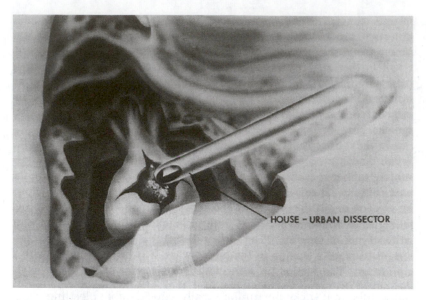

Figure 9–13. House-Urban rotating vacuum dissector starts gutting the tumor within its capsule.

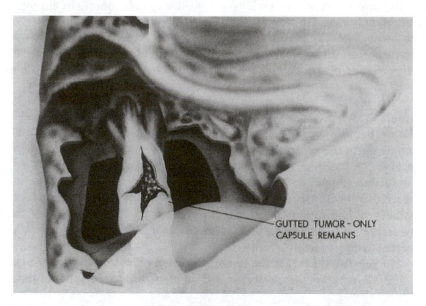

Figure 9–14. Tumor gutted. Only the capsule remains. Note the size of tumor as compared to Figure 9–12.

out, as first advocated by Dandy (1925). Development of the capsule is begun posteriorly and inferiorly. As long as work is confined to the exact plane between the arachnoid sheath and the tumor capsule, major bleeding is avoided. This dissection is facil-

itated greatly by placing small cottonoids in the plane and advancing them forward, and also by using a fenestrated suction tip, as developed by Dr. Brackmann (Figure 9–12). Use of this type of tip avoids the tumor being sucked up into the end of the suction, thus shutting it off. The tip is used to push cottonoids ahead into the tumor-arachnoid plane.

Since the tumor is extensively gutted, the capsule can be pushed into the interior space to collapse it. The surface of the capsule then is followed down to the brainstem. We try to develop the posterior aspect of the tumor to the point where it can be seen at the brainstem tumor plane. Cottonoids are placed over the surface of the cerebellum to maintain this plane, while the tumor is developed inferiorly down to the brainstem.

In developing the inferior aspect of the tumor, be alert for the ninth nerve. Since the cochlear aqueduct is a landmark of the approximate position of the ninth nerve, the surgeon knows to look for the ninth nerve in the region close to the porus acusticus. The ninth nerve fibers on larger tumors usually are stretched over the surface of the tumor, allowing development of the plane between the ninth nerve and the tumor surface.

During this development, the pulse may slow because of nerve irritation. There is a tendency to use atropine to prevent this slowing. However, we do not advocate use of this drug because it reduces one of the parameters used to measure damage from surgical trauma. We prefer to stop what is being done and wait for the pulse to return to normal.

Large vessels also appear around the inferior surface of the tumor, since the usual location of the anterior-inferior cerebellar artery is inferior and anterior to the tumor. These vessels are separated off carefully, and branches of the vessels that penetrate the tumor are cauterized bipolarly. Choroid plexus tissue seen coming out of the foramen of Luschua also can be separated off the tumor. When the posterior and inferior aspects of the capsule are developed down to the brainstem, additional capsule can be removed to reduce the overall bulk of the tumor.

An attempt now is made to develop the superior aspect of the capsule. This part of the tumor has to be approached with considerable caution because large veins—the petrosal veins and their branches extending up to the superior petrosal sinus—transverse the superior aspect. Because the facial nerve may extend over the top of the tumor, it is important not to push cottonoids blindly around the tumor in the superior aspect. However, it is advisable to develop some of this area to achieve mobility of the tumor. Once the posterior and inferior aspects of the tumor are well developed, we turn to development of the tumor in the internal auditory canal.

In general, the larger the tumor, the longer the time required to gut it and develop the posterior and inferior aspects of the capsule. However, any size tumor can be developed in the way described above. Also, maneuvers for separating the facial nerve off the tumor are the same for medium to very large tumors.

During the skeletonization and the removal of the bone on the posterior half of the internal auditory canal, a very accurate dissection of the superior vestibular nerve and the facial nerve canals is carried out, as noted previously. This dissection exactly locates the exit of the facial nerve from the internal auditory canal at a point of bone called Bill's bar (the vertical crest). Also, the transverse crest that separates the superior and inferior compartments of the lateral part of the internal auditory canal has been carefully dissected out, so that the lateral inferior part of the canal is widely opened. The operating table is rolled away from the surgeon slightly, so that the lateral aspect of the internal auditory canal comes into view. With use of a hook to push the dura of the internal auditory canal away, Bill's bar again is identified. The hook then is inserted into the superior vestibular nerve canal to pull the total superior vestibular nerve out of its canal. Without wide opening of the vestibule and proper skeletonization of the facial nerve above it, the lateral extent of the internal auditory canal may not be well visualized. Thus, Bill's bar will be difficult to identify. At Bill's bar, the surface of the facial nerve comes into view (Figure 9–15).

Again I emphasize that this procedure for identifying the facial nerve is the same

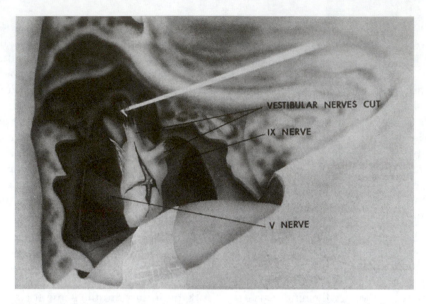

Figure 9–15. Superior and inferior vestibular nerves cut above level of transverse crest. Note the ninth nerve and fifth nerve in the posterior fossa.

for tumors of all sizes. One of the principal advantages of the translabyrinthine approach is that it permits this positive, consistent means of exact identification of the facial nerve.

All of the superior vestibular nerve fibers are removed completely to identify the exact surface of the facial nerve. The dura of the internal auditory canal is the structure that narrows down to surround the facial nerve and become its epineurium. Therefore, the dura of the internal auditory canal must be reflected away from the facial nerve to visualize accurately the surface of the facial nerve where it exits the internal auditory canal. The arachnoid sheath completely surrounds the tumor and encompasses the facial nerve as well as the cochlear nerve, since the tumor started inside the arachnoid sheath that surrounds the seventh and eighth nerve bundle. Separating the facial nerve off the surface of the tumor requires separating the arachnoid sheath along the length of the facial nerve (Figures 9–16 and 9–17). For this reason, the plane between the facial nerve and the tumor must be developed, and the edges of the facial nerve

must be identified accurately on its superior and inferior aspects. The arachnoid sheath is divided as the tumor is removed from the internal auditory canal.

The tumor must be mobilized at the lateral part of the internal auditory canal so that the tumor can be pushed posteriorly toward the surgeon. This push brings the exact plane between the facial nerve and the acoustic tumor into view. As soon as a few millimeters of the facial nerve have been developed at the lateral end of the internal auditory canal, the portion of the tumor in the lateral part of the internal auditory canal is developed carefully. To avoid tumor remnants in the lateral portion of the internal auditory canal, all tumor is swept out of the inferior compartment below the transverse crest. Check for smooth surface of the tumor at this point to ensure total removal.

Removal of the tumor from the inferior part of the canal also can include the removal of cochlear nerve, if it is very thin. In every case, it includes the inferior vestibular nerve. In some cases, a plane is developed between the tumor and the cochlear nerve. This plane gives further protection

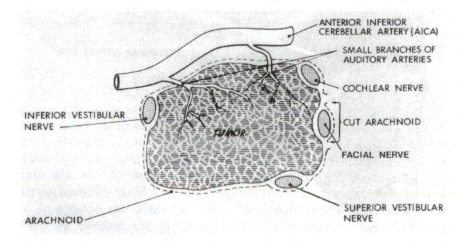

Figure 9–16. Schematic illustration showing the relationship of the tumor capsule to the anterior-inferior cerebellar artery, vestibular nerve, facial nerve, and surrounding arachnoid sheath. Arrows indicate where the arachnoid sheath is cut to separate the tumor capsule from facial nerve.

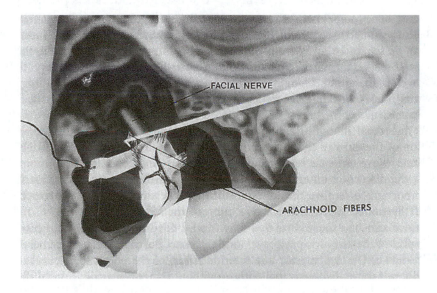

Figure 9–17. Tumor capsule separated from facial nerve by careful cutting of arachnoid sheath.

against the surgeon's penetrating the anterior-inferior cerebellar arteries on the inferior and anterior aspect of the tumor. How

ever, there usually is a tongue of tumor that extends up between the facial nerve and the cochlear nerve. This entire section of tumor must be removed totally, and the plane along the inferior part of the facial nerve must be developed carefully.

At this point, the arachnoid is dissected, allowing the tumor to be pulled posteriorly away from the facial nerve (Figure 9–17). The portion of the tumor in the internal auditory canal now is pulled toward the surgeon. The plane between the facial nerve, especially the arachnoid sheath along the edges of the facial nerve, is divided so that the facial nerve can be separated away from the tumor. It is important not to stretch the facial nerve during these maneuvers. Usually, it is relatively easy to develop the plane along the facial nerve within the internal auditory canal, but considerable difficulty arises when the porus acusticus is reached.

Around the entire circumference of the porus acusticus is an adhesion of the dura to the surface of the tumor, as noted earlier. This adhesion, whose presence remains unexplained, is found consistently. As soon as the dissection along the facial nerve reaches the porus acusticus, it is important to remove the adhesions of the dura along the superior aspect of the tumor. Since the exact location of the facial nerve is known, removal can be executed safely. This is why development of the superior aspect of the tumor is postponed until the exact position of the facial nerve is known. On the anterior and inferior aspect of the porus acusticus, the adhesions also are separated with or without the cochlear division of the nerve. A blunt instrument, such as a Rosen dissector, is used to avoid damage to the anterior-inferior cerebellar artery, which may loop up into the internal auditory canal between the seventh and eighth nerves. If a hook or other instrument is pushed out into the cerebellopontine angle, this artery, which usually is lying on the anterior surface of the cochlear nerve close to the tumor, can be damaged. Therefore, the tumor is pushed carefully toward the surgeon, and the adhesions inferior to the facial nerve are divided carefully. The surgeon must watch constantly for the anterior-infe-

rior cerebellar artery to avoid damaging it.

Once all the adhesions at the porus acusticus are divided, the tumor becomes mobile. Then, it is possible to continue to follow the plane along the facial nerve, but it is at the same time easy to push the tumor forward, stretching the facial nerve. Therefore, avoid excess pushing of the tumor until the facial nerve is completely separated away, and the tumor is retracted away from facial nerve.

After the facial nerve leaves the internal auditory canal and progresses over the surface of the tumor down toward the brainstem, it is spread over the surface of the tumor, because it is not surrounded by an epineurium in the cerebellopontine angle. This spread, of course, makes it difficult to dissect the thinned-out nerve off the tumor. To eliminate or minimize damage to the facial nerve, the tumor is pushed posteriorly toward the surgeon, the plane between the facial nerve and tumor capsule is continually developed, and the arachnoid sheath, which extends on each side of the facial nerve onto the surface of the tumor, is severed. If the arachnoid sheath is thick, the facial nerve simply can be left on the arachnoid sheath so that the plane between the facial nerve and tumor and between the arachnoid sheath and tumor can be developed adequately.

One of the principal problems at this point is staying in the exact plane between the facial nerve and the surface of the tumor. Once tumor substance is entered, which is easy to do, it is difficult to return to the proper plane. Remaining in the proper plane demands wide experience or observation of experienced surgeons making this maneuver. Although the facial nerve may wind anterior to the tumor or go over the top of the tumor, it tends to go over the anterior aspect of the tumor more than over the very superior aspect of the tumor. One can avoid damaging the facial nerve by following it.

One problem encountered is the presence of small blood vessels that run in the substance of the facial nerve and branch out onto the surface of the tumor. Forming a barrier, these vessels make a dissection difficult when the plane between the facial nerve and the surface of the tumor is followed. Sometimes, a sharp hook must be used to dissect the small vessels, producing bleeding that, of course, further obscures the development of the planes. In rare cases, bipolar cautery is necessary along the facial nerve, but it is to be avoided if possible.

The facial nerve plane then leads down to the brainstem. The facial nerve is compressed into the surface of the brainstem by the expanding tumor. The fifth nerve also is encountered over the top at the brainstem tumor junction. In most cases, development of the plane between the fifth nerve and the superior aspect of the tumor is easy. By the time the fifth nerve is encountered, the brainstem tumor plane is the major focus of the dissection.

Once the facial nerve has been developed down to the brainstem, it is important to remove the major bulk of tumor, leaving only a small portion of the tumor attached to the brainstem. This allows greater visibility of the development of the brainstem tumor plane, a critical part in the removal of the tumor. In rare cases, the anterior-inferior cerebellar artery will be trapped in this plane between tumor and brainstem. In many cases, a number of large veins along this plane seem to be trapped between the brainstem and the tumor. Large tumors that distort and indent the brainstem make development of this plane difficult, if major adhesions occur. Fortunately, adhesions between brainstem and tumor capsule usually are not dense, permitting removal of the tumor without major damage to the surface of the brainstem.

The facial nerve plane is followed down along the brainstem, and the tumor is separated superior to inferior. Once the facial nerve is cleared completely, the inferior aspect of the tumor may be elevated (Figure 9–18). Blood vessels, usually veins, attached firmly to the tumor capsule are dissected away. If the veins are large and difficult to control with bipolar cautery, they are clipped. Obviously, any artery of significant size that does not actually penetrate the tumor should be carefully separated off the tumor to avoid thrombosis and the necessity of clipping. Finally, with careful maneuvering and elevation of the tumor off the brainstem, a total removal can be accomplished in almost every case.

Once the tumor is removed totally, bleeding must be controlled. It is obviously essential to control all bleeding before the cerebellopontine angle is closed. The wound is irrigated liberally with Ringer's solution, which brings into view small oozing vessels. They can be controlled by bipolar cautery. When cottonoids are removed, a large vessel that was controlled by the pressure of the cottonoid sometimes is encountered. A large vessel usually is a venous bleeder that can be controlled by packing with Surgicel, by clipping, or by bipolar cautery. Ample time should be taken to ensure good control of bleeding and to ensure that as many clots as possible have been washed out of the cerebellopontine angle. Then, closure can be accomplished.

A word of caution about Surgicel. If this oxidized cellulose is used to pack venous bleeding, only small pieces must be left in the cerebellopontine angle. This material tends to expand due to absorption of fluid. Its size usually doubles in the hours following surgery. Large amounts of Surgicel in the wound obviously can cause pressure on surrounding vessels, consequent brainstem ischemia, or even thrombosis. In the future, it is hoped that better materials to control venous bleeding will be developed.

We use fat from the abdomen to close the cerebellopontine angle. No attempt is made to suture the dura. Fat is placed in the opening in the cerebellopontine angle posterior fossa dura. Some fat is placed in the vestibule of the inner ear and in the middle ear attic above the incus and malleus. The remaining cavity is filled with a fat plug up to the surface of the cortex of the temporal bone.

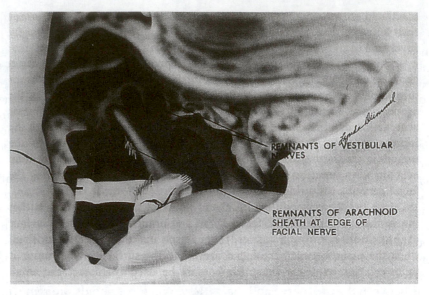

Figure 9–18. Tumor capsule carefully separated from facial nerve.

The postauricular incision now is closed with subcuticular gut sutures, and the abdominal incision is closed. The patient is allowed to react on the table and is transferred directly to the intensive care unit.

CONCLUSIONS

In this chapter, we have provided an overall view of the technical details of acoustic tumor removal through the translabyrinthine approach. Fortunately, most of the techniques involving the temporal bone itself can be learned by dissecting temporal bones in the laboratory. The tumor removal and the dissection of the facial nerve, however, must be learned at the operating table. It has been our experience that observation of a number of acoustic tumor procedures gives a good basis for the young surgeon to proceed with tumor removal. This observation should be in the operating room.

We feel that surgeons interested in acoustic tumor surgery should be capable of performing the procedure from beginning to end, regardless of their particular background. For the neurosurgeon, additional training in the translabyrinthine approaches through the temporal bone is necessary. The otologist will require additional training in the cerebellopontine angle removal of the acoustic tumor. If the operating team, ideally composed of a neurosurgeon and an otologist, is well versed in all phases of the procedure, one member can relieve the other in order to avoid fatigue during long procedures. In this way, the team accomplishes the best possible result for the patient.

ACKNOWLEDGMENTS

The illustrations are by Reda Ibrahim, M.D., Research Fellow, Ear Research Institute, and Lynda Dümmel, Medical Illustrator.

REFERENCE

Dandy, W. E. (1925). An operation for total removal of cerebellopontine (acoustic) tumors. *Surgery, Gynecology, and Obstetrics, 41,* 129.

CHAPTER 10

A Neurosurgical Perspective on the Translabyrinthine Approach

C. Keith Whittaker, M.D.

This chapter will expound on what I consider to be important points of the translabyrinthine approach, and will proceed chronologically from prior to the start of the operation to its completion.

Bill House reported excising his 1,000th acoustic tumor at the time (1977) of the publication of the two-volume predecessor of this book. Now, the House Ear Clinic has over 3,500 such cases. Bill, in his direct way, said, "Drilling can be learned in the temporal bone lab, but tumor removal and handling of the facial nerve must be learned in the operating room." I agree. Although I seldom do the drilling any more, I feel competent to drill out the facial nerve in the temporal bone, expose the internal auditory canal, or plug the Eustachian tube by opening the facial recess. This confidence fulfills the House dictum, namely, that the otologist and the neurosurgeon should be co-surgeons, each capable of doing the entire operation. Likewise, I have no hesitancy in turning over the soft tissue dissection near

the brainstem to the otologist who is working with me, if I have grown tired. (My impression is that fatigue can be detected by a certain hesitancy, that is, a tendency to dawdle and not progress steadily or to pick at the tissue. When I note this in myself, I know it is time to change operators. I tend to watch the clock and become suspicious of myself after 2–3 hours.)

The neurosurgeon should participate in the pretreatment planning. The first decision is whether to simply observe the tumor or treat it. Many tumors may be watched safely for a time. Neurofibromatosis type 2, with bilateral acoustic tumors, often demands observation of the second tumor if hearing is still present (see Chapter 20). The second decision, after the decision for treatment, is whether to use surgery or stereotaxic radiation, which is gaining in popularity and apparent success (see Chapter 21). If surgery is the choice for treatment, I always advise translabyrinthine surgery unless hearing preservation is to be attempted, in which case I have come to believe that the middle fossa approach is preferable to the posterior fossa approach (retrosigmoid, transmeatal, etc.). I do not like the retrosigmoid operation, because it leaves tumor behind in the lateral aspect of the internal auditory canal, and it puts the facial nerve in greater jeopardy—in my hands.

Intravenous antibiotics, usually a penicillinase-resistant penicillin, are given before the incision is made. For all but small tumors, autologous blood is prepared for possible transfusion or, rarely, for use as fibrin glue. I like to give steroids for 48 hours before surgery and for a short time afterward, because I think it helps facial nerve integrity.

Positioning can be important. I do not like too much soft padding under the patient's head, because the up-and-down motion of the head can throw the tissue of interest into and out of the plane of focus of the microscope. Earlier, we had some loss of hair from the scalp, presumably from pressure ischemia on the down side. Now, we avoid this hair loss by using a sheepskin under the head. The common bulky plastic sponge for the head is too unstable for me. If the Greenberg retractor is needed, I like to make sure it is solidly attached to the skull by using the Mayfield head holder with skull pins. This can interfere with access and mobility a bit, but if the temporal lobe is to be lifted rostrally or the cerebellum and sigmoid pulled backwards, the Greenberg, or a similar retractor, is very helpful and attaches to the Mayfield head rest securely. In neurosurgery, nothing is worse than a brain retractor cutting the brain when it or the brain moves and the other does not. Generally, we do not use skeletal fixation of the head for routine translabyrinthine exposure. We elevate the patient's legs about 6 inches on a wedge-like cushion and use elastic hose. We use an electromyographic-style monitor of facial nerve/muscle with double needle electrodes in the orbicularis oris and oculi. We have not monitored cranial nerves V, IX, X, XI, or XII.

I have learned to let the family in the waiting room know when the preparations are complete and the operation has begun to prevent them from thinking the operation is going faster than it actually is. Likewise, about every hour, a short message is sent from the operating room to the family; nothing has met with more appreciation than this one courtesy.

Extreme temperatures in the operating room, especially when the room is too cold, can hasten the fatigue of the surgeon. The surgeon's comfort is essential. The chair we use has a backrest and is able to be raised or lowered by simple rotation on a screw in its base. I am uncomfortable only when I am attempting to pull forward a far posterior pole of a large acoustic tumor. Then, even with the head rotated more "nose-up," the tumor may retreat behind the line of vision that one can achieve by looking from in front of the sigmoid sinus. This can be an awkward problem. I have solved this by lowering the table as far as possible and, if that is not enough, I then place the table in Trendelenberg (head-down) position; this position may be hard on my knees, but it is necessary. I like to pull this posterior capsule forward and gut the posterior tumor until I have worked forward to the choroid plexus or the eighth nerve. If this is done, the table can then be taken out of Trendelenberg and, from that point onward, the surgeon's comfort again rules. I have not encountered any serious venous bleeding by dropping the head into Trendelenberg position.

Sloppiness about residual oozing of blood from drilled bone surfaces is not good. Finishing off the drilling with a polishing diamond burr completes the job and avoids contamination of the working area by blood running in from ragged raw bone.

We routinely expose the Eustachian orifice by way of the facial recess and always plug it with tissue, usually temporal fascia and muscle. After 6 months or so, the middle ear becomes re-aerated, and delayed CSF leak has not occurred at all.

I have learned never to cut the capsule of the tumor without exploring the area with a stimulating electrode probe. On the posterior capsule, the facial nerve practically is never seen, except in meningiomas. However, superiorly, the facial nerve can be lurking just in front of a vein or two of the petrosal vein of Dandy, surprisingly rostral and near the trigeminal nerve. Now, I like to divide the vein of Dandy cautiously early on and use the electrode to explore in front of this vein for about 5–10 mm, searching for the facial nerve.

We usually obtain a frozen section on a biopsy of the tumor after an incision into the posterior capsule. (This biopsy is largely a waste of money; we should stop this practice on economic grounds.) Then, we use the House-Urban rotary dissector to gut the tumor, saving the capsule until last. We have used an ultrasonic aspirator and a carbon dioxide laser, but we have returned to the simplicity of the House-Urban, the setup time for which is negligible. Unfortunately, this beloved instrument is no longer manufactured.

When the remaining tumor is judged to be small and mobile, or when I am afraid to continue gutting because of a thin capsule or squawking facial nerve monitor, I proceed to the work in the canal. I know I sometimes go to the canal too soon, but I prefer to see the facial nerve, usually positioned forward, and safely remove the tumor posteriorly, rather than proceed blindly too far and injure the facial nerve.

Seeing the facial nerve in the lateral end of the canal at Bill's bar is essential. Do not leave little filaments of the superior vestibular nerve attached and intact next to the facial nerve here; the temptation is great to do so and to stay slightly away from the facial nerve, but this later can lead to mistakes, as the nerves wind around each other as they traverse medially. Thus, keep both sides of the intact facial nerve clean. Do not cauterize vessels in the canal on the facial nerve. Instead, use Avitene or just leave them

alone to bleed a little. Experience with middle fossa or suboccipital attempts to save hearing have shown me that cautery can be avoided in the internal auditory canal; cautery is very hazardous to the cochlear nerve and probably also to the facial nerve. I always do this dissection—and almost any really delicate dissection—with running irrigating solution (pH adjusted to about 7.2–7.4) and the finest, smallest Brackmann suction-irrigator. I like high magnification. The water adds to the magnification and keeps even the tiniest amount of blood washed away for good vision. (I have adopted this same technique for dissecting out aneurysms, a spin-off of neurotology that I appreciate.) The tumor is almost always firm and solid in the canal and usually comes away from the facial nerve easily. I like to sweep everything, including the arachnoid but not the dura, away from the facial nerve, working from lateral to medial. Some "anastomotic" fibers between the facial and vestibular nerves may need to be cut. I seldom recognize the nervus intermedius as a separate bundle in the internal auditory canal.

Fisch's angle is treacherous, where the facial nerve angulates sharply forward against the petrous bone's posterior face, especially in large tumors. Do not push cottonoids blindly over the superior surface of the tumor. At this point, searching with the stimulating electrode probe also is a good idea. Having the most thorough drilling away of the anterior superior lip of the internal auditory canal will be much appreciated at this time; sometimes, additional drilling can be done after the tumor is removed from the canal and porus in order to see the facial nerve anteriorly. This is still the area in the translabyrinthine dissection where the surgeon gets stuck most often. Millimeters of additional exposure make a big difference here. Sometimes, I will go to the brainstem, divide the eighth nerve, find the facial nerve at the brainstem, and trace it distally, so as to meet my dissection anteriorly, where I became stuck. This may help. While it is possible to stay patiently in the correct plane between tumor and nerve, and gradually roll the tumor backward away from the facial nerve, even when it is out of sight and straight ahead of the surgeon, I have come to prefer an attack that is slightly from the side of the nerve. It is precisely here where early taking down and dividing the petrosal vein of Dandy may give just exactly that amount of sideways movement of the tumor to allow a visual inspection of one side of the facial nerve as it goes forward along the petrous face and encircles the remaining anterior tumor. If, as usually happens, the side of the facial nerve can be seen, it can be dissected free. Once the anterior pole of the tumor is free, the surgeon can be a little more forceful in retracting the tumor, but not the facial nerve, posteriorly. The capsule of the tumor should not be cut near the line of surgical attention as the tumor is pulled away from the facial nerve or the brainstem; this capsule's integrity can be preserved often by placing a flat, cottonoid patty over the tumor surface and retracting on the cottonoid. Soon, the facial nerve is seen to go deep to the pia-arachnoid, just in front of its root exit zone. However, this root exit zone can have a vessel here alongside the facial nerve or between the facial and the cochleovestibular nerve right at the brainstem. Special care must continue until only the eighth nerve remains as the last stalk of the tumor. Doing vestibular nerve sections for Ménière's disease familiarizes the surgeon with the microanatomy of the eighth cranial nerve's root exit area.

Otologists may not know what neurosurgeons do about cottonoids. Cottonoids can be used for suctioning onto delicate tissue and blotting or tamponading bleeders, but I also use them liberally as markers of where I have been. For example, if I leave the superior aspect of the tumor near the trigeminal nerve to work on the inferior side, near the jugular bulb, I place cottonoids on the exposed brainstem as far as I have dissected near the trigeminal nerve; when blood clot

fills the area, and I must return, it is comforting to be able to remove the cottonoids and recognize the former site of dissection. Cottonoids should always have strings; if the string is accidentally cut off a cottonoid while dissecting, the cottonoid should immediately be searched out and removed.

I have come to wonder if, as some tumors grow, the vein of Dandy somehow tethers the facial nerve close to the tentorium, keeping the facial nerve in proximity to the trigeminal nerve. The vein may crease the tumor, carrying the facial nerve into a crevice within the tumor, which itself may grow outward to surround the nerve and vein. If the nerve is not accompanied by a vessel, it is much less likely to be in the situation. Facial function should be assessed as early as possible, either in the operating room or the recovery room. Of course the John House/Brackmann classification scale should be used.

We routinely use both abdominal fascia (as the deeper layer) and abdominal fat for closure of these wounds. Our rate of cerebrospinal fluid (CSF) leak is low, but not zero.

When CSF leak occurs in the first week, and if the leak is in the wound, suturing the wound usually suffices. If rhinorrhea is the problem, we now try a lumbar catheter for CSF drainage; formerly, we were inclined to repack the wound with fresh fat. I am convinced that CSF leak can be present but undetected and undetectable. I believe that various reported incidence rates of postoperative CSF leaks must be taken as minimal estimates, with broad ranges of possible error.

In my experience, a headache is much more likely to occur following suboccipital operations, and subsequent cranioplasty has not provided a cure. Middle fossa operations have minor postoperative problems, but the translabyrinthine method has the fewest problems of all the methods of dealing with tumors in the cerebellopontine angle and environs.

Large tumors (30–55 mm in diameter) definitely are treated best by the translabyrinthine exposure, perhaps enlarged by a transcochlear addition or even the addition of a middle fossa craniotomy with division of the tentorium and backward retraction of the cerebellum with the tentorium. Petroclival meningiomas and chordomas especially are nicely exposed in this latter manner.

Retrolabyrinthine vestibular nerve section is a wonderful operation because, besides curing the patient with Ménière's syndrome of vertigo, it teaches the neurosurgeon the normal anatomy of the cerebellopontine angle. After 80 vestibular nerve sections and 300 translabyrinthine tumor removals, I continue to be impressed with the value of this translabyrinthine collaborative technique. Direct facial-to-facial neuroanastomosis has always been accomplished when needed at the same sitting, thanks to the full exposure of the facial nerve provided by the translabyrinthine exposure. Meningiomas that grow into the internal auditory canal probably cannot be removed completely with certainty except with the translabyrinthine exposure. I have not clipped aneurysms or performed microvascular decompressions with this technique, because hearing loss is too big a price to ask the patient to pay.

In summary, in my experience, handling the facial nerve in the cerebellopontine angle is most happily done with the translabyrinthine approach.

CHAPTER 11

Middle Fossa Approach

Charles A. Syms, III, M.D.
Derald E. Brackmann, M.D., F.A.C.S.

HISTORY

The middle fossa approach, although popularized by Dr. William House (1961) over three decades ago, was first described by Hartley (1892) as an approach for the surgical treatment of trigeminal neuralgia. In the middle of this century, this approach was used for the treatment of petrous apicitis, prior to the availability of antibiotics. At various times, this approach has been used for sectioning the vestibular and cochlear nerves (Parry, 1904), sectioning the greater superficial petrosal nerve in an attempt to relieve unilateral headaches (Gardner, Stowell, & Putlinger, 1947), fenestration of the superior semicircular canal to destroy vestibular function, and for facial nerve decompression and grafting (Parisier, 1977).

House (1961) presented his Triologic thesis on the middle fossa approach to the internal auditory canal, and it was nothing short of revolutionary. The principles of skull-base surgery that are now taken for granted were introduced, such as the use of the operating microscope, continuous suction-irrigation, diamond stone drill bits, an intimate knowledge of the anatomy of the temporal bone, and, most importantly, the team approach, combining the separate skills of the neurotologist and the neurosurgeon. In subsequent publications (House, Gardner, & Hughes, 1968; House & Luetje, 1979), he refined and popularized a systematic approach to patients with acoustic tumors, and this chapter provides an update of that approach.

PATIENT SELECTION

The middle fossa approach is suited best for patients with good hearing and a small acoustic tumor that extends no more than 1 cm into the cerebellopontine angle. This generally limits the tumor's greatest dimension to less than 2 cm. More important than absolute size, however, is the position of the tumor. If the bulk of the tumor is situated medially and does not extend into the internal auditory canal, we prefer the retrosigmoid approach. In our experience, however, this is an uncommon constellation of circumstances.

There are several major advantages that the middle fossa approach has over the retrosigmoid approach. The middle fossa approach is entirely extradural until the tumor is removed, thereby limiting the exposure time of the brain and contamination of the cisterns with bone dust. Acoustic tumors commonly extend to the fundus of the internal auditory canal, and removal of tumor in this region can be accomplished under direct vision with the middle fossa approach, ensuring total tumor removal. The lateral aspect of the internal auditory canal is hidden from view with the retrosigmoid approach, and tumor removal from this area must be accomplished either blindly or with the aid of endoscopes. Perhaps the most important advantage is that the middle fossa approach allows identification of the facial nerve distal to the tumor. Identification of Bill's Bar establishes a plane among the superior vestibular nerve, the tumor, and the facial nerve. The extension of this facial-tumor interface facilitates removal of the tumor and preservation of the facial nerve (Brackmann, Hitselberger, Beneke, & House, 1985).

We do not use any strict criteria for offering the middle fossa approach for acoustic tumor removal. We look at the favorable and unfavorable data from the patient's preoperative assessment and, once the potential outcomes are understood, the patient chooses on the basis of his or her own risk benefit analysis. Favorable characteristics for successful hearing preservation include a smaller tumor (especially <1.5 cm in greatest dimension), a pure-tone average better than 50 dB HL and speech discrimination scores better than 50%, normal auditory brainstem response (ABR) findings or preservation of normal waveform morphology with only a slightly prolonged latency, and absent or reduced vestibular responses on caloric testing. Tumors arising from the superior vestibular nerve will have less tendency to involve the cochlear nerve. Superior nerve tumors usually will displace the facial nerve anteriorly, and there is a relationship between a reduced vestibular response on caloric testing and tumors arising from the superior aspect of the internal auditory canal. Tumors arising from the inferior compartment need to be removed from underneath the facial nerve and, not infrequently, involve the cochlear nerve or its blood supply.

There are no consistent, reliable predictors of hearing preservation. For those individuals in whom sound localization was important, we have preserved hearing that, for binaural input, was poor before surgery. We also have preserved hearing in patients with inferior vestibular nerve tumors and grossly abnormal ABRs. The most reliable predictors for saving useful hearing are the size and location of the tumor. Patients with small tumors situated in the medial aspect of the superior internal auditory canal have the best chance for hearing preservation.

We prefer that patients undergoing middle fossa craniotomy be less than 65 years of age, as the dura is thinner and more adherent in patients older than this. This is not a strict guideline, and we have performed middle fossa craniotomies in older patients. We do, however, discourage this option in older patients, because these anatomic changes add risk to the procedure.

PREOPERATIVE EVALUATION

Once the diagnosis of acoustic neuroma is made, the evaluation is completed, if it was not part of the assessment prior to the magnetic resonance imaging (MRI) with gadolinium. We obtain ABR and electronystagmography (ENG) data, and a complete general physical examination is conducted by the internist who will be assisting in the postoperative care of the patient. Diagnostic laboratory tests and chest radiographs are obtained on the basis of coexisting disease, the patient's history, and age. We encourage autologous blood donation with an adequate time interval before surgery. In our experience, the blood loss from the middle fossa approach consistently is greater than with the translabyrinthine approach. Although homologous transfusion is infrequently necessary, it is enough of a risk that it is preferable to have the patient's own blood available prior to surgery.

Counseling for the patient with a small tumor and relatively good hearing should address the issue of hearing conservation. Based on results of our most recent series (Brackmann, House, & Hitselberger, 1994), we inform the patient that we can preserve hearing at or near preoperative levels in two thirds of patients and that, additionally, one patient in eight retains some residual hearing. The patient also is informed that there is a one in six chance of losing all hearing. With regard to the facial nerve, patients are told that they have a greater than 90% chance of eventually having normal or near normal facial nerve function, and that less than 50% of patients have a temporary weakness or paralysis that develops after surgery. The patient is told that facial nerve function immediately after surgery is the best predictor of the eventual facial nerve outcome. Many patients ask about the influence of surgery on tinnitus. They are told that, in all likelihood, it will improve but will not go away. Patients who do not have tinnitus before surgery are counseled that they stand a 25% chance of developing it after the operation. The other possible complications, such as meningitis, cerebrospinal fluid leak, central nervous system problems, and even death are reviewed with the patient. Patients frequently ask about the risk of tumor recurrence. They are told that, in the House Ear Clinic's (formerly the Otologic Medical Group) series, there has been not a single recurrence in patients who have undergone the middle fossa approach, which is used only in patients with small acoustic tumors. The average postoperative course is reviewed so that the patient knows what to expect. In particular, the ENG is examined, and the patient with no reduction of caloric response is warned of the possibility of significant postoperative dizziness.

SURGICAL APPROACH

Preoperative Preparation

The patient always is shaved in the preoperative holding area while awake, offering reassurance that the preparation is on the correct side. The shave encompasses a postauricular area that extends 6 cm from the external ear canal to nearly the vertex. Plastic adhesive drapes, acting as a barrier to the residual hair-bearing scalp, are applied prior to moving the patient to the operating suite.

Except for the induction period, general endotracheal anesthesia is used, avoiding muscle relaxation agents. Thus, accurate facial nerve monitoring is insured, and the monitoring electrodes are applied immediately after intubation is accomplished. Insert earphones and recording electrodes then are placed for far-field ABR recording. Placement of an eighth nerve recording electrode within the internal auditory canal is done after bone removal. The pinna, external auditory canal, and insert earphones then are covered with adhesive drapes. To avoid both the surgical wound and the course of the greater auricular nerve (availing a nerve graft donor site), careful arrangement of the line delivering the auditory input is necessary. Patient positioning and operating room setup (see Figure 11–1) is different from other neurotologic procedures. No external head fixation devices are necessary. We routinely administer preoperative mannitol and furosemide to enhance brain relaxation, reducing the amount of temporal lobe retraction that is necessary. Decadron is given routinely as a single preoperative dose and is continued postoperatively if the tumor is very adherent to the nerves in the internal auditory canal or if excessive brain retraction is required. We now routinely employ the use of a single dose of preoperative antibiotics, since a meta analysis of the topic demonstrated its efficacy even when the surgeon's infection rate is low (Barker, 1994). A routine Betadine scrub then is performed.

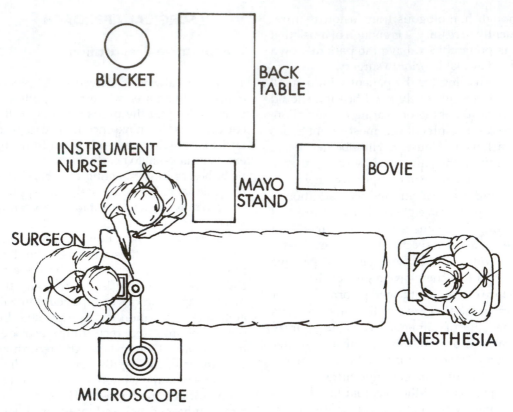

Figure 11–1. The operating room arrangement. The surgeon is seated at the head of the table.

Technique

The surgical technique of the middle fossa approach can be divided into six steps, each of which will be addressed separately.

Soft Tissue

The incision starts in the patient's hairline, the inferior aspect of which is just anterior to the junction of the root of the helix and the tragal cartilage. This area is approximated roughly by a line that crosses a plane between the lateral canthus and the external auditory canal. Our current incision forms an open question mark (see Figure 11–2), rather than the previously used vertical incision. Branches of the superficial temporal vessels usually are encountered in the soft tissue under the vertical part of the question mark. The artery and vein are ligated separately with silk sutures to avoid

the late complication of subcutaneous hematoma formation. The temporalis muscle then is incised to form an inferiorly based flap with an upside down J-shaped incision. A cuff of muscle and periosteum is left along the insertion of the muscle into the squamous portion of the temporal bone to facilitate closure. Elevation then is accomplished, with a Lempert or Langenbeck periosteal elevator, in a superior to inferior direction until the muscle passes inferior to the zygomatic arch. The muscle then is held in place with stay sutures and, if necessary, a self-retaining retractor.

Extracranial Bone Dissection

The craniotomy then is fashioned with a high-speed drill and a 4-mm cutting burr. The bone flap is approximately 5.5 cm (anterior-posterior) by 5.0 cm (inferior-superior), located two-thirds anterior to and one-

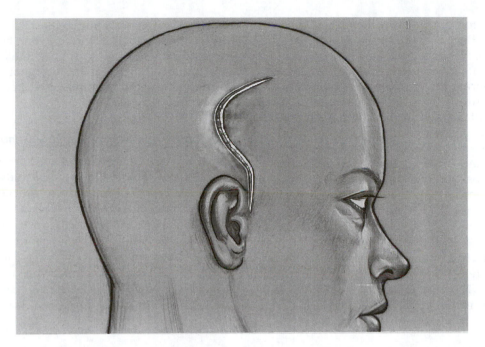

Figure 11–2. Our current procedure utilizes a longer, curved incision, rather than the previous vertical incision.

third posterior to the external auditory canal. The inferior aspect of the craniotomy must be flush to the floor of the middle cranial fossa, which usually necessitates retraction of the muscle by an assistant. Care must be taken to avoid lacerating the dura, since temporal lobe herniation can occur subsequently through the defect. The squamous temporal bone, is thinner at its inferior aspect than at the squamo-parietal suture. Skeletonizing the bone, so that the dura and vessels are visible through the residual bone, is the best way to preserve dural integrity and yet allow for easy removal of the bone flap. The dura is separated from the bone flap with a "joker" (Adson periosteal) elevator. The bone is marked, sharp edges removed, and passed off to the scrub nurse for storage in normal saline prior to replacement at the conclusion of the procedure.

Dural Elevation and Exposure of Landmarks

The dura is separated from the bone edges, and bleeding is controlled with bone wax and oxidized cellulose (Surgicel) packing. If the inferior aspect of the craniotomy is not flush with the floor of the middle cranial fossa, the intervening bone is removed with a drill, with a cutting burr, or a rongeur. The dura then is elevated from the floor of the middle cranial fossa with either the joker or House narrow elevator, until the middle meningeal artery is identified. The House-Urban middle fossa retractor is positioned and locked in place along the margins of the craniotomy. The blade of the retractor is inserted, and elevation along the floor of the middle cranial fossa is continued. At its exit from the foramen spinosum, the middle meningeal artery marks the anterior limit of dissection. If its identification is in doubt, it can be confirmed by exposing the gasserian ganglion. Venous bleeding from the foramen is not uncommon and can be controlled with Surgicel packing. It is important then to start dissecting from a posterior-to-anterior direction, while moving progressively medial. Elevation of the greater superficial petrosal nerve would be possible, if the dissection was done in an anterior-to-posterior direction. Damage to the facial nerve could ensue and, in the worst case, the geniculate ganglion itself could be elevated, because it is devoid of any bone covering in approximately 5–15% of cases. Additionally, it is not uncommon to encounter a dehiscent carotid artery, and the surgeon must be cognizant of the critical anatomy of this region. The posterior petrous ridge is identified, and the superior petrosal sinus is elevated carefully out of its semicanal. The blade of the House-Urban retractor then is placed medial to the true petrous ridge, centered over the plane of a line extended from the external auditory canal (see Figure 11–3). Proper placement of the retractor avoids excessive brain retraction. The arcuate eminence usually is easily identifiable at this point. It is important to

spend the time obtaining hemostasis from any definite vessels at this juncture, before proceeding with the exposure of the internal auditory canal. It is best to ignore diffuse oozing from multiple sites, because this will stop on its own.

Exposure of the Internal Auditory Canal

There are three methods that have been described to identify the internal auditory canal. Dr. House first described the route to the internal auditory canal by following the greater superficial petrosal nerve to the geniculate ganglion and, hence, to the labyrinthine segment of the facial nerve (House, 1961). We still use this method when we approach pathology of the facial nerve that requires a middle fossa approach. Dr. Ugo

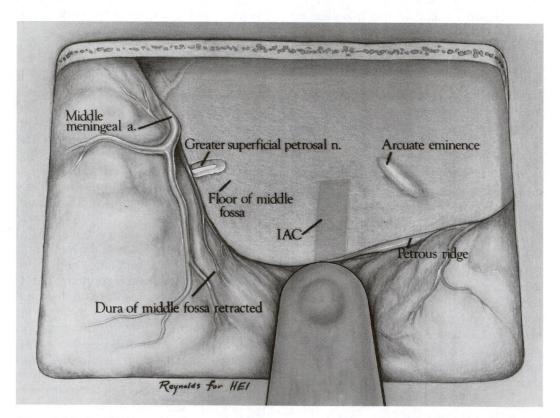

Figure 11–3. The internal auditory canal (IAC) is visualized using the technique of Garcia-Ibánez. The angle formed by the greater superficial petrosal nerve and the arcuate eminence is bisected to give the location at its medial aspect. Drilling is started medially in this safe area.

Fisch next described a process by which the internal auditory canal is identified by removing bone from the arcuate eminence until the superior semicircular canal is "blue-lined." The internal auditory canal is located at a 60° angle to the superior canal ampulla (Fisch, 1970). We presently use the method popularized by Garcia-Ibánez and Garcia-Ibánez (1980). They described the internal auditory canal as being located at the bisection of an angle formed by the greater superficial petrosal nerve and the arcuate eminence. The bone removal commences at the most medial aspect of the petrous ridge in the plane of this angle and proceeds from a medial-to-lateral direction. Therefore, this dissection proceeds from the safest to the most critical area. The bone removal is 270° at the porus and narrows to

only 90° at the fundus in order to avoid inadvertent entry into the cochlea or ampulla of the superior semicircular canal (see Figure 11–4). This additional bone removal was advocated by Wigand (Wigand, Haid, Berg, Schuster, & Goertzen, 1991), and allows for easier tumor removal. The entire labyrinthine segment of the facial nerve is decompressed to allow for swelling that may occur following surgery. This completes the bone removal and exposure of the internal auditory canal (see Figures 11–5a and 11–5b). The direct-nerve monitoring electrode, consisting of a Teflon-coated silver wire that is uncoated for its final 1–2 mm and an attached cotton wick, then is placed extradurally in the anterior-inferior aspect of the internal auditory canal. This enables direct eighth nerve or near-field ABR recordings to check the

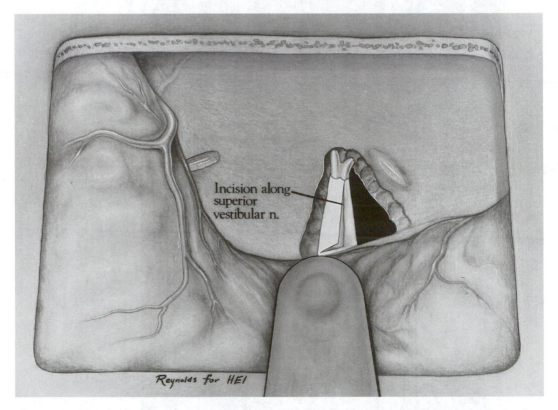

Incision along superior vestibular n.

Reynolds for HEI

Figure 11–4. The exposure at the porus acousticus is 270°. After completing the bone work, the dura is incised posteriorly and reflected anteriorly.

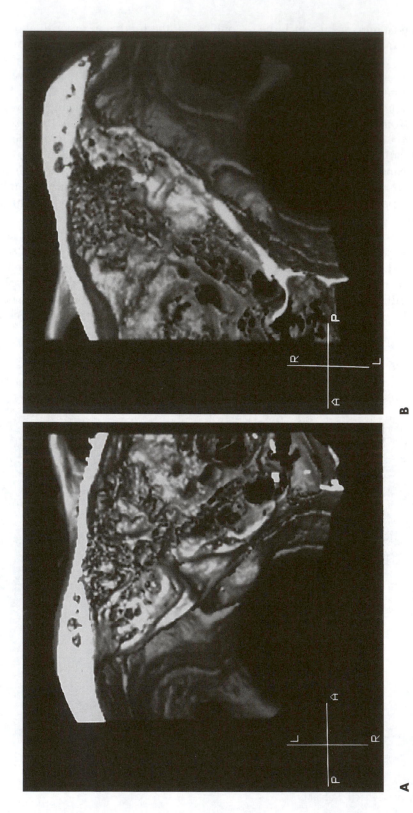

A

B

Figure 11–5. A. Three dimensional computerized tomography reconstruction, demonstrating the bone removal in a patient who had undergone a left middle fossa approach. The bone removal is 270° at the porus and 90° at the fundus. **B.** Three dimensional computerized tomography reconstruction, demonstrating the normal right temporal bone in the same patient, for comparison.

status of the cochlear nerve and cochlea, either on a real-time basis or with a delay of less than 5 seconds.

Tumor Removal

The main objectives in acoustic tumor surgery are to remove all of the tumor and preserve facial nerve function. The dura of the internal auditory canal is incised along the posterior aspect and reflected anteriorly (see Figure 11–4). The facial nerve is dissected free from the tumor starting at Bill's bar, using sharp dissection. It is sometimes helpful to use high power (40×) magnification to ensure preservation and accurate separation of the facial nerve. Prior to tumor dissection from the contents of the internal auditory canal, intracapsular debulk-

ing is accomplished, if necessary. Removing the tumor is always accomplished in a medial-to-lateral direction (see Figure 11–6). When dissecting on the medial aspect of the tumor, the anterior-inferior cerebellar artery is identified carefully and dissected free from the tumor to avoid posterior fossa hemorrhage. The cochlear nerve divides into many different fibers as it enters the modiolus and is vulnerable to avulsion or damage in this area. In addition, it would be possible to injure the delicate branches of the labyrinthine artery with a lateral-to-medial dissection. If the tumor arises from the superior vestibular nerve, we now leave the inferior vestibular nerve intact in order to preserve the blood supply. With this preserved function, there is the jeopardy of an uncompensated vestibulopathy. In a previ-

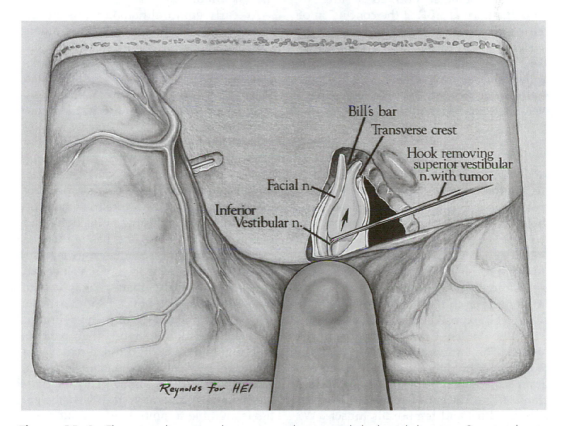

Figure 11–6. The tumor dissection always proceeds in a medial-to-lateral direction. Care is taken to avoid any medial traction of the nerves in the area of the fundus.

ous series, a patient required a complete nerve section, because the inferior nerve was preserved. This is an acceptable risk, since we believe this modification has enhanced our rate of hearing preservation (Brackmann, House, & Hitselberger, 1994). Any changes in the direct eighth nerve recordings prompt us to cease tumor dissection and traction immediately. If there is not prompt return of the action potential, we apply papaverine to the eighth nerve. Because this additional maneuver causes prompt return of the action potential, we believe that, the majority of the time, the trauma of dissection is inducing vasospasm. After the tumor is completely removed, we customarily place papaverine-soaked Gelfoam on the eighth nerve. Final direct nerve recordings and facial nerve stimulation are performed at this point, and meticulous hemostasis is obtained prior to closure. Although a normal ABR at the conclusion of the procedure is favorably predictive of postoperative hearing, the reverse is not. We have seen patients with an absent ABR at the conclusion of surgery who had normal hearing during audiometric testing 6 weeks after the operation.

Closure

Abdominal fat is harvested by an assistant during the bone or tumor removal. Minimal electrocautery is used so that facial nerve monitoring can continue uninterrupted. The free graft of abdominal fat is much smaller than that necessary to close a translabyrinthine approach, as the bone removal is correspondingly less. After adequate closure of the internal auditory canal with fat, and sealing all exposed cell tracts with bone wax, the House-Urban retractor is removed. The temporal lobe will promptly re-expand to hold the fat in place. A Penrose drain is placed along the floor of the middle cranial fossa. The bone flap then is replaced, held by dura and temporalis muscle. We purposely do not fix the bone flap with wires or miniplates. The wound is closed in a layered fashion, and a sterile pressure dressing is applied.

POSTOPERATIVE COURSE

The patient is monitored in the intensive care unit for 24 to 48 hours after the procedure. The facial nerve grade is checked when the patient is following commands. Prior to this state of arousal, nasal flaring, if observed, is indicative of good facial nerve function. The abdominal wall and craniotomy wound drains are removed on the first postoperative day, along with the nasogastric tube and the Foley catheter. The morning after surgery, the patient is almost always out of bed, sitting in a chair. Early ambulation is encouraged, depending on the amount of dizziness.

An early epidural hematoma is an uncommon and life threatening complication. Patients with deteriorating neurologic status, in whom signs of increased intracranial pressure are present, should be suspected of having this complication. The treatment includes opening the wound in the intensive care unit in order to release the increased intracranial pressure. This maneuver is accomplished prior to any imaging, as delay may result in permanent sequelae. We believe that rigid fixation simply prolongs the time required to release the pressure from the epidural collection, and nonunion of the bone flap has not been a problem. Temporal lobe injury always is a concern in these patients. We have not had any patients with hemiparesis or aphasia in our series. We have noticed some patients who, for the first several days after surgery, appear to be more lethargic than patients who undergo translabyrinthine removal of their tumors. It is the rare patient, however, who is not ready for discharge by the fifth-to-seventh postoperative day. Usually, patients are able to ambulate without assistance by this time and have only minimal unsteadiness. Patients may get their wounds wet by the seventh postoperative day. On discharge from the hospital, patients are instructed to take their temperature four times a day and call if it is greater than 101°F on two consecutive readings. They also are informed of the signs of a cerebrospinal fluid leak and instructed to avoid heavy lifting, straining, and vigorous activity for 1 month. When dizziness has resolved, and the patient can turn the head quickly without any disorientation, driving may be resumed. Most patients are back to work 6 weeks after the operation, providing their occupation is not balance-dependent.

RESULTS

Since the introduction of magnetic resonance imaging with paramagnetic contrast, the percentage of tumors presenting for removal at the House Ear Clinic in the small size group has increased considerably. As a consequence of better detection of smaller tumors, a higher percentage of our acoustic neuroma operations have been accomplished by the middle fossa approach. Increased experience and technical modifications have resulted in improved facial nerve and hearing results. For tumors 1.5 cm or smaller, the latest series revealed no difference in facial nerve function between the middle fossa and translabyrinthine approaches (Arriaga, Luxford, & Berliner, 1994). Ninety-six percent of patients had normal or near normal (House-Brackmann Grade I or II) facial nerve function (Arriaga, Luxford, & Berliner, 1994). During 1992, a series of 24 consecutive patients yielded 17 patients (71%) with hearing preserved at near-preoperative levels, 3 patients (12%) with some measurable hearing, and 4 patients (16%) without any measurable hearing. On the basis of these results, we believe that the middle fossa approach is the best method for removing small acoustic tumors if attempting to conserve hearing.

ACKNOWLEDGMENTS

The authors would like to thank Dr. Karen I. Berliner, Ms. Stacy Dorcas, and Ms. Liz Gnerre for their assistance in the preparation of this manuscript, Dr. William Lo for the postoperative imaging, and Mr. Butch Welch for his preparation of the figures.

REFERENCES

Arriaga, M.A., Luxford, W.M., & Berliner, K.I. (1994). Facial nerve function following middle fossa and translabyrinthine acoustic tumor surgery: A comparison. *American Journal of Otology, 15*, 620–624.

Barker F.G. (1994). Efficacy of prophylactic antibiotics for craniotomy. *Neurosurgery, 35*, 484–492.

Brackmann, D.E., Hitselberger, W.E., Beneke, J.E., & House, W.F. (1985). Acoustic neuromas: Middle fossa and translabyrinthine removal. In R.W. Rand (Ed.), *Microsurgery* (pp. 311–334). St Louis: C.V. Mosby.

Brackmann, D.E., House, J.R. III, & Hitselberger, W.E. (1994). Technical modifications to the middle fossa craniotomy approach in removal of acoustic neuromas. *American Journal of Otology, 15*, 614–619.

Fisch, U. (1970). Transtemporal surgery of the internal auditory canal: Report of 92 cases, technique indications, and results. *Advances in Otorhinolaryngology, 17*, 203–240.

Garcia-Ibánez, E. Garcia-Ibánez, J.L. (1980). Middle fossa vestibular neurectomy: A report of 373 cases. *Archives of Otolaryngology—Head and Neck Surgery, 88*, 486–490.

Gardner, W.J., Stowell, A., & Putlinger, R. (1947). Resection of the greater superficial petrosal nerve in the treatment of unilateral headaches. *Journal of Neurosurgery, 4*, 105–114.

Hartley, F. (1892). Intracranial neurectomy of the second and third divisions of the fifth nerve. A new method. *New York Medical Journal, 55*, 317–319.

House, W.F. (1961). Surgical exposure of the internal auditory canal and its contents through the middle, cranial fossa. *Laryngoscope, 71*, 1363–1385.

House, W.F., Gardner, G., & Hughes, R.L. (1968). Middle cranial fossa approach to acoustic tumor surgery. *Archives of Otolaryngology—Head and Neck Surgery, 88*, 631–641.

House, W.F., & Luetje, C.M. (Eds.). (1979). *Acoustic tumors: Management* (Vol. 2). Baltimore: University Park Press.

Parisier, S.C. (1977). The middle cranial fossa approach to the internal auditory canal—An anatomical study stressing critical distances between surgical landmarks. *Laryngoscope, 87*(Suppl. 4), 1–20.

Parry, R.H. (1904). A case of tinnitus and vertigo treated by division of the auditory nerve. *Journal of Laryngology, Rhinology, and Otology, 19*, 402–406.

Wigand, M.E., Haid, T., Berg, M., Schuster, B., & Goertzen, W. (1991). Extended middle cranial fossa approach for acoustic neuroma surgery. *Skull Base Surgery, 1*, 183–187.

CHAPTER 12

Suboccipital Approach

Michael E. Glasscock, III, M.D.
Pamela S. Bohrer, M.D.

The history chapters in this book follow the development of the suboccipital approach for removal of cerebellopontine angle (CPA) lesions. They describe its evolution from a wide, bilateral exposure to the unilateral craniotomy that it is today. These chapters also address the political controversy that has surrounded cerebellopontine angle surgery, and the polarity between neurosurgery and neurotology regarding the most appropriate method for addressing this region. The following paragraphs will discuss tailoring of the surgical plan and identify the characteristics that are most appropriately addressed via the suboccipital technique.

There are several advantages to the suboccipital approach. First, it may be used for any size lesion, from a tiny intracanalicular tumor to huge tumors greater than 4 cm. Although many neurotologists would choose the middle fossa approach for intracanalicular tumors, or the translabyrinthine approach for lesions greater than 2 cm (Jackler & Pitts, 1992), it cannot be denied that it is feasible to address any size tumor via the suboccipital exposure. This is the philosophy of the majority of neurosurgeons

who choose this technique for all acoustic neuromas (Ojemann & Martuza, 1990).

Another advantage is the excellent exposure seen from the suboccipital viewpoint with smaller tumors (Rhoton, 1993). It provides a panoramic view of the posterior fossa. After decompression of cerebrospinal fluid (CSF) and lysis of arachnoid adhesions, the cerebellum falls posteriorly, widely exposing the cerebellopontine angle. In the early days of acoustic neuroma surgery, partial resection of the cerebellum was used to increase exposure. The advent of the operating microscope has allowed excellent visualization without cerebellar excision in most cases. The line of sight extends along the cerebellum and brainstem, anteriorly toward the clivus. If tumor bulk does not obstruct the view, cranial nerves IV through XII may be identified, and the posterior fossa vasculature is well seen.

A third advantage of the suboccipital method is the possibility of hearing conservation. Preservation of hearing also is possible by the middle fossa route, but the labyrinth is destroyed intentionally with the translabyrinthine and transcochlear approaches.

One of the primary disadvantages of sub-occipital surgery is the occurrence of post-operative headaches. These occur in a large percentage of patients and can be very debilitating. Multiple modalities are used to treat the so-called "suboccipital headaches," but these headaches may be recalcitrant and severe. In addition, the surgical exposure is not particularly well suited to address far anterior extensions of cerebellopontine angle tumors that reach toward the clivus. As an alternative, the transcochlear approach allows more direct access to the anterior skull base.

HEARING PRESERVATION

The suboccipital technique is an excellent choice when an attempt to preserve hearing is desired. Three criteria are suggested for patients to be selected for hearing preservation via the suboccipital approach. They are good preoperative hearing, tumor size smaller than 1.5 cm, and a tumor placed medially in the internal auditory canal (Josey, Glasscock, & Jackson, 1988).

First, the patient should have serviceable hearing preoperatively. The determination of "serviceable" hearing depends on both the patient and the surgeon. Most neurotologists would like to see a pure tone average better than 30–50 dB HL and speech discrimination better than 30–50%, but these general guidelines must be modified to fit the situation. Particularly, with poor speech discrimination, patients with a normal contralateral ear do not benefit from hearing conservation. Even with hearing aid augmentation of pure tone thresholds, speech understanding is poor, and they do not have functional improvement. Some patients state that, even though they can hear sounds in the affected ear, the sounds are distorted and annoying. The distortion is caused as the tumor compresses and stretches the cochlear nerve. It may be more comfortable to have a deaf ear, rather than an ear that causes severe sound distortion.

The second criterion for hearing preservation surgery is tumor size less than 1.5 cm. Although successful hearing preservation has been reported for tumors as large as 3 cm, surgeons generally agree that this is an unusual occurrence. Even with tumors less than 1.5 cm, the overall success rate for hearing preservation is only 35% in most hands.

Third, the anatomic configuration of the tumor is important. Hearing is more likely to be conserved when the tumor is located medially in the internal auditory canal (Figure 12–1). A laterally placed tumor (Figure 12–2) is more challenging to dissect from the cranial nerves, and more trauma is sustained where the nerves insert into the labyrinth. A medially located lesion is easier to remove while maintaining neural continuity.

Other indicators predict potentially successful hearing preservation surgery, including good waveform morphology on the preoperative auditory brainstem response (ABR) and a reduced caloric response on electronystagmography (ENG). The ABR is useful on two accounts. In addition to the correlation between good preoperative ABR waveform morphology and successful hearing preservation, the ABR tracing also serves as a baseline for intraoperative monitoring of auditory function. During surgery, the ABR may be followed, and deterioration of the waveform alerts the surgeon that the cochlear nerve is sustaining damage. This allows modification of the surgical technique, as appropriate.

The ENG also is useful as a preoperative indicator in predicting hearing preservation. In this case, "bad is good"; that is, a reduced caloric response in the affected ear correlates with successful maintenance of hearing. Figure 12–3 shows the configuration of the seventh and eighth cranial nerves in the internal auditory canal as they enter the bony labyrinth. A typical acoustic neuroma will emanate from either the superior or inferior branch of the vestibular nerve. A poor caloric response is indicative of a malfunction of the horizontal semicircular canal, suggesting a tumor of the *supe-*

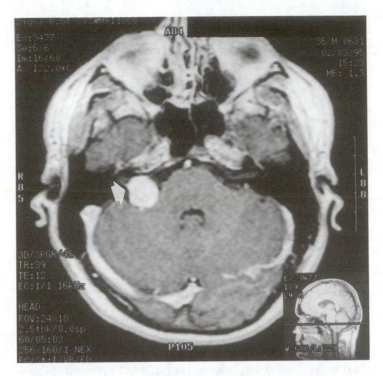

Figure 12–1. Tumor in the medial internal auditory canal (*arrow*).

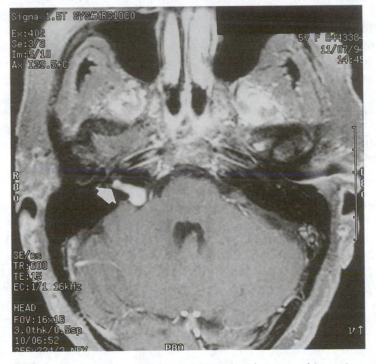

Figure 12–2. Tumor in the lateral internal auditory canal (*arrow*).

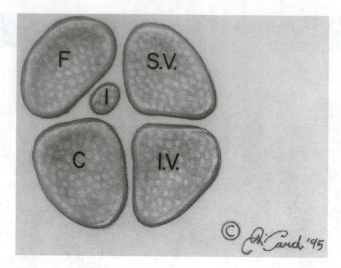

Figure 12–3. The configuration of the internal auditory meatus, right ear, showing the superior vestibular (SV), facial (F), inferior vestibular (IV), and cochlear (C) nerves.

rior vestibular nerve. Since the superior vestibular nerve is located at the furthest possible location from the cochlear nerve, it is less likely to cause compression and damage of the cochlear nerve and, thus, hearing may be more likely to be preserved.

No single testing modality can tell the surgeon whether or not hearing conservation attempts, in particular, the suboccipital approach, are appropriate for a given patient. The available information must be integrated, and the options should be discussed thoroughly with the patient to determine the optimal treatment plan.

SURGICAL TECHNIQUE

The first step in suboccipital surgery pertains to patient positioning. The "park bench," or three-quarters lateral position (Figure 12–4), allows excellent access to the occipital area, with minimal neck torsion. The standard otologic position of supine with the head to the side also may be used, but it is difficult to achieve sufficient neck rotation to allow the appropriate viewing angle of the posterior fossa. The head is placed in the Mayfield headrest with pinions to assure a secure placement and to allow the surgeon to be seated close to the operative site. Several key procedures must be undertaken during positioning. First, the patient must be strapped securely to the operating table to prevent slippage. This allows the bed to be rolled toward and away from the surgeon, optimizing the angle of exposure. Second, the patient must be padded properly to prevent pressure damage to the skin and nerves. Third, the neck should be maintained in a straight line with the spine. Finally, the shoulder on the operative side may be depressed gently with taping to increase access to the occiput, but too much pull may result in brachial plexus injury.

The second step in the suboccipital approach is monitoring. Both facial nerve and ABR monitors are applied and secured. When the nerve can be exposed properly, some surgeons use direct monitoring via an electrode placed on the cochlear nerve.

Next, the operative site is prepared by shaving the surrounding hair and injecting with 2% xylocaine with 1:100,000 epineph-

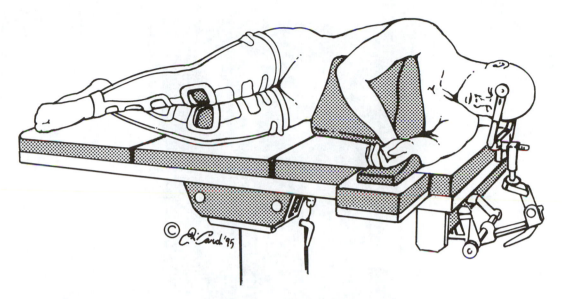

Figure 12–4. The park bench position.

rine (for hemostasis). The site then is scrubbed with sterile solution, and surgical drapes are applied. The ear canal is cleaned and inspected with the operating microscope, and the ABR stimulus probe is inserted. An occlusive dressing is placed over the external auditory canal to prevent fluid from interfering with the ABR probe. Mannitol is administered intravenously (1–2 gm/kg) to encourage cerebellar decompression.

Surgery itself begins with an inverted hockey stick incision three-to-four finger breadths behind the postauricular crease (Figure 12–5). This is carried down through the subcutaneous tissues, and the edges are undermined approximately 1.5 cm. A stair step incision then is made 1 cm anterior to the skin incision, through the muscle and periosteum, down to the skull. The anteriorly based, postauricular flap is elevated forward and held in position with self-retaining retractors.

The remainder of the work is performed with the assistance of the operating microscope. The craniotomy (using the craniotome) or craniectomy (using burrs and suction-irrigation) then is performed, removing bone

to the level of the dura. The limits of the bony dissection (Figure 12–6) extend to uncover the posterior edge of the sigmoid sinus (anteriorly) and the inferior edge of the transverse sinus (superiorly); additionally they extend around the curve of the skull base to allow easy access to the cisterna magna (inferiorly), as well as 4–5 cm in the anterior-posterior dimension.

When bone removal is complete, the dura is incised in an inverted "T" shape, with a curved inferior limb and the base of the "T" at the junction of the sigmoid and transverse sinus (Figure 12–7). The CSF is decompressed via the cisterna magna and cerebellopontine angle cistern. Arachnoid adhesions are lysed. As the cerebellum falls posteriorly, it is covered by a protective pad, then lightly retracted. The cochleovestibular/facial nerve complex is visualized, with the tumor at the porus acousticus (Figure 12–8). The trigeminal nerve is seen superiorly, and the glossopharyngeal/vagus/accessory nerve complex is seen inferiorly.

The next step is removal of the bone over the internal auditory canal (Figure 12–9). First, the dura on the posterior face of the

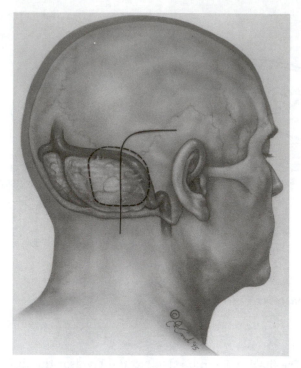

Figure 12–5. The incision for the suboccipital approach.

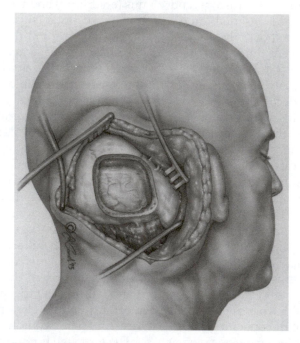

Figure 12–6. The craniotomy, showing the sigmoid sinus (SS), with mastoid air cells (AC) anteriorly and the transverse sinus superiorly (TS).

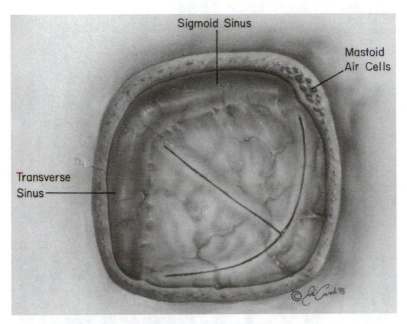

Figure 12–7. The dural incision.

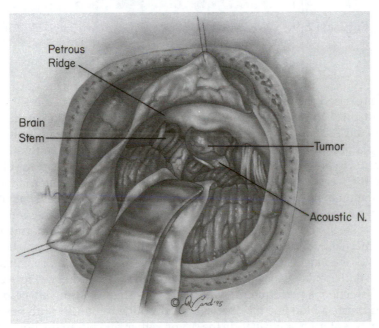

Figure 12–8. Exposure of the cerebellopontine angle, showing the petrous ridge (PR), tumor (T), brainstem (BS), and cochleovestibular nerve complex (N).

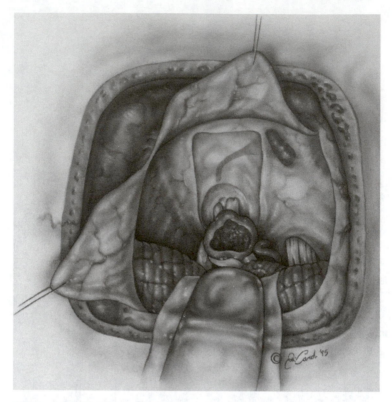

Figure 12–9. Dissection of the internal auditory canal, showing the inverted "J" of the endolymphatic duct (ED).

petrous ridge is excised, then small diamond burrs are used until the internal auditory canal is uncovered 180° from superior to inferior. It is important to use continuous suction and irrigation to prevent bone dust from collecting in the cerebellopontine angle. There is speculation that this bone dust may be the inciting source of suboccipital headaches. During dissection of the most lateral extent of the internal auditory canal, care is taken not to enter the inner ear, in particular, the posterior semicircular canal and vestibule. If the dissection is performed slowly with diamond burrs, a blue line may be visualized prior to entering the canal. If the labyrinth is breached, total sensorineural hearing loss is the likely result. Dissection following the "inverted J" shape of the endolymphatic duct will help prevent entry into the posterior semicircular canal.

The CT scan is useful to assess the anatomic configuration of the internal auditory canal, which may limit the ability of the surgeon to remove the tumor and successfully maintain hearing (Blevins & Jackler, 1994). In a long internal auditory canal with very lateral extension of tumor, it is more difficult to obtain complete exposure of the tumor without entering the labyrinth. In addition, if defects in the bone surrounding the internal auditory canal are encountered during surgery (Figures 12–10 and 12–11), the CT scan can help the surgeon determine if the labyrinth has been entered or, rather, air cells in the bone. This can help guide the continued exposure.

The dura covering the canal is removed, and the nerves are identified as they enter the labyrinth. At this juncture, it is important to visualize the most lateral extent of

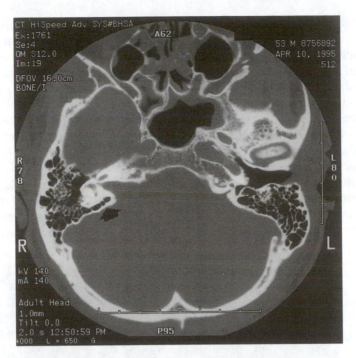

Figure 12–10. The pneumatized posterior petrous apex around the internal auditory canal (*arrow*).

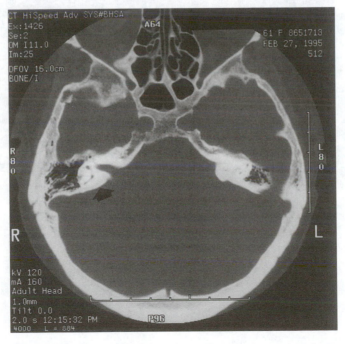

Figure 12–11. Solid bone surrounding the internal auditory canal (*arrow*).

the tumor so that complete tumor excision is assured.

During the subsequent dissection, the facial and cochlear nerves are monitored and preserved. The superior vestibular and facial nerves are identified at Bill's bar (Figure 12–12). The superior vestibular nerve is removed from its lateral attachment and retracted medially. The superior vestibular nerve and tumor then are freed from the facial and cochlear nerves as dissection proceeds in a lateral-to-medial direction.

If the tumor is large, its contents are debulked, while the capsule is left intact. At the discretion of the surgeon, debulking may be performed by a variety of methods, including cold steel and bipolar cautery, the ultrasonic aspirator, and the laser. Careful dissection lifts the tumor capsule off the brainstem and preserves all essential vascular structures. Tumor removal proceeds from medial to lateral at the brainstem, and from lateral to medial in the internal auditory canal. Eventually, the facial and cochlear nerves are identified both proximal and distal to the tumor, and the final dissection separates the tumor from them. The vestibular nerve is transected at the brainstem (Figure 12–13).

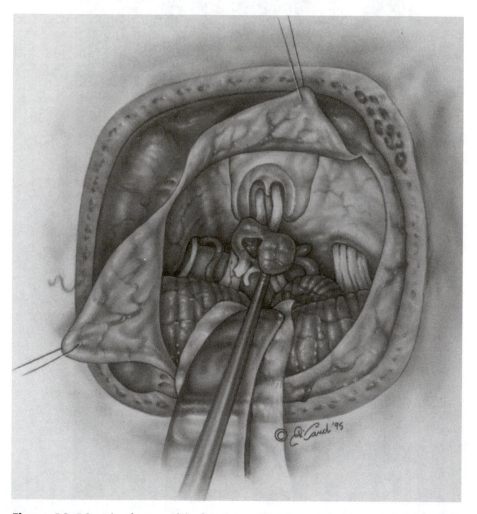

Figure 12–12. Identification of the facial nerve (FN) in the lateral internal auditory canal. The superior vestibular (SV) nerve has been retracted. The tumor (T) has been debulked.

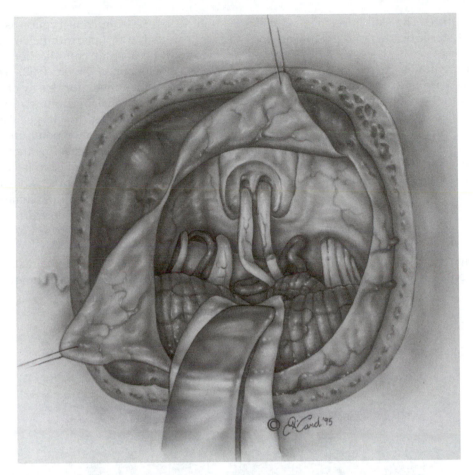

Figure 12–13. After tumor removal, showing the facial (F), cochlear (C), and trigeminal (T) nerves and the glossopharyngeal/vagus/accessory nerve complex (X).

In order to preserve hearing and facial function, care is taken in hemostasis. Use of cautery is minimized, because it can cause irreversible neural damage. Instead, Gelfoam®, Surgicel®, Avitene®, or other hemostatic agents are used to control bleeding.

The goals of acoustic neuroma surgery include total tumor excision and preservation of facial function. With the suboccipital approach, hearing conservation is attempted if there is serviceable hearing preoperatively. In difficult cases, microscopic tumor capsule may be left on the facial nerve in order to preserve function. However, when attempting to save hearing, subtotal exci-

sion with tumor left on the cochlear nerve is not an acceptable outcome.

After tumor removal is completed, the integrity of the facial and cochlear nerves is tested and recorded. Hemostasis is secured. Bone wax is used to seal completely any air cells that have been exposed around the internal auditory canal or sigmoid sinus. This prevents a cerebrospinal fluid leak through the middle ear and eustachian tube. The dura is closed in a watertight fashion with interrupted silk sutures. If a bone flap was retained, it is replaced and stabilized. The muscle and subcutaneous layers then are closed watertight with interrupted absorbable suture. The skin is secured with staples. A sterile headwrap is left in place for 4 to 6 days.

Postoperative care is provided in the intensive care unit, and the patient is transferred to the neurosurgical floor after 24 to 48 hr. There are several issues that should receive particular postoperative attention, including neurological status, vital signs, and eye care with facial paralysis. Further discussion may be found in Section V.

DISCUSSION

In our series, the suboccipital approach is used only for attempts at hearing conserva-

tion. When hearing conservation is not a surgical goal, translabyrinthine surgery is preferred, because its complication rate is lower (Brackmann & Green, 1992). The facial nerve is identified more easily and preserved via the translabyrinthine route, especially when addressing larger tumors. From the suboccipital viewpoint, the facial nerve is on the far surface of the tumor and is difficult to reach if the lesion is large. In contrast, the translabyrinthine exposure allows direct access to the intracanalicular segment of the nerve and more direct visualization of the anterior surface of the tumor (Figure 12–14).

It is somewhat difficult to compare complication rates for these two techniques, be-

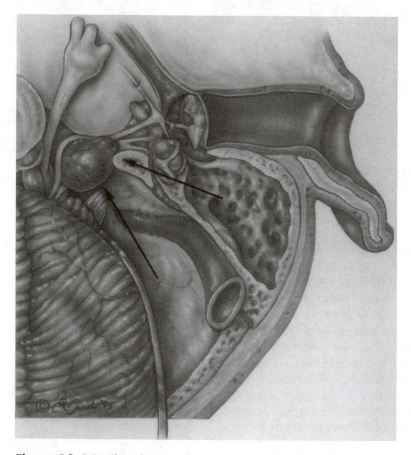

Figure 12–14. The suboccipital (SO) and translabyrinthine (TL) viewpoints of the acoustic neuroma (AN) and facial nerve (FN).

cause the suboccipital approach is used for small and medium size tumors, while the translabyrinthine approach is used for all tumor sizes (and has a much higher incidence of large tumors) (Table 12–1). Since the rate of complications (e.g., cerebrospinal fluid leak) increases as tumor size increases (Table 12–2), one would expect that the rate of complications would be higher for the translabyrinthine series than for the suboccipital series. In fact, our complication rates for translabyrinthine and suboccipital cases are similar (Table 12–3). Since the translabyrinthine series contains a much higher percentage of large tumors, these numbers suggest that lower morbidity is seen in our hands with the translabyrinthine approach. Therefore, the suboccipital approach is used in our practice primarily for attempted hearing conservation.

If it were possible to conserve hearing in a large portion of patients, the higher morbidity of suboccipital surgery might be more acceptable. However, the success of attempted hearing preservation is approximately 35% in most series (Cerullo, Grutsch, Heiferman, & Osterdock, 1993; Glasscock, McKennan, & Levine, 1987; Mazzoni, Calabrese, Danesi, & DeNigris, 1993; Sterkers, Morrison, Sterkers, & El-Dine, 1994; Thomsen & Tos, 1993). Preoperative factors, such as hearing, size of tumor, location of tumor, ABR waveform, and ENG calories can help predict whether a hearing conservation attempt will be successful, but these predictive indicators are not always accurate. Intraoperative ABR is useful to assess cochlear nerve integrity, but the information provided by the ABR lags behind the surgical events. If the ABR deteriorates, it will be noted several seconds after

TABLE 12–1. Tumor size by approach (N = 1330).

Approach	<1.5 cm	>1.5 cm
Suboccipital	77%	23%
Translabyrinthine	23%	77%

TABLE 12–2. CSF leaks by tumor size.

	<1.5 cm	1.5 cm–2.9 cm	>3.0 cm
CSF Leaks	13%	13%	21%

TABLE 12–3. CSF leaks by approach.

Approach	CSF leaks
Suboccipital	15%
Translabyrinthine	13%

the injury occurred. Some authors describe an electrode placed directly on the cochlear nerve for real time feedback of nerve injury. This technique can be awkward at times and has not been shown to improve hearing conservation rates (Nedzelski, Chiong, Cashman, Stanton, & Rowed, 1994; Silverstein, McDaniel, Norrell, & Haberkamp, 1986). The relatively low success rate of hearing preservation surgery of acoustic neuroma is unfortunate, especially since magnetic resonance imaging with gadolinium currently allows diagnosis of tiny tumors before cranial nerve VIII is damaged. Therefore, treatment technology is challenged to find a way to preserve hearing while curing the tumor.

Postoperative or "suboccipital" headaches are unique to the suboccipital approach (Schessel, Rowed, Nedzelski, & Feghali, 1993). Possible theories regarding the origin of the pain include bone dust in the cerebellopontine angle, traction of the occipital musculature on the dura, neuralgia of the occipital nerve, and spasm of the occipital musculature. The headaches usually begin within a few weeks after surgery and, often times, meningitis must be ruled out. The headaches may be unilateral on the side of surgery, generalized, or retro-orbital in location. They often are incited by activity or change in position. The headaches usually are very difficult to control. One of the more successful treatment strategies is scheduled dosing of nonsteroidal antiinflammatory medications. Other modalities, such as heat, ice, massage, and exercise meet with variable success. The headaches generally subside or decrease in intensity over a period of months to years. It is important to include a discussion of these headaches in the preoperative consent process, because they can be of enormous postoperative concern.

The suboccipital approach is a versatile surgery that is applicable to a variety of clinical situations. It is an important addition to the armamentarium of the well-rounded acoustic neuroma surgeon.

REFERENCES

Blevins, N.H., & Jackler, R.K. (1994). Exposure of the lateral extremity of the internal auditory canal through the retrosigmoid approach: A radioanatomic study. *Archives of Otolaryngology—Head and Neck Surgery, 111,* 81–90.

Brackmann, D.E., & Green, J.D. (1992). Translabyrinthine approach for acoustic tumor removal. *Otolaryngologic Clinics of North America, 25,* 311–329.

Cerullo, L.J., Grutsch, J.F., Heiferman, K., & Osterdock, R. (1993). The preservation of hearing and facial nerve function in a consecutive series of unilateral vestibular nerve schwannoma surgical patients (acoustic neuroma). *Surgical Neurology, 39,* 485–493.

Glasscock, M.E., McKennan, K.X., & Levine, S.C. (1987). Acoustic neuroma surgery: The results of hearing conservation surgery. *Laryngoscope, 97,* 785–789.

Jackler, R.K., & Pitts, L.H. (1992). Selection of surgical approach to acoustic neuroma. *Otolaryncolocic Clinics of North America, 25,* 361–387.

Josey, A.F., Glasscock, M.E., & Jackson, C.G. (1988). Preservation of hearing in acoustic tumor surgery: Audiologic indicators. *Annals of Otology, Rhinology and Laryngology, 97,* 626–630.

Mazzoni, A., Calabrese, V., Danesi, G., & DeNigris, M. (1993). La via sub-occipitale nella chirurgia funzionale del neurinoma dell'viii nervo cranico. *Acta Otorhinolaryngologica Italica, 13,* 3–11.

Nedzelski, J.M., Chiong, C.M., Cashman, M.Z., Stanton, S.G., & Rowed, D.W. (1994). Hearing preservation in acoustic neuroma surgery: Value of monitoring cochlear nerve action potentials. *Archives of Otolaryngology—Head and Neck Surgery, 111,* 703–709.

Ojemann, R.G., & Martuza, R.L. (1990). Acoustic neuroma. In J.R. Youmans (Ed.), *Neurological surgery* (pp. 3316–3350). Philadelphia: W.B. Saunders.

Rhoton, A.L. (1993). Microsurgical anatomy of acoustic neuromas. In L.N. Sekhar & I.P. Janecka (Eds.), *Surgery of cranial base tumors* (pp. 687–713). New York: Raven Press.

Schessel, D.A., Rowed, D.W., Nedzelski, J.M., & Feghali, J.G. (1993). Postoperative pain following excision of acoustic neuroma by the suboccipital approach: Observations on possible cause and potential amelioration. *American Journal of Otology, 14,* 491–494.

Silverstein, H., McDaniel, A., Norrell, H., & Haberkamp, T. (1986). Hearing preservation after acoustic neuroma surgery with intraoperative direct eighth cranial nerve monitoring: Part II. A classification of results. *Archives of Otolaryngology—Head and Neck Surgery, 95,* 285–291.

Sterkers, J.M., Morrison, G.A., Sterkers, O., & El-Dine, M.M. (1994). Preservation of facial, cochlear, and other nerve functions in acoustic neuroma treatment. *Archives of Otolaryngology—Head and Neck Surgery, 110,* 146–155.

Thomsen, J., & Tos, M. (1993). Management of acoutic neuromas. *Annales d' Oto-Laryngologie et de Chirurgie Cervico-Faciale, 110,* 179–191.

CHAPTER 13

Partial Versus Total Removal of Acoustic Tumors

Leigh Anne Dew, M.D.
Clough Shelton, M.D.
William Hitselberger, M.D.

Modern acoustic tumor surgery has several objectives. The first and foremost objective is the preservation of life with total removal of the tumor. The second objective is the preservation of the facial nerve, and the final objective, when appropriate, is the preservation of hearing. Many advances have significantly lowered the morbidity and mortality of acoustic tumor surgery. Early diagnosis, advances in neuroanesthetic techniques, the use of the operating microscope, and intraoperative facial nerve monitoring have made preservation of brainstem and lower cranial nerve functions routine. In addition, hearing preservation results continue to improve. In carefully selected patients, useful hearing can be maintained one third of the time (Gardner & Robertson, 1988; Nadol, Levine, Ojemann, Martuza, Montgomery, & de Sandoval, 1987; Brackmann, House, & Hitselberger, 1989).

These advances also facilitate the primary objective of surgery, which is the complete removal of tumor. Historically, how-

ever, this has not always been the case. In the early 1900s, when the symptoms of intracranial tumors were first recognized, the sole aim of surgical management was to reduce the intracranial pressure. In 1913, the mortality rate of acoustic tumor resection approached 80% (Glasscock, 1968). Because of these appalling statistics, Cushing recommended bilateral suboccipital decompressive craniectomies and extensive intracapsular removal of the tumor by finger dissection, reducing surgical mortality to 40%. His ultimate case mortality, however, must have approached 100%, since the tumor inevitably recurred when a major portion of the capsule was left intact. In 1925, Dandy described the unilateral suboccipital approach for total removal of tumor. With improved methods to control hemorrhage and meticulous dissection of the tumor capsule, he was able to perform intracapsular enucleation followed by careful excision of the tumor capsule (Dandy, 1925). He reported an operative mortality rate of 22% for total tumor resections (House, 1979).

The rate of total tumor removal has risen from 60% in the 1960s (House & Hitselberger, 1964) to 88% to 100% (Abramson, Stein, Pedley, Emerson, & Wazen, 1985; Baldwin, King, & Morrison, 1990; Cannoni, Pech, & Pellet, 1989; Cohen, Hammerschlag, Berg, & Ransohoff, 1986; Ekvall & Byncke, 1988; Glasscock, Kveton, Jackson, & McKennan, 1986; Hardy, MacFarlane, Baguley, & Moffat, 1989; Harner, Beatty, & Ebersold, 1990; House & Hitselberger, 1985; Kemink, La Rouere, Kileny, Telian, & Hof, 1990; Mangham, 1988; Mercke, Harris, & Sundbarg, 1988; Nadol et al., 1987, 1992; Nystrom, Palva, & Jokinen, 1988; Samii, Turel, & Penkert, 1985; Shelton, Brackmann, House, & Hitselberger, 1989b; Sterkers, Sterkers, & Maudlelonde, 1984; Sugita & Kobayashi, 1982; Thomsen, Tos, & Harmsen, 1989; Tos, Thomsen, & Harmsen, 1982; Whittaker & Luetje, 1985; Wigand, Haid, & Berg, 1989). Although subtotal removal is still performed in certain circumstances, total removal of acoustic tumors is now the norm (Long, 1992).

Many different terms are used to describe the completeness of tumor removal, often causing confusion in reporting and discussing surgical results. For partial removal, terms such as "subtotal" (Wazen, Silverstein, Norrel, & Besse, 1985), "near total" (Kemink, Langman, Niparko, & Graham, 1991), and "radical intracapsular removal" (Lowrie & Drake, 1991) have been used. There is even some ambiguity regarding the concept of total tumor removal. Cases in which tiny fragments of tumor are left attached to critical structures are regarded by some as "complete" removals (Dutton et al., 1991; Lye, Pace-Balzan, Ramsden, Gillespie, & Dutton, 1992).

SUBTOTAL VERSUS TOTAL REMOVAL

The most common reason for subtotal resection is intraoperative vital sign changes that indicate potential brainstem ischemia. The second most common reason is tumor adherence to the brainstem, vital vascular structures, or the facial nerve (Shea, Hitselberger, Benecke, & Brackmann, 1985). Although Cushing's work in the 1930s alerted physicians to the early symptoms of acoustic tumors, many patients were not diagnosed until they had reached an advanced stage or had developed symptoms of increased intracranial pressure. Because these tumors generally have a slow growth rate, and significant morbidity was once associated with surgical removal of the tumor, many physicians adopted a "watch and wait" policy for patients who had an asymptomatic cerebellopontine mass (Shelton & Hitselberger, 1991). Surgical resection often was delayed until the expanding tumor caused compressive symptoms, thus increasing surgical morbidity and mortality. In addition, the incidence of injury to the facial nerve was as high as 50–70% (House & Luetje, 1979), and many patients were unwilling to accept disfiguring facial paralysis as a consequence of total tumor removal (Lownie & Drake, 1991).

Vital sign change can be manifested by changes in pulse or blood pressure. Pulse changes are less significant and merely may represent manipulation of the eleventh and twelfth cranial nerves. Increases in pulse and blood pressure also may be seen when working around the fifth nerve.

When the dissection is near the brainstem, a change in blood pressure (usually elevation) can be an ominous sign, reflecting brainstem ischemia. Initially, cottonoids should be removed from the posterior fossa, and tumor removal should stop. If the blood pressure abnormalities persist, the rocedure should be terminated and the operation staged. The second stage procedure usually is carried out 6 months later. During the second operation, the tumor usually is found to be less adherent to the brainstem and blood vessels, probably due to the tumor decompression and disengagement from the brainstem.

A review of 3,123 acoustic tumor cases at the House Ear Clinic revealed 28 patients who underwent a staged tumor removal (Shelton, in press). Most of these staged removals were performed in the 1960s and 1970s and required staging due to intraoperative vital sign changes. The majority had successful tumor removal at the second stage. Currently, staged tumor removal seldom is required. The decreased incidence of staging is probably due to improvement in anesthesia techniques and increased experience of the operative team.

Some authors assert that there are several cases in which planned subtotal resection is a valid surgical option (Jackler & Pitts, 1990; Kemink et al., 1991; Phillippon, 1992). In cases of bilateral acoustic tumors or patients with tumors in the only-hearing ear, the option of partial resection with the goal of hearing preservation, rather than eradication of tumor, could seem attractive. Other factors that are considered to be important when selecting subtotal removal are the patient's age, general medical condition, and ability to accept facial paralysis in exchange for total tumor removal.

In constrast, many do not consider these factors to take precedence over total tumor removal. Some maintain that patients with a small tumor and rapidly deteriorating hearing in their only-hearing ear may benefit from middle fossa decompression of the internal auditory canal (Gadre, Kwartler, Brackmann, House, & Hitselberger, 1990). This is thought to relieve pressure on the cochlear nerve and blood supply and has resulted in hearing improvement in some patients (usually improvement of speech discrimination). Unfortunately, decompression only defers the inevitable, and these patients experience continued tumor growth with associated hearing deterioration. They eventually need definitive tumor removal, usually in 12 to 18 months.

Patients with neurofibromatosis type 2 (NF-2) require special consideration regarding recurrence. The tumor behavior can be quite different for these tumors compared to unilateral acoustic schwannomas. The NF-2 tumors have been observed to be in-

nately more invasive and tend to infiltrate the cochlear nerve (Linthicum & Brackmann, 1980; Perre, Viala, & Foncin, 1990; Shelton, 1992). This cochlear nerve infiltration probably is responsible for the poor hearing success rate with partial tumor removal in patients with NF-2. Also, in these patients, a "recurrent" tumor actually could represent a new tumor on a different cranial nerve, rather than a true recurrence (Thedinger, Whittaker, & Luetje, 1991). For patients with NF-2 and bilateral acoustic tumors, some surgeons prefer to defer surgery in the better-hearing ear, perform a translabyrinthine removal when required, and rehabilitate the patient with a brainstem implant which, in the past, yielded results similar to a single-channel cochlear implant (Shelton, 1992). Recently, for some patients, the multi-channel brainstem implant has provided open-set speech discrimination (see Chapter 20).

RECURRENCE

Tumor regrowth is reported infrequently. Of those cases reported in the literature, most were originally removed by the suboccipital/retrosigmoid approach. Some feel that many of these "recurrences" actually represent the residual tumor left in the internal auditory canal at the initial surgery (Beatty, Ebersold, & Harner, 1987; Thedinger et al., 1991). One commonly acknowledged limitation of the suboccipital approach is that the intracanicular portion of the tumor is more difficult to expose, which increases the difficulty of exposing the lateral portion of the facial nerve (Mangham, 1988).

Roberson and co-workers reviewed 35 cases of "recurrent" acoustic tumors after initial suboccipital removal at an outside institution (Roberson, Brackmann, & Hitselberger, 1996). The recurrences subsequently were removed through the translabyrinthine approach. The majority of recurrences were centered on the lateral internal auditory canal, an area not visible through the suboccipital approach without violating the labyrinth. It was concluded in this study that, after initial surgery, any residual tumor left in the lateral internal auditory canal was responsible for the majority of observed recurrences.

Tumor regrowth has been described as "recurrence," irrespective of the degree of the original tumor removed (Shea et al., 1985). However, according to Thedinger, Glasscock, Cueva, and Jackson (1992), the term "residual tumor" is synonymous with subtotal excision. Thus, if the initial tumor removal was partial, the regrowth of the tumor is best described as persistent, or residual, tumor. For our purposes, if all visible tumor (using the surgical microscope) is removed, including any fragment in the internal auditory canal, and there is tumor regrowth, it is considered a true recurrence.

There have been several reports of long-term follow-up of patients with acoustic tumors, specifically evaluating them for recurrence. These series evaluated patients who had undergone cochlear nerve preservation in an attempt to preserve hearing and, therefore, were postulated to be at risk for recurrence. In a follow-up study of 28 patients who had undergone attempted hearing preservation via the suboccipital approach, no recurrent acoustic tumors were identified (Schessel, Nedzelski, Kassel, & Rowed, 1992). This group had a minimum follow-up of 5 years, an average follow-up of 7.5 years, and patients were evaluated primarily by contrast-enhanced CT scan. In another series of 18 patients who had undergone complete tumor removal for attempted hearing preservation, no recurrences were identified (Rosenberg, Cohen, & Ranshoff, 1987). Atlas and colleagues studied a group of 159 patients undergoing acoustic tumor removal and identified two recurrent tumors (Atlas, Harvey, & Fagen, 1992). Experience with 23 recurrent acoustic tumors originally removed predominantly by the suboccipital approach was reviewed by Beatty and colleagues (1987). Eleven patients were identi-

fied who had complete tumor removal at the primary surgery but suffered a recurrence, with a median time interval to recurrence of 78 months. The most common symptoms at recurrence were ataxia, facial paresthesia, headaches, dysphagia, and dysarthria. As most patients have lost function of the eighth cranial nerve, symptoms at recurrence were dependent on other residual neurologic function. In another study of 25 patients who underwent middle fossa approach acoustic tumor removal and who had a minimum of 3 years of follow-up, no recurrent tumors were identified (Shelton, Hitselberger, House, & Brackmann, 1990).

Unilateral acoustic tumor recurrence after presumed total removal through the translabyrinthine approach has been reported only rarely. Thedinger and colleagues (1991) reviewed 999 acoustic tumor surgeries and identified three patients with recurrent acoustic tumors, for a recurrence rate of 0.5%. Of the three patients, only one was not afflicted by NF-2. This patient underwent a complete translabyrinthine removal of a unilateral acoustic tumor and developed a recurrence 9 years later, necessitating removal again through the translabyrinthine approach.

The surgical records of the House Ear Clinic were reviewed for patients with a diagnosis of acoustic neuroma between 1961 and 1993. During this time, 3,123 acoustic tumors were removed, the majority by the translabyrinthine approach. Subsequently, 76 of these patients developed "recurrent" tumors. Of these patients, 28 had a staged tumor removal, most of which were conducted in the 1960s and 1970s and were staged because of intraoperative vital sign changes. Thirteen patients had a complete suboccipital tumor removal performed at another institution and developed a recurrence that was removed by the translabyrinthine approach; three of these patients required two translabyrinthine removals each to achieve total removal. Two patients developed recurrent tumors after complete tumor removal by the translabyrinthine approach performed elsewhere, and the recurrences were removed again through the translabyrinthine approach.

Ten patients who underwent their initial surgery at the House Ear Clinic were identified with recurrent tumors. Five of these patients had NF-2 and were excluded from the study. The remaining five patients developed a recurrence after initial total removal through the translabyrinthine approach, for a total recurrence rate of approximately 0.3%. No pre- or postoperative factors were identified to predict recurrence, although the initial tumor size in these patients was large. Both the operating neurotologist and neurosurgeon felt that all tumor was removed in the initial operation. The average time interval from initial removal to recurrence was approximately 10 years, ranging from 109 to 151 months. The growth rate of the recurrent tumors, measured as the diameter divided by the years passed since the initial surgery, ranged from 0.79 mm to 5.2 mm per year (Table 13–1). Flow cytometric analysis did not reveal any fundamental differences between the recurrent acoustic tumor group and a larger group of 112 patients with acoustic tumors (Shelton, in press). This indicates that the recurrent tumors are not uniquely aggressive neoplasms, and other mechanisms may explain the recurrence.

The initial tumors in these patients were large, with only one of five tumors measuring less than 3.5 cm. The recurrences theoretically could represent viable cells spilled into the operative field, because such large tumors are removed in piecemeal fashion. This is unlikely, because this mechanism also could produce recurrences remote from the operative site, which was not observed. However, careful irrigation and inspection of the cerebellopontine angle after tumor removal is recommended to disperse any viable tumor cells from the operative field.

Histologic evidence supports three areas where microscopic tumor could persist at initial operation, including the eighth nerve stump at the brainstem, the lateral end of the internal auditory canal, and the facial nerve (see Figure 13–1). Microscopic intraneural tumor invasion and multicentric eighth nerve origin of acoustic tumors have been described in patients who do not have NF-2 (Luetje, Whittaker, Callaway, & Veraga, 1983; Neely, 1981, 1984; Perre et al., 1990). The abundant blood supply of the brainstem would sustain tumor growth in the area of the eighth nerve stump, but tumor presence may not be apparent at surgery. This is supported by one of the recur-

TABLE 13–1. Recurrent acoustic tumors in patients who underwent translabyrinthine removal at The House Ear Clinic from 1961–1993.

Case	Symptoms at Recurrence	Initial Tumor Size (cm)	Recurrent Tumor Size (cm)	Interval Between Surgery (cm)	Growth Rate (mm/year)
1	Headache	4.5	3	132	2.73
2	None	4	2.5	134	2.23
3	Headache	4.5	1	151	0.79
4	Trigeminal nerve numbness	2	3.2	109	3.52
5	Trigeminal nerve numbness	3.5	5	116	5.17

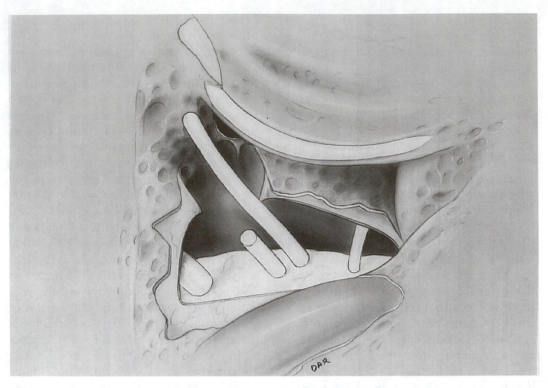

Figure 13–1. Three likely areas as sources for recurrence: eighth nerve stump, facial nerve, and lateral internal auditory canal (Reprinted with permission from Unilateral Acoustic Tumors: How Often Do They Occur After Translabyrinthine Removal? by C. Shelton, 1996. *Laryngoscope, 107.*)

rences in the current series, in which tumor clearly was found to be originating from this site. Tumor also may be left in the lateral end of the internal auditory canal. Visualization of this area requires removal of part of the bony partition between the vestibule and the lateral internal auditory canal. In some cases, the tumor will be adherent in this area, known as "Bill's tongue" (see Figure 13–2). Failure to sever this attachment can lead to residual tumor. Histologically, this was shown in a postmortem study of a temporal bone from a patient who had undergone a complete translabyrinthine removal of an acoustic tumor 11 years prior to his demise of unrelated causes. The operating surgeon believed that all tumor had been removed at the time of surgery. The postmortem exam of the temporal bone revealed a tumor fragment on the superior vestibular nerve at "Bill's

tongue" (House & Belal, 1980). Finally, there may not be a definite plane between tumor and facial nerve. At surgery, it may be very difficult to separate tumor from nerve, especially when the facial nerve is attenuated. In one of the recurrent cases, a small recurrent tumor was found attached to the facial nerve, presumably arising from a small scrap of tumor unknowingly left behind at the initial surgery.

Based on the observed, average, tumor growth rate of 2.8 mm per year, a single, postoperative, gadolium-enhanced MRI scan conducted 5 years after complete translabyrinthine tumor removal is recommended. If a tumor is present at that time, it would average 15 mm, which would be large enough to be detected easily by MRI, but still small enough to be managed surgically without excessive difficulty. After 5 years, even the slowest growing tumor in

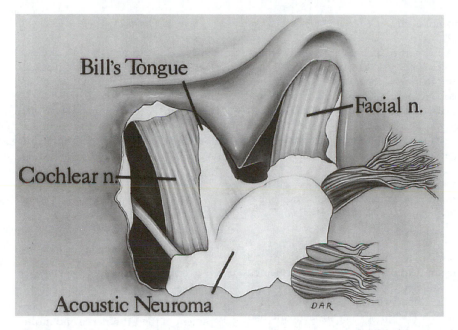

Figure 13-2. Tumor adherent to the lateral internal auditory canal (Bill's tongue). (Reprinted with permission from Unilateral Acoustic Tumors: How Often Do They Occur After Translabyrinthine Removal? by C. Shelton, 1996. *Laryngoscope, 107.*)

this series (0.75 mm increase in diameter per year) would be approximately 4 cm in diameter and also could be detected easily. If ambiguous areas of enhancement are present, serial MRIs should be performed to exclude growing tumor. This recommendation must be individualized to the findings and clinical course of each patient. For patients who undergo a planned, subtotal resection of tumor, or for those in whom a small amount of tumor is left attached to vital neurovascular structures, annual MRIs are recommended for postoperative surveillance.

REFERENCES

Abramson, M., Stein, B., Pedley, T., Emerson, R., & Wazen, J. (1985). Intraoperative BAER monitoring and hearing preservation in the treatment of acoustic neuromas. *Laryngoscope, 95,* 1318–1322.

Atlas, M., Harvey, C., & Fagen, P. (1992). Hearing preservation in acoustic neuroma surgery: A continuing study. *Laryngoscope, 102,* 779–783.

Baldwin, D, King, T., & Morrison, A. (1990). Hearing conservation in acoustic neuroma surgery via the posterior fossa. *Journal of Laryngology and Otology, 104,* 463–467.

Beatty, C., Ebersold, M., & Harner, S. (1987). Residual and recurrent acoustic neuromas. *Laryngoscope, 97,* 1168–1171.

Cannoni, M., Pech, A., & Pellet, W. (1989). Experiences at the Timone Hospital, Marseille in acoustic neuroma surgery. *Archives of Otolaryngology, 246,* 297–298.

Cohen, N., Hammerschlag, P., Berg, H., & Ransohoff, J. (1986). Acoustic neuroma surgery: An eclectic approach with emphasis on preservation of hearing. The New York University-Bellevue experience. *Annals of Otology, Rhinology and Laryngology, 95,* 21–27.

Dandy, W. (1925). Operation for total removal of cerebellopontine (acoustic) tumors. *Surgery, Gynecology and Obstetrics, 41,* 129–148.

Dutton, J., Ramsden, R., Lye, R., Morris, K., Keith, A., Page, R., & Vafadis, J. (1991). Acoustic neuroma (schwannoma) surgery. 1978–1990. *Journal of Laryngology and Otology, 105,* 165–173.

Ekvall, L., & Bynke, O. (1988). The translabyrinthine approach in 100 patients with acoustic tumors. *Acta Otolaryngologica (Stockh.), 559,* 213–216.

Gadre, A., Kwartler, J., Brackmann, D., House, W., & Hitselberger, W. (1990). Middle fossa decompression of the internal auditory canal in acoustic neuroma surgery: A therapeutic alternative. *Laryngoscope, 100,* 948–952.

Gardner, G., & Robertson, J. (1988). Hearing preservation in unilateral acoustic neuroma surgery. *Annals of Otology, Rhinology and Laryngology, 97,* 55–56.

Glasscock, M. E., III. (1968). History of the diagnosis and treatment of acoustic neuromas. *Archives of Otolaryngology—Head and Neck Surgery, 88,* 578–585.

Glasscock, M. E., III, Kveton, J., Jackson, C., & McKennan, K. (1986). A systematic approach to the surgical management of acoustic neuroma. *Laryngoscope, 96,* 1088–1094.

Hardy, D., MacFarlane, R., Baguley, D., & Moffat, D. (1989). Surgery for acoustic neuroma. *Journal of Neurosurgery, 71,* 799–804.

Harner, S., Beatty, C., & Ebersold, M. (1990). Retrosigmoid removal of acoustic neuroma: Experience 1978-1988. *Archives of Otolaryngology—Head and Neck Surgery, 103,* 40–45.

House, W. (1979). A history of acoustic tumor surgery: 1917-1961, the Dandy era. In W. House & C. Luetje (Eds.), *Acoustic tumors.* Baltimore: University Park Press.

House, W., & Bellal, A., Jr. (1980). Translabyrinthine surgery: Anatomy and pathology. *Journal of Otology, 1*(4), 189–198.

House, W., & Hitselberger, W. (1964). Total versus subtotal removal of acoustic tumors. *Archives of Otolaryngology—Head and Neck Surgery, 80,* 751–752.

House, W., & Hitselberger, W. (1985). The neuro-otologist's view of the surgical management of acoustic neuromas. *Clinical Neurosurgery, 32,* 214–222.

House, W., & Luetje, C. (1979). Evaluation and preservation of facial function: Postoperative results. In W. House & C. Luetje (Eds.), *Acoustic tumors.* Baltimore: University Park Press.

Jackler, R., & Pitts, L. (1990). Acoustic neuroma. *Neurosurgery Clinics of North America, 1,* 199–223.

Kemink, J., Langman, A., Niparko, J., & Graham, M. (1991). Operative management of acoustic neuromas: The priority of neurologic function over complete resection. *Archives of Otolaryngology—Head and Neck Surgery, 104,* 96–99.

Kemink, J., LaRouere, M., Kileny, P., Telian, S., & Hoff, J. (1990). Hearing preservation following subtotal removal of acoustic neuromas. *Laryngoscope, 100,* 597–601.

Linthicum, F., & Brackmann, D. (1980). Bilateral acoustic tumors: A diagnostic and surgical challenge. *Archives of Otolaryngology—Head and Neck Surgery, 106,* 729–733.

Long, D. (1992). Non-glial tumors of the brain: Tumors of the cerebellopontine angle and meningiomas. *Current Opinions in Neurology and Neurosurgery, 5,* 813–817.

Lownie, S., & Drake, C. (1991). Radical intracapsular removal of acoustic neurinomas: Long-term follow-up review of 11 patients. *Journal of Neurosurgery, 74,* 422–425.

Luetje, C., Whittaker, C., Callaway, L., & Veraga, G. (1983). Histologic acoustic tumor involvement of the VIIth nerve and multicentric origin in the VIIIth nerve. *Laryngoscope, 93,* 1133–1139.

Lye, R. H., Pace-Balzan, A., Ramsden, R. T., Gillespie, J. E., & Dutton, J. M. (1992). The fate of tumour rests following removal of acoustic neuromas: An MRI Gd-DTPA surgery: An eclectic approach with an emphasis on preservation of hearing. The New York University-Bellvue experience. *Annals of Otology, Rhinology and Laryngology, 95,* 21–27.

Mangham, C. (1988). Complications of translabyrinthine vs. suboccipital approach for acoustic tumor surgery. *Archives of Otolaryngology—Head and Neck Surgery, 99,* 396–407.

Mercke, U., Harris, S., & Sundbarg, G. (1988). Translabyrinthine acoustic neuroma surgery as performed by the otoneurosurgical group at Lund University Hospital. *Acta Otolaryngologica, 452*(Suppl.), 34–37.

Nadol, J., Jr., Chiong, C., Ojemann, R., McKenna, M., Martuza, R., Montgomery, W., Levine, R., Ronner, S., & Glynn, R. (1992). Preservation of hearing and facial nerve function in resection of acoustic neuroma. *Laryngoscope, 102,* 1153–1158.

Nadol, J., Jr., Levine, R., Ojemann, R., Martuza, R., Montgomery, W., & de Sandoval, P. (1987). Preservation of hearing in surgical removal of acoustic neuromas of the internal auditory canal and cerebellopontine angle. *Laryngoscope, 97,* 1287–1294.

Neely, J. (1981). Gross and microscopic anatomy of the eighth cranial nerve in relationship to the solitary schwannoma. *Laryngoscope, 91,* 1512–1531.

Neely, J. (1984). Is it possible to totally resect an acoustic tumor and conserve hearing? *Archives of Otolaryngology—Head and Neck Surgery, 92,* 162-167.

Nystrom, S., Palva, A., & Jokinen, K. (1988). Acoustic neuroma surgery in northern Finland. *Acta Otolaryngologica (Stockh.), 452* (Suppl.), 52–56.

Perre, J., Viala, P., & Foncin, J. (1990). Involvement of cochlear nerve in acoustic tumors. *Acta Otolaryngologica (Stockh.), 110,* 245–252.

Phillippon, J. (1992). Reoperation for extra-axial brain tumors. *Clinical Neurosurgery, 39,* 212–232.

Roberson, J. B., Jr., Brackmann, D. E., & Hitselberger, W. E. (1996). *Acoustic neuroma recurrence following suboccipital resection: Management with translabyrinthine resection.* Manuscript submitted for publication.

Rosenberg, R., Cohen, N., & Ranshoff, J. (1987). Long-term hearing preservation after acoustic neuroma surgery. *Archives of Otolaryngology—Head and Neck Surgery, 97,* 270–274.

Samii, M., Turel, K., & Penkert, G. (1985). Management of seventh and eighth nerve involvement by cerebellopontine angle tumors. *Clinical Neurosurgery, 32,* 242–272.

Schessel, D., Nedzelski, J., Kassel, E., & Rowed, D. (1992). Recurrence rates of acoustic neuroma in hearing preservation surgery. *American Journal of Otology, 13,* 233–235.

Shea, J., Hitselberger, W., Beneke, J., & Brackmann, D. (1985). Recurrence rate of partially resected acoustic tumors. *American Journal of Otology, 5*(Suppl.), 107–109.

Shelton, C. (1992). Hearing preservation in acoustic tumor surgery. *Otolaryngology Clinics of North America, 25*(3), 609–621.

Shelton, C. (in press). Unilateral acoustic tumors. How often do they recur after translabyrinthine removal? *Laryngoscope.*

Shelton, C., Brackmann, D., House, W., & Hitselberger, W. (1989a). Acoustic tumor surgery: Prognostic factors in hearing conservation. *Archives of Otolaryngology—Head and Neck Surgery, 115,* 1213–1216.

Shelton, C., Brackmann, D., House, W., & Hitselberger, W. (1989b). Middle fossa acoustic tumor surgery: Results in 106 cases. *Laryngoscope, 99,* 405–408.

Shelton, C., & Hitselberger, W. (1991). The treatment of small acoustic tumors: Now or later? *Laryngoscope, 101*(9), 925–928.

Shelton, C., Hitselberger, W., House, W., & Brackmann, D. (1990). Hearing preservation after acoustic tumor removal: Long term results. *Laryngoscope, 100,* 115–119.

Sterkers, J., Sterkers, O., & Maudlelonde, C. (1984). Preservation of hearing by the retrosigmoid approach in acoustic neuroma surgery. *Advances in Otology, Rhinology, and Laryngology, 34,* 187–192.

Sugita, K., & Kobayashi, S. (1982). Technical and instrumental improvements in the surgical treatment of acoustic neuromas. *Journal of Neurology, 57,* 747–752.

Thedinger, B., Glasscock, M., III, Cueva, R., & Jackson, C. (1992). Postoperative radiographic evaluation after acoustic neuroma and glomus jugulare tumor removal. *Laryngoscope, 102,* 261-266.

Thedinger, B., Whittaker, C., & Luetje, C. (1991). Recurrent acoustic tumor after suboccipital removal. *Neurosurgery, 29*(5), 681–687.

Thomsen, J., Tos, M., & Harmsen, A. (1989). Acoustic neuroma surgery: Results of translabyrinthine tumor removal in 300 patients. Discussion of chioce of approach in relation to overall results and possibility of hearing preservation. *British Journal of Neurosurgery, 3,* 349–360.

Tos, M., Thomsen, J., & Harmsen, A. (1988). Results of translabyrinthine removal of 300 acoustic neuromas related to tumor size. *Acta Otolaryngologica (Stockh.), 452*(Suppl.), 38–51.

Wazen, J., Silverstein, H., Norrell, H., & Besse, B. (1985). Pre-operative and post-operative growth rates in acoustic neuromas documented with CT scanning. *Archives of Otolaryngology—Head and Neck Surgery, 93,* 151–155.

Whittaker, C., & Luetje, C. (1985). Translabyrinthine removal of large acoustic tumors. *American Journal of Otology, 6*(Suppl.), 155–160.

Wigand, M., Haid, T., & Berg, M. (1989). The enlarged middle cranial foss approach for surgery of the temporal bone and of the cerebellopontine angle. *Archives of Otorhinolaryngology, 246,* 299–302.

CHAPTER 14

Management of Giant Acoustic Neuroma

Robert Thayer Sataloff, M.D., D.M.A.
Donald L. Myers, M.D.
Mary J. Hawkshaw, R.N., B.S.N.

The management of acoustic neuromas depends upon many issues discussed elsewhere in this book. Tumor size is one of the most important factors. Most small, medium, or large acoustic neuromas can be resected completely, with minimal morbidity, through a middle fossa, translabyrinthine, or suboccipital approach, as detailed in previous chapters. Tumors larger than 5 or 6 cm present special problems, particularly if they cross the midline anterior to the brainstem or extend in an unusual fashion into brain structures. This chapter reviews the surgical treatment of such tumors through combined and novel approaches.

SURGICAL PHILOSOPHY

Certain aspects of acoustic tumor management are controversial and remain in the realm of "the art of medicine." Consequently, it is important for readers to know authors' biases so that recommendations can be interpreted appropriately. Some of the procedures discussed in this chapter are extensive, some might even be called heroic, and there are those who would consider some of them excessive.

We feel that every effort should be made to completely resect even the very large acoustic neuromas in most patients. Signs of recent tumor growth, as evidenced by progression of neurological symptoms or signs, make this effort even more imperative. We do not consider advanced chronological age a contraindication to surgery so long as the patient is in good medical condition and able to tolerate prolonged anesthesia with acceptable risk. Except under extraordinary circumstances, we do not believe in planned partial resection (debulking alone), even in "elderly" patients. The fact that a patient is in his or her seventies or eighties does not mean necessarily that the patient will not live for another 20 or 30 years. The best opportunity for cure occurs at the time of the first surgical procedure. Consequently, in virtually all cases, we design a treatment plan directed toward total tumor removal. In general, we plan to resect even giant acoustic neuromas in one stage. We continually monitor physiologic conditions intraoperatively, and we may opt to convert to a staged procedure if brain swelling or vital sign changes warrant alteration in strategy.

Most medium and even some large acoustic neuromas can be resected through a translabyrinthine or suboccipital approach in 3 to 10 hours. However, safe resection of giant tumors with preservation of cranial nerves occasionally may take 18–30 hr. We have developed protocols for planned prolonged surgery and have 15 years of close collaboration with an excellent anesthesia department. When we anticipate that prolonged surgery may be necessary for problems such as a giant acoustic neuroma or extensive cancers involving the skull base, we schedule the case for 24 hr, and the prolonged surgery protocols automatically go into effect. Anesthesia and nursing staffing are planned well in advance, preoperative patient padding and other precautions are taken to avoid decubitus ulcers, intravenous infiltration, thrombophlebitis, and so on; and the intensive care unit nurses, cardiologist, deep venous thrombosis team, and other associates are made aware of the scheduled procedure. Prolonged use of nitrous oxide is avoided. In recent years, we have had no complications related to the duration of the surgical procedure except occasional cases of thrombophlebitis of the lower extremity.

Intraoperative developments have required us to terminate the surgical procedure prior to completion on only two occasions. We perform the second stage within 10 days to 2 weeks, if possible. Although some surgeons advocate a 6-month interval, we have found this much less satisfactory. At 6 months, there may be substantial scar. Consequently, the difficulty of surgery and the risk of cranial nerve injury are increased, and the chance for total tumor resection is decreased. At about 10 days, the residual tumor may be necrotic, and we

have found that resection can be conducted more easily than at the time of the initial procedure. Bits of tumor that were stuck under draining veins of the brainstem usually can be dissected and aspirated more readily. Moreover, by 10 days to 2 weeks, the brain has reexpanded significantly from its initial tumor-compressed position, and vital sign changes are less likely. If the initial procedure produced any significant transient cerebral edema (usually this is not a problem, if surgery and retraction are gentle), the edema should have resolved sufficiently by this time. However, with a second stage, the brain may be soft and less able to sustain retraction. Some bits of adherent tumor capsule may no longer be accessible because the expanded brainstem now has everted the tumor cavity, and the full tumor bed can no longer be visualized readily. Of course, imaging studies are performed shortly before the second stage in order to assess the brain, ventricles, and residual tumor.

When prolonged surgery is planned, the condition of the surgeons also must be recognized as an important factor in determining success. The authors (a neurotologist and a neurosurgeon) were medical school roommates. We have operated together since our careers began. The neurosurgeon has taken temporal bone courses and is comfortable operating anywhere in the skull base, and the neurotologist is comfortable operating in the posterior fossa. For procedures of this magnitude, it is highly desirable for all members of the team to be able to take over and perform any portion of the case at any time. It is crucial to remember that operative time is of the essence, and a surgeon must be aware of his own physical limitations. During the early debulking phase, steady, continued reduction in tumor mass is essential. Sometimes it is poor judgment to extensively dissect (suboccipitally) in one small area early in the procedure, while fighting for retraction against the mass of tumor. Having the support of a surgical team and the ability to move comfortably to different surgical areas, at any time makes a tremendous difference in these massive tumors. The surgeon knows that he can rest for a few hours and later revisit a troublesome area. We also work with an excellent staff of resident physicians. From a personal standpoint, we plan in advance for such cases, making certain that we are rested the day before the case and that no patients are scheduled for at least 1 or 2 days after the case. The pressures of imminent office hours or another planned surgical procedure are deleterious. Moreover, patients undergoing resection of very large tumors sometimes need close attention in the neurosurgical intensive care unit within the first 24 hr. We consider attending-level postoperative care part of our surgical responsibility, and we schedule it into our surgical agenda.

PRESERVATION OF CRANIAL NERVES

We believe that it is worth taking extra time and precautions intraoperatively in order to preserve cranial nerve function whenever possible. It usually is possible to preserve anatomically all cranial nerves except for VIII, even in giant acoustic neuromas. In a couple of cases, we have attempted hearing preservation with large acoustic neuromas. So far, the attempts have been unsuccessful and have added considerable time to already lengthy cases. Although we always are ready to reexamine this issue, we believe that hearing preservation generally is not practical when attempting total resection of very large acoustic neuromas. However, anatomic preservation of the facial nerve is generally possible and worthwhile. A high incidence of temporary facial paralysis is to be expected, but routine permanent facial paralysis is unnecessary. Occasionally, there is no surgically apparent cleavage plane between the tumor and the facial nerve. Jaaskelainen et al. (1994) confirmed histologically that the cleavage plane

may be absent. Such cases usually result in at least temporary facial paralysis but, even in this situation, we generally have found it possible to avoid transecting the nerve by cutting the tumor away circumferentially and leaving the fascicles intact, as described for selected facial neuromas (Sataloff, Fratalli, & Myers, 1995). Even temporary injury to other cranial nerves generally can be avoided.

SURGICAL APPROACHES

The surgical approach to very large acoustic neuromas is selected on the basis of several factors. Tumor size, shape, position, temporal bone invasion, and brainstem compression are paramount. Once the tumor has been mapped, we try to select an approach that will provide optimal exposure with minimal brain retraction. This is especially important for tumors that extend anterior to the brainstem because compressed brainstem in this region is very intolerant of manipulation. We are willing to retract (or occasionally, even resect) portions of the cerebellum. We prefer not to retract the brainstem (even with a cottonoid) under most circumstances. Rather, we modify the exposure so that we can gain access to the tumor in and around the brainstem directly, without the need for retraction. In some cases, even very large acoustic neuromas can be resected safely through either a suboccipital or translabyrinthine approach. When this is not possible, resection of these large tumors may become technically feasible through use of combined approaches. This chapter reviews some of the approaches utilized, including one approach discussed here for the first time.

The Suboccipital Approach

The suboccipital approach also is discussed elsewhere in this book, and initial surgical details will not be reviewed here. This approach remains the main route for resection and initial debulking of massive tumors. It provides extensive access to the posterior fossa, the ability to visualize the brain structures, and access superiorly into the incisura, as well as inferiorly into the foramen magnum. When the tumor can be accessed and collapsed through a suboccipital approach, the surgeon essentially converts a giant acoustic neuroma to a medium-sized acoustic neuroma. However, tumor collapse may not be feasible using this approach; for example, if there is a large bulk of tumor anterior to the brainstem. The operating laser, House-Urban rotary dissector, CUSA, or other devices may be extremely helpful for debulking within the tumor capsule and al-

so may save a great deal of intraoperative time. Debulking must be done gently and with caution, because these large tumors produce extreme brainstem compression and distortion. Tumor debulking allows shifting of the brain to occur, which occasionally may cause devastating hemorrhage deep within the brain substance. The only death of a patient with an acoustic neuroma in over 15 years of our experience occurred for this reason during rapid debulking of a large acoustic neuroma early in our careers (Figure 14–1). Great care must be taken to avoid this complication, and other brainstem catastrophes, such as peduncular hemiplegia (Desgeorgas & Sterkers, 1984).

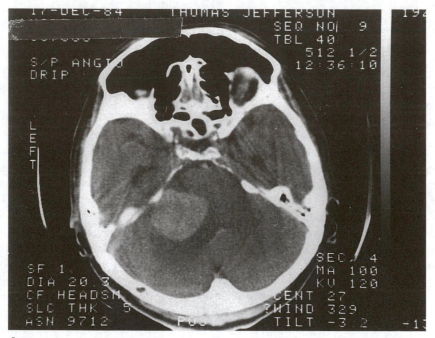

A

Figure 14–1. A, CT and **B,** MR of a 61-year-old female with a large acoustic neuroma crossing the midline. She had a 55 dB HL hearing loss in the speech frequencies in the left ear, dropping to 90 dB HL at 8000 Hz. Her discrimination score was 12%. Her tumor was approached through a suboccipital route. Surgery seemed to be going very smoothly, when her pulse suddenly stopped and blood pressure dropped to zero. Intraoperative efforts at resuscitation were unsuccessful. Autopsy revealed intracerebral hemorrhage 1 to 2 cm medial to the tumor, an area that had not been approached surgically. It was due to rapid re-expansion of the brain.

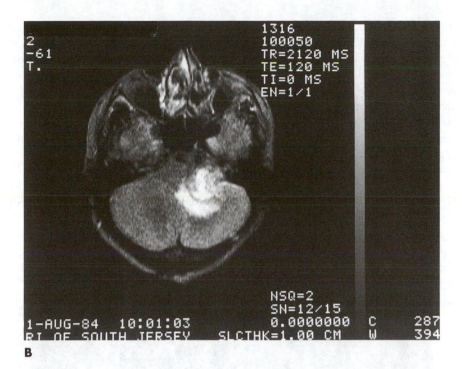

B

A few key details of operative technique help facilitate safe excision of large and giant tumors. The importance of maintaining tumor capsule integrity cannot be overemphasized, particularly with very large tumors. This is the optimal technique in most tumor resection; however, in giant tumors, it may be critical. Entry through the capsule may be performed in a moderately lateral and well visualized area. We debulk extensively, then thin the tumor within the capsule wall. Once the capsule is thin and fairly mobile, we partially bipolar cauterize the outside surface gently, allowing the capsule to shrivel up slightly. As the tumor is debulked partially, very gentle, sustained retraction of the tumor from the brainstem using broad based pressure on areas of the intact capsule may assist in tumor separation. It also is helpful to work around the different margins of the tumor in sequence in order to identify optimal tumor separation planes. Neural structures generally are so severely distorted that the usual anatomic relationships may be quite difficult to recognize. For example, the distance between the fifth nerve root entry zone and the seventh nerve entry zone may seem enormous when the brainstem is stretched and draped across a giant tumor. The basilar artery may lie twisted and almost fully exposed, with tumor lifting it away from the brainstem. One must be ever vigilant of the two planes of vasculature: the brainstem vessels and the tumor vessels. One pitfall of violation of the brainstem plane is that the vessels dive straight into the brainstem and are not bipolared readily. In this circumstance, the hole in the brainstem keeps getting deeper as the bleeding continues. Every effort should be made to avoid brainstem transgression and to minimize even "minor" brainstem surface trauma.

The suboccipital approach offers the possibility of preserving cranial nerve function (including hearing), even in selected large tumors (Strauss, Fahlbusch, Berg, & Haid, 1989). If the cranial nerves have been *pushed* by tumor capsule, rather than *encompassed* within the substance of the tumor, then they can be identified and preserved in the customary fashion. After suboccipital debulking, the remaining intracanalicular portion of tumor can be resected completely through the posterior fossa by using a drill to expose the contents of the internal auditory canal. Occasionally, in schwannomas and certain other large tumors (meningiomas) with minimal symptoms and signs, cranial nerves actually may lie within the tumor. This situation makes it less safe to use rapid debulking instruments, such as the laser or House-

Urban rotary dissector, during much of the case. Under these circumstances, it still may be possible to preserve the cranial nerves by meticulous dissection, a fraction of a millimeter at a time (Figure 14–2).

The Translabyrinthine Approach

Some surgical teams, including ours, usually would not select a translabyrinthine approach for very large tumors. However, in a

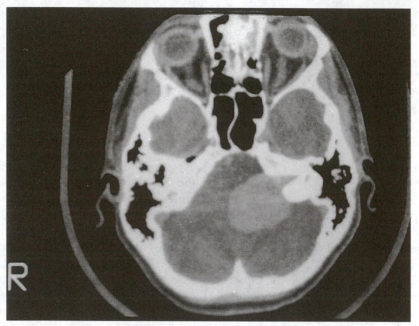

A

Figure 14–2. A. This 34-year-old white female complained of left-sided tinnitus. Her hearing was normal below 2000 Hz. At 3000 Hz, it dropped to 50 dB HL, decreasing to 65 dB HL at 8000 Hz. Discrimination was 64%, and there was a reduced vestibular response on the left side. However, all other cranial nerves were intact. The tumor was removed entirely through a suboccipital approach. The lower cranial nerves ran directly through the tumor substance. Thirteen years later, the patient has had no recurrence and has grade II/VI facial nerve function with no neurological deficits, except hearing loss, on the operated side. **B.** The cochlear nerve, prepared with Bodian stain (stains neurons, but not Schwann cells), is seen coursing uninterrupted through the substance of a neurofibroma. This is common in neurofibromas and occurs occasionally with acoustic neurons, as was the case for the patient described in Figure 14–2 A. (From *An Atlas of Micropathology of the Temporal Bone*, by F. H. Linthicum and J. A. Schwartzman, 1994, p. 75. San Diego: Singular Publishing Group. Copyright 1994 by Singular Publishing Group, Inc. Reprinted with permission.)

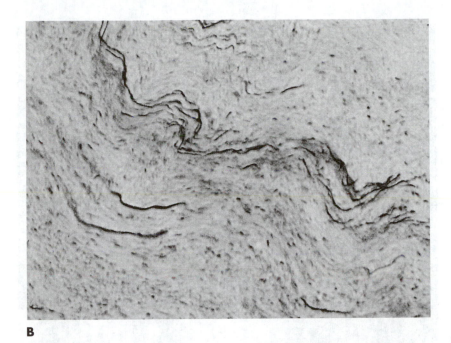

B

patient with a large, well pneumatized mastoid and a tumor that extends primarily medially, the translabyrinthine approach may provide satisfactory exposure and actually may be advantageous (Figure 14–3). For such tumors, the suboccipital approach often requires prolonged cerebellar retraction, whereas the translabyrinthine approach may require none. Any safe approach that decreases brain retraction and manipulation is likely to minimize morbidity and enhance rapid recovery. Some surgical teams have favored the translabyrinthine approach for the majority of their patients with large tumors and have reported success with this approach, even in some very large tumors (Briggs, Luxford, Atkins, & Hitselberger, 1994; Dyck, 1977). The translabyrinthine approach is discussed in detail elsewhere in this book.

The Combined Translabyrinthine— Suboccipital Approach

Combining the suboccipital and translabyrinthine approaches provides a much broad-

er exposure and better anterior visualization than the suboccipital approach alone. Crucial elements of this approach include identification of the facial nerve in the temporal bone, as well as excellent access for resection of tumor that has extended laterally into the interstices of the temporal bone. This combination of surgical approaches is a natural extension of each, and Hitselberger and House (1966a, 1966b) emphasized the value of this combined approach as early as 30 years ago. In 1979, Glasscock and Dickins (1979) reported 69 large tumors, 36 of which were managed through combined translabyrinthine/suboccipital approaches. If the size of the mastoid, position of the tumor, and shape of brainstem compression are suitable, even giant tumors may be resectable using this straightforward combined approach (Figure 14–4).

The Transcochlear Approach

The transcochlear surgical approach to the skull base was introduced in 1976 (House, De la Cruz, & Hitselberger, 1978; House &

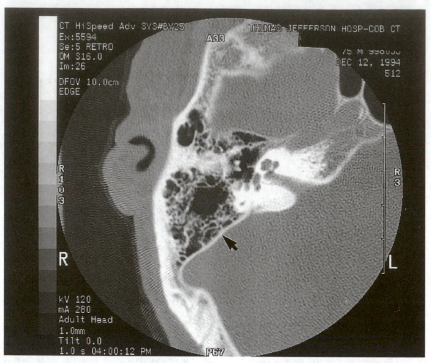

A

Figure 14–3. This 75-year-old male was discovered to have a large acoustic neuroma while he was being evaluated following a head injury. Although this patient's large tumor does not fall into "giant" category, it illustrates anatomic relationships that are particularly favorable for the selection of a translabyrinthine approach, rather than an occipital approach. **A.** CT reveals that the mastoid is adequately pneumatized. **B.** MR shows the tumor extending medially, pushing into the brain so that the cerebellum essentially is wrapped around the tumor posteriorly and laterally (*arrows*). In this case, the suboccipital approach requires considerably more cerebellar retraction, and the translabyrinthine approach represents the most direct, safe access to this large tumor. We have seen similar anatomy with considerably larger tumors, as well.

Hitselberger, 1976; Sanna, Mazzoni, Saleh, Taibah, & Russo, 1994). The technique involves an anterior extension of the translabyrinthine approach. Bone removal is carried through the cochlea to the internal carotid artery after transposing the facial nerve posteriorly (Figure 14–5). Medially, bone removal can extend into the lateral aspect of the clivus. Originally, this approach was introduced for lesions based anteriorly in the posterior fossa, such as meningiomas of the petrous tip and clivus. For some very large acoustic neuromas, it is useful to add

the transcochlear approach to a translabyrinthine or combined translabyrinthine/suboccipital exposure. This especially is helpful for tumors that extend anteriorly to the brainstem, crossing the midline at the clivus, particularly if the tumor is firm, vascular, and does not dissect or collapse easily (Figure 14–6). Combining the three approaches permits wide exposure of the posterior fossa and allows access to the anterior reaches of the posterior fossa from almost a direct, lateral perspective. When tumor has compressed the brainstem ante-

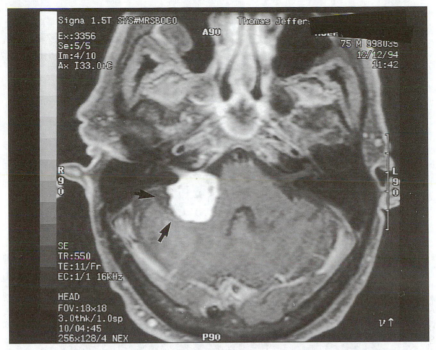

B

riorly, this approach has allowed even direct visualization into the internal auditory canal on the opposite side (Antonio De la Cruz, personal communication, 1984). Such direct access without retraction permits safe resection of tumors that often have been classified as "unresectable."

The Infratemporal Fossa Approach

The infratemporal fossa approach will not be described in detail in this chapter, because it is almost never necessary for resection of acoustic neuromas. It was designed to allow resection of anterior skull base lesions, such as clival chordoma (Fisch, 1977; Fisch, 1978; Fisch, Oldring, & Senning, 1980). However, it does provide another angle of access to the anterior portion of the posterior fossa, which conceivably could be useful in rare instances of resection of giant acoustic neuromas, and the surgical team should be skilled at this approach and prepared to use it, when appropriate.

The Translabyrinthine— Transtentorial Approach

The translabyrinthine-transtentorial combined approach to the cerebellopontine angle also is rarely needed for resection of acoustic neuromas (Figure 14–7). However, some authors have found it advantageous. The idea of approaching the posterior fossa from the middle fossa through the tentorium was reported first in 1896 (Stieglitz, Gerster, & Lilienthal, 1896). This approach was discussed again by several authors during ensuing decades (Bonnal, Louis, & Combalbert, 1964; Fay, 1930; Naffziger, 1928). Rosomoff (1971) introduced this concept in the otolaryngologic literature 25 years ago. Additional reports by Morrison and King (1973) highlighted the potential usefulness of the technique and also cited important unpublished contributions in 1965 by J.K. Henderson. The procedure combines the translabyrinthine approach with a large, middle fossa craniotomy and transtentorial approach to the posterior fos-

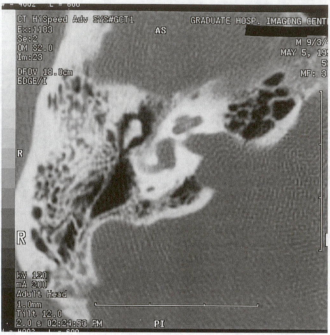

A

Figure 14–4. This 49-year-old male had undergone partial excision of a right acoustic neuroma 7 years prior to our evaluation and the imaging studies shown here. A staged removal had been planned by the neurosurgeon at that time, but the patient had refused to proceed with the second stage. Six months prior to our evaluation, he developed posterior headache aggravated by coughing and straining, rapidly worsening disequilibrium, and pulsatile tinnitus. In the few months preceding his visit with us, he also had developed difficulty holding a pen, deterioration of his penmanship, intermittent slurring of speech, deteriorating coordination of the fine movements in his right hand, and aspiration while eating. Audiogram revealed total deafness on the right and moderate-to-severe high-frequency hearing loss on the left. He had right beating nystagmus, decreased fifth nerve sensation, decreased gag sensation, decreased tenth nerve function, and normal function in the distribution of his facial and lower cranial nerves. **A.** CT scan revealed erosion of the internal auditory canal. **B, C, D,** and **E,** MR scans at several levels revealed a giant acoustic neuroma. It was removed entirely through a combined translabyrinthine-suboccipital approach. The lower cranial nerves were preserved, and tenth nerve function returned to normal. The facial nerve could not be saved, and the patient suffered a stroke (the only patient with this complication in our acoustic neuroma series), prolonging his hospitalization before he was discharged and returned home.

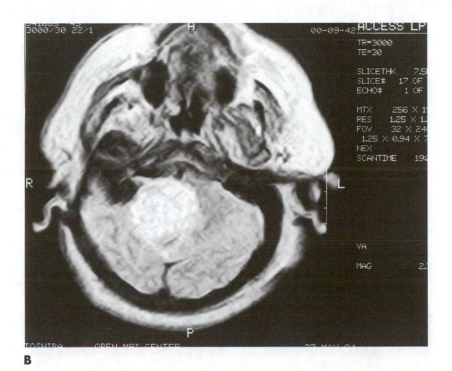

B

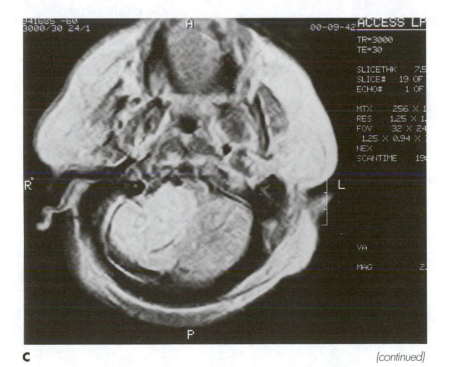

C

(continued)

Figure 14–4. *(continued)*

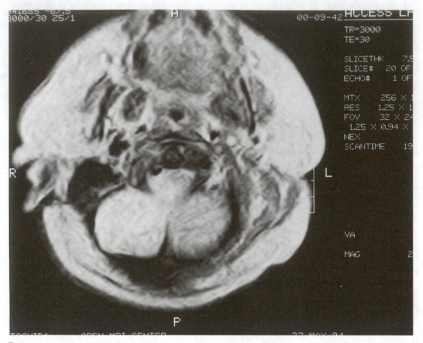

D

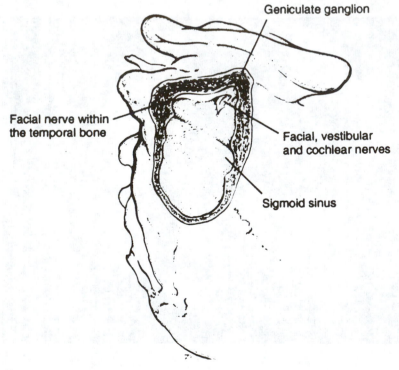

E

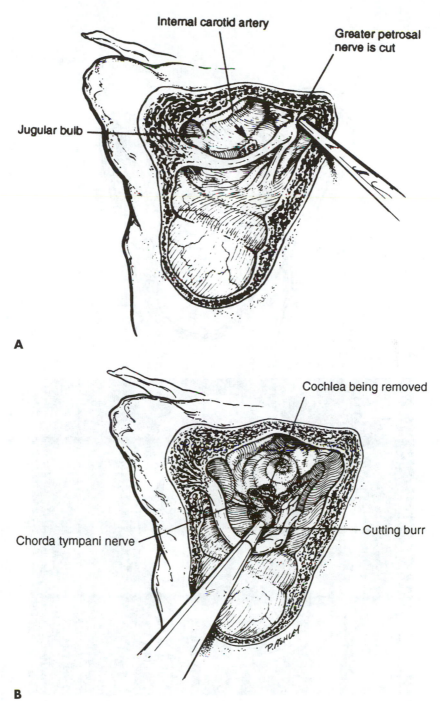

A

B

Figure 14–5. The transcochlear approach. **A.** After completing the translabyrinthine approach and entry into the internal auditory canal, the facial nerve is decompressed throughout its course, and the greater superficial petrosal nerve is divided. The external auditory canal has been removed, and the stapes (*arrow*) is visible. **B.** The facial nerve is transposed posteriorly, providing access to the cochlea, which is resected with a drill. **C.** The temporal bone is drilled away to the level of the carotid artery and eustachian tube anteriorly and the jugular bulb inferiorly, completing the transcochlear approach. The superior petrosal sinus can be seen. The posterior fossa dura then can be entered, allowing access to the anterior portion of the posterior fossa. Care must be taken to avoid the intracranial venous sinus system.

(continued)

Figure 14–5. *(continued)*

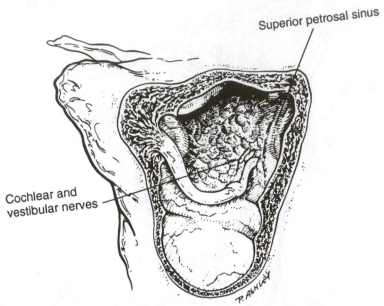

C

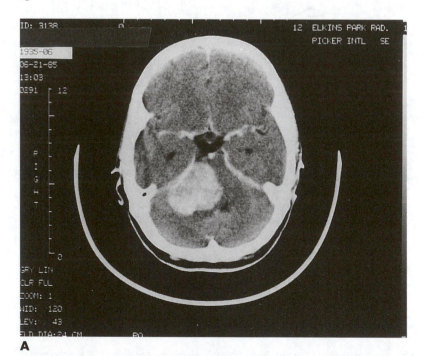

A

Figure 14–6. This 51-year-old female presented with a primary complaint of right facial numbness. She also had active chronic otitis media on the left, with a draining mastoid cavity and threshold of 80 dB HL in the speech frequencies. The hearing in her right ear was 55 dB HL at 8000 Hz, 30 dB HL at 4000 Hz, and normal below 4000 Hz. **A.** Axial MRI scan showed a large acoustic neuroma crossing the midline.

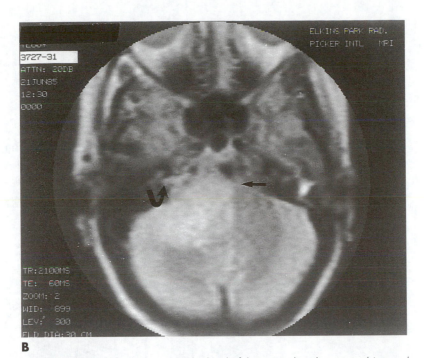

B

Figure 14–6. B. Axial scan at the level of the internal auditory canal (*curved arrow*) shows the anterior extent of the lesion across the midline (*straight arrow*).

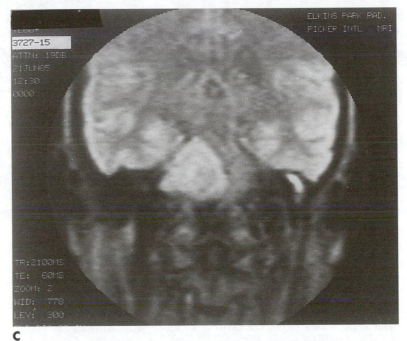

C

Figure 14–6. C. Coronal MR shows marked brainstem shift and tumor extending well across the midline. The tumor was extremely fibrous and difficult to dissect. The portion of the tumor that extended across the midline, anterior to the brainstem, required surgery in an area that could not be visualized easily through the combined translabyrinthine/sub-occipital approach alone. Adding the transcochlear perspective permitted excellent visualization. The facial nerve was paralyzed, but all other cranial nerves were preserved. She has had no recurrence in the subsequent 10 years.

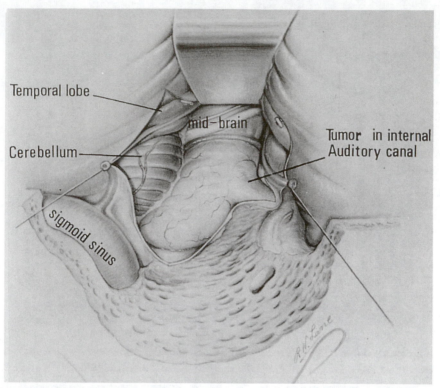

Figure 14–7. The translabyrinthine-transtentorial approach to the cerebellopontine angle. This combined middle fossa and translabyrinthine approach, with division of the superior petrosal sinus (*arrows*), provides excellent exposure of the superior and anterior portions of the tumor without significant brainstem retraction. It may be helpful for selected tumors with significant brainstem compression high in the anterolateral region of the posterior fossa or near the midline adjacent to the clivus. We have modified this approach by adding a retrosigmoid (suboccipital) craniotomy for tumors with much greater posterior extent than the one illustrated here. (From Experiences with a translabyrinthine-transtentional approach to the cerebellopontine angle, by A.W. Morrison and T.T. King, 1973, *Journal of Neurosurgery, 38,* p. 386. Copyright 1973 by American Association of Neurological Surgeons. Reprinted with permission.)

sa. Retracting the temporal lobe and entering the posterior fossa from above permits excellent access to tumors that compress or adhere to the tentorium and parts of the anterior portion of the posterior fossa. The technique also may facilitate facial nerve preservation (Tator & Nedzelski, 1982). We have extended this technique, combining it with a suboccipital craniotomy, and we have found that it provides extraordinary exposure and control. We have used it primarily for meningiomas and total temporal bone resection for carcinoma. We uncommonly have found it to be necessary in the resection of even giant acoustic neuromas

but, for some tumors, it may be helpful (Figures 14–8 and 14–9).

The Combined Suboccipital-Midline Transvermis-Transventricular Approach: A New Technique

Occasionally, tumors are so large or inconveniently positioned that none of the published surgical approaches will suffice. Under these circumstances, the surgeons must depend on their knowledge of anatomy, understanding of tumor location and biology,

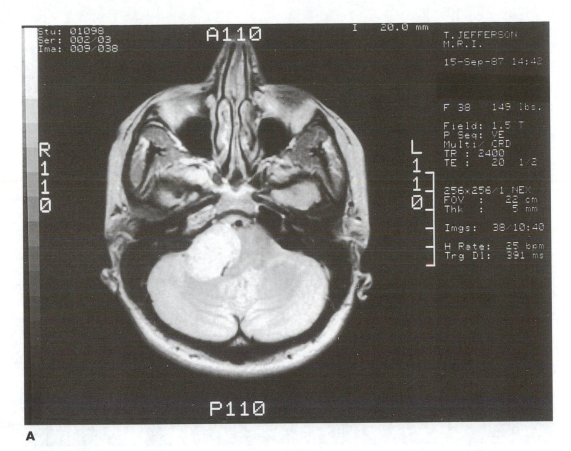

A

Figure 14–8. Axial (**A** and **B**) and coronal, **C**, MR scans of a large acoustic neuroma extending across the midline. It also extends anteriorly in the posterior fossa to approach the clivus. In addition, the coronal section reveals that the neuroma is in contact with the tentorium and is compressing the brainstem at a relatively high level. At the time of presentation, this 37-year-old female had a 6-year history of right facial numbness, a 1-year history of mild hearing loss, and a 1-month history of tinnitus. In this setting, combining the transtentorial and posterior fossa approaches enhances visibility and tumor access and minimizes the need for retraction.

(continued)

and creative imagination. In fact, these principles led to the development of all of the aforementioned approaches. In 1993, we encountered a patient with such a tumor (Figure 14–10). We currently are preparing a paper on this approach (unique, to the best of our knowledge), and this chapter represents an initial discussion of our experience combining lateral and midline approaches. The 37-year-old female who led us to this procedure had undergone partial tumor removal at another institution, complicated by stroke and injury to cranial nerves VI through XII. She still had an extremely large tumor that extended medially into the brainstem and also protruded into the fourth ventricle. In order to resect this tumor safely, we began by reopening the original, large, lateral suboccipital approach, having prepared to add a midline approach, if necessary. Extensive dense scar made it quite dangerous to try to develop dissection planes. It was not possible even to access the central part of this tumor without risking unacceptable

Figure 14–8. *(continued)*

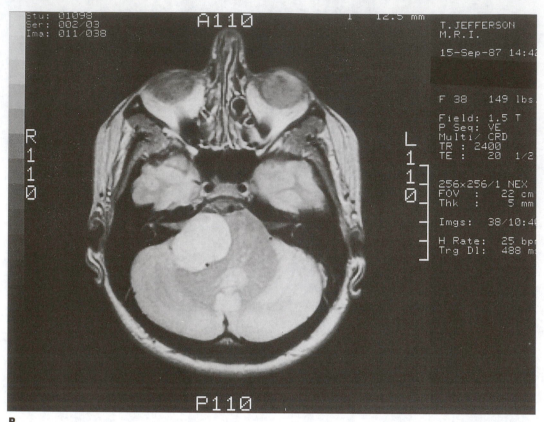

B

trauma to the deep cerebellar nuclei. Consequently, we made a second incision in the midline, removed the arch of the first cervical vertebra (CI), performed a craniectomy, opened the cisterna magna, opened the vermis, and entered the fourth ventricle. The tumor was visible immediately on the floor of the lateral recess of the fourth ventricle. Under direct vision, the tumor capsule was entered directly, then debulked with the laser centrally. As the tumor shrank under the effects of the laser, it then was dissected from the fourth ventricle and elevated away from the brainstem through the fourth ventricle. Using this approach, we were able to clearly visualize the tumor capsule and, working from the outside of the capsule, we were able to dissect it safely and

entirely from the brainstem and deliver it into the region of the suboccipital exposure. Thus, we were able to remove the tumor in its entirety. Had the cranial nerves not been injured already, we are confident that we would have been able to preserve them using this approach. MR has confirmed that the patient is free of tumor 2½ years following surgery, and she has no additional morbidity or neurological deficit from our procedure.

CONCLUSIONS

Extremely large acoustic neuromas present imposing surgical challenges. These tumors are not "inoperable." They do not require

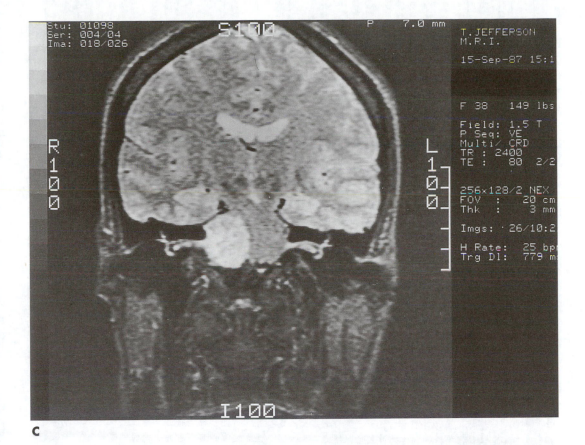

C

only partial resection, nor do they mandate significant postoperative neurological deficit. However, performance of these strenuous and demanding procedures does require full and complete neurotological and neurosurgical collaboration, as well as total commitment of the surgeons during the operative procedure. In most cases, surgical procedures are not substantially prolonged. However, the entire medical team (especially the patient) must be prepared fully for lengthy operating times. Experience with prolonged procedures has shown that they can be carried out safely and may permit resection of very large acoustic neuromas without cranial nerve sacrifice and without the problems associated with planned residual tumor or the risks of repeated surgical procedures. Hearing preservation has not proven practical. However, permanent facial

injury usually can be avoided, and damage to other cranial nerves should be uncommon, even when operating upon the largest of tumors. It generally is possible to completely resect even giant acoustic neuromas with acceptable morbidity and low mortality.

REFERENCES

Bonnal, J., Louis, R., & Combalbert, A. (1964). L'abord temporal transtentorial de l'angle ponto-cérébelleux et du clivus. *Neurochirurgie, 10,* 3–12.

Briggs, R.J., Luxford, W.M., Atkins, J.S., Jr., & Hitselberger, W.E. (1994). Translabyrinthine removal of large acoustic neuromas. *Neurosurgery, 34,* 785–790.

Desgeorges, M., & Sterkers, J.M. (1984). La chirurgie des gros neurinomes de l'acoustic operes uniquement par voie translabyrin-thique. A propos de 50 cas. *Neurochirurgie, 30,* 355–364.

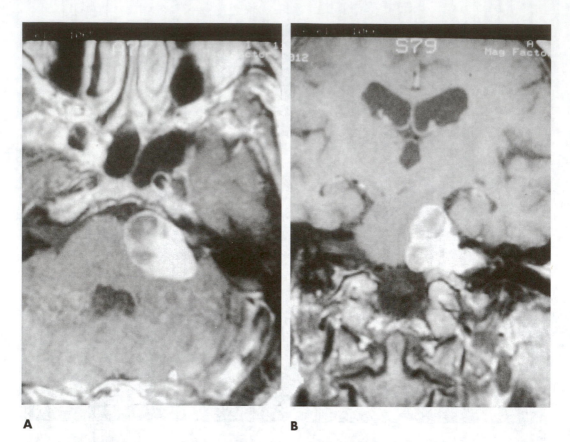

A

B

Figure 14–9. The 51-year-old male whose tumor is pictured here also is well suited for the combined translabyrinthine-transtentorial approach. Like the patient whose tumor is pictured in Figure 14–8, axial **A.** MR shows the tumor extending fairly far into the anterior portion of the posterior fossa. The tumor also extends medially, compressing the brain, so that there is cerebellum directly lateral to the tumor. A suboccipital approach would require substantial cerebellar retraction, which can be avoided almost entirely through a translabyrinthine approach. The transtentorial component improves visibility, assists in easy removal of the anterior extension of the tumor, and provides easier access to the superior portion of the tumor seen on the coronal image **B.** Certainly, many similar tumors can be removed with a translabyrinthine or suboccipital approach alone. However, the transtentorial approach should be kept in mind when visibility is limited or dissection is difficult, especially when there is extensive anterior tumor involvement. The wide decompression and visibility is especially helpful for tumors that are based fairly high in the anterior portion of the posterior fossa, but the transcochlear approach may be better for tumors that approach the foramen magnum at or across the midline. Such anatomically difficult tumors are not infrequent.

Dyck, P. (1977). Peduncular hemiplagia following removal of large cerebellopontine angle tumors: Discussion of a mechanism of brain stem injury. *Bulletin of the Los Angeles Neurological Society, 42,* 8–15.

Fay, T. (1930). The management of tumors of the posterior fossa by a transtentorial approach. *Surgical Clinics of North America, 10,* 1427–1459.

Fisch, U. (1977). Infratemporal approach for extensive tumors of the temporal bone and base of skull. In H. Silverstein & H. Norell (Eds.), *Neurological surgery of the ear* (pp. 34–53). Birmingham: Aesculapius Publishing.

Fisch, U. (1978). Infratemporal fossa approach to tumors of the temporal bone and base of the skull. *Journal of Laryngology and Otology, 92,* 949–967.

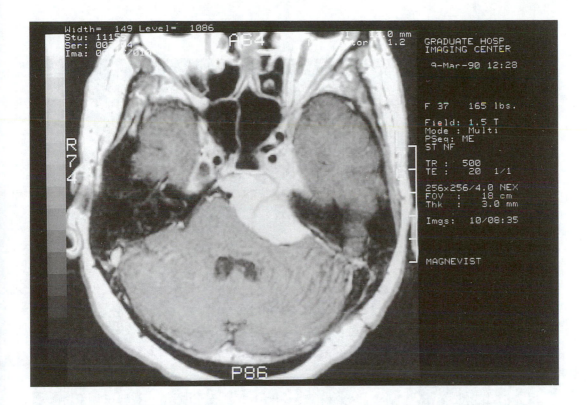

C

Figure 14–9. For example, **C.** (*axial*) and **D.** (*coronal*) images show tumor extending anteriorly across the midline on another patient, a 37-year-old female. These images were taken at the time of our initial examination, 3 years after the tumor had been excised partially by another surgeon.   *(continued)*

Fisch, U., Oldring, D.J., & Senning, A. (1980). Surgical therapy of internal carotid artery lesions of the skull base and temporal bone. *Archives of Otolaryngology—Head and Neck Surgery, 88,* 548–554.

Glasscock, M.E., & Dickins, J.R.E. (1977). Cerebellopontine angle tumors: Results of the combined translabyrinthine–suboccipital approach. In H. Silverstein & H. Norell (Eds.), *Neurological surgery of the ear* (Vol. 2, pp. 260–261). Birmingham: Aesculapius Publishing.

Hitselberger, W.E., & House, W.F. (1966a). A combined approach to the cerebellopontine angle. *Archives of Otolaryngology, 84,* 49–67.

Hitselberger, W.E., & House, W.F. (1966b). Surgical approaches to acoustic tumors. *Archives of Otolaryngology, 84,* 68–73.

House, W.F., & Hitselberger, W.E. (1976). The transcochlear approach to the skull base. *Archives of Otolaryngology, 102,* 334–342.

House, W.F., De la Cruz, A., & Hitselberger, W.E. (1978). Surgery of the skull base: Transcochlear

Figure 14–9. *(continued)*

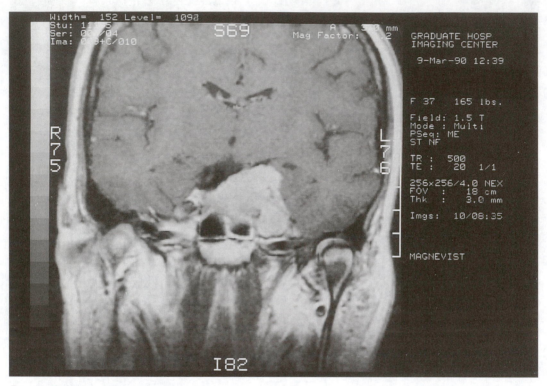

D

approach to the petrous apex and clivus. *Otolaryngology, 86,* 770–779.

Jaaskelainen, J., Paetu, A., Pyykko, I., Blomstedt, G., Palva, T., & Trouup, H. (1994). Interface between the facial nerve and large acoustic neurinomas. Immunohistochemical study of the cleavage plane in NF2 and non-NF2 cases. *Journal of Neurosurgery, 80,* 541–547.

Morrison, A.W., & King, T.T. (1973). Experiences with a translabyrinthine—transtentorial approach to the cerebellopontine angle. *Journal of Neurosurgery, 38,* 382–390.

Naffziger, H.C. (1928). Brain surgery with special reference to exposure of the brain stem and posterior fossa; the principle of intracranial decompression, and the relief of impactions in the posterior fossa. *Surgery, Gynecology, and Obstetrics, 46,* 241–248.

Rosomoff, H.L. (1971). The subtemporal transtentorial approach to the cerebellopontine angle. *Laryngoscope, 81,* 1448–1454.

Sanna, M., Mazzoni, A., Saleh, E.A., Taibah, A.K., & Russo, A. (1994). Lateral approaches to the median skull base through the petrous

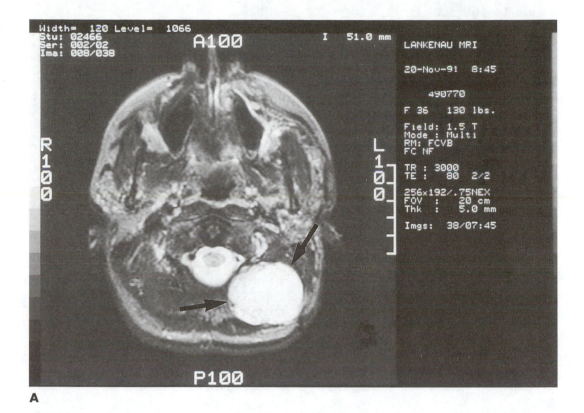

A

Figure 14–10. This 37-year-old female presented 1 year and 8 months following acoustic neuroma surgery, during which she had suffered a stroke and permanent injury to cranial nerves VI through XII. **A.** The anatomic consequences of her stroke were obvious on MR (*arrows*). **B, C,** and **D.** MR views at several levels revealed an extensive tumor crossing the midline and extending laterally toward the carotid artery **B.** Tumor invasion into the fourth ventricle was obvious on axial (**E**) and coronal (**F**) images (*arrows*). The tumor was removed in its entirety through a combined suboccipital-midline/ transvermis/transventricular approach. The patient has had no recurrence in the subsequent 2½ years. *(continued)*

bone: The system of the modified transcochlear approach. *Journal of Laryngology and Otology, 108,* 1036–1044.

Sataloff, R.T., Fratalli, M.A., & Myers, D.L. (1995). Intracranial facial neuromas: Total tumor removal with facial nerve preservation: A new surgical technique. *ENT Journal, 74,* 244–256.

Stieglitz, L., Gerster, A.G., & Lilienthal, H. (1896). A study of three cases of tumor of the brain in which operation was performed:

One recovery, two deaths. *American Journal of Medical Science, 111,* 509–531.

Strauss, C., Fahlbusch, R., Berg, M., & Haid, T. (1989). Funktionserhaltende mikrochirurgie bei der suboccipitalen entfernung grosser akustikusneurinome. *Hals-Nase-Ohren, 37,* 281–286.

Tator, C.H., & Nedzelski, J.M. (1982). Facial nerve preservation in patients with large acoustic neuromas treated by a combined middle fossa transtentorial translabyrinthine approach. *Journal of Neurosurgery, 57,* 1–7.

Figure 14–10. *(continued)*

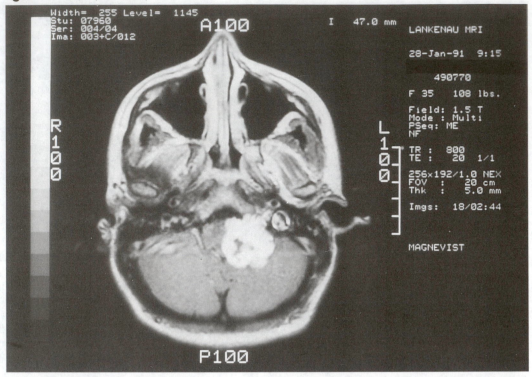

B

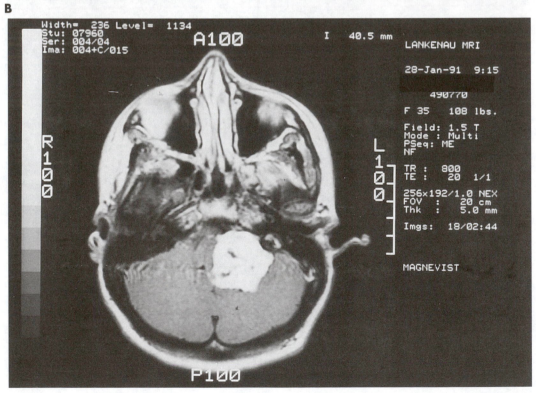

B

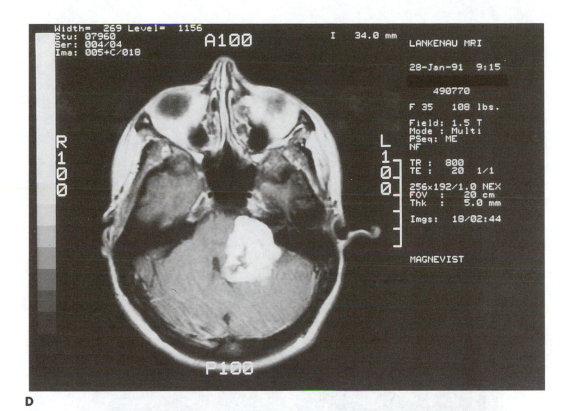

D

E

(continued)

Figure 14–10. *(continued)*

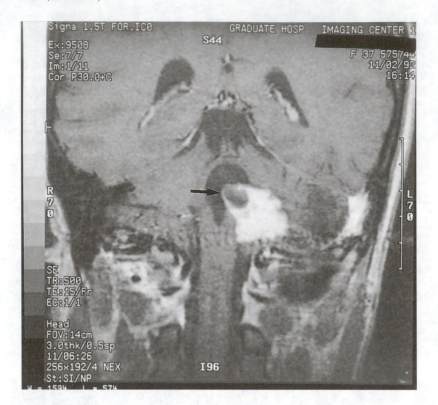

F

CHAPTER 15

Intraoperative Cranial Nerve Monitoring

P. Gerard Reilly F.R.C.S.Ed.(ORL)
Anil K. Lalwani, M.D.
Charles D. Yingling, Ph.D.

The application of microsurgical techniques to acoustic neuroma surgery has led to a steady decrease in the mortality and morbidity associated with the procedure. One factor that has helped to decrease the morbidity associated with postsurgical facial nerve palsy is intraoperative cranial nerve monitoring. Hearing conservation also can be attempted with more confidence using intraoperative auditory brainstem response (ABR) monitoring.

Cranial nerve stimulation during posterior fossa surgery first was conducted in 1894 by Krause, who performed a cochlear nerve section for tinnitus and noted that unipolar faradic stimulation of the facial nerve trunk led to contraction of the ipsilateral facial musculature (Krause, 1912). However, Frazier (1912) was the first to point out that this phenomenon could be used to identify the position of the facial nerve. Initially, a basic procedure was used during which an observer, often the anesthesiologist, was asked to look for movement of the facial muscula-

ture on stimulation of the nerve trunk. A significant advance was introduced by Delgado in 1975, when he reported use of facial nerve electromyography (Delgado, Buchheit, Rosenholtz, & Chrissian, 1979). The use of facial nerve monitoring to reduce the morbidity of acoustic neuroma surgery has been well documented and now is standard practice in most centers (Jellinek, Tan, & Symon, 1991; Lalwani, Butt, Jackler, Pitts, & Yingling, 1994).

Other cranial nerves also can be monitored during surgery. These include the cochlear nerve (by observing the auditory brainstem responses), the motor component of the trigeminal nerve, and the lower cranial nerves.

INSTRUMENTATION

The basic requirements for successful motor cranial nerve monitoring are a stimulator that preferably can provide a constant voltage that can be adjusted precisely at levels from 0–2 V, a low noise amplifier that is capable of amplifying microvolt level signals, an oscilloscope, and an audio monitor. The latter should be fitted with a squelch circuit to mute the output during use of electrocautery. Commercial devices are available or they can be custom-made. The latter include the advantages of being able to be fitted with as many channels as necessary, and they can be calibrated exactly according to needs. The authors prefer a six-channel system with amplifiers and stimulator (Grass, Quincy, Mass.), an oscilloscope (Tektronix, Beaverton, Ore.), and a custom-built audiomonitor (see Figures 15–1 and 15–2).

Auditory brainstem responses can be measured using an averaging computer with high gain, low noise electroencephalogram (EEG) amplifiers, and an acoustic stimulus generator that can be programmed to deliver clicks of calibrated intensity at controlled polarity and known, adjustable repetition rates. Most commercially available ABR equipment is suitable for these needs. The best method for delivering sound to the ear is through a short, plastic tube extending from an earphone placed away from the ear. The resulting acoustic delay separates any electrical stimulus artifact from the response. The tube is terminated with a foil-covered sponge that is inserted into the ear canal and that provides an acoustic seal against extraneous noise. This sponge also serves as one of the recording electrodes for the ABR.

A variety of electrodes is necessary for stimulation and recording during monitoring. Recording can be conducted using either needle or surface electrodes. Needle electrodes have the advantages of being re-

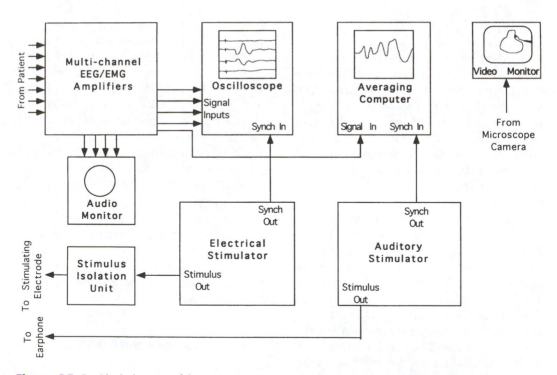

Figure 15–1. Block diagram of the monitoring circuitry used in intraoperative cranial nerve monitoring during acoustic neuroma surgery. (From *Neurotology*, by R. K. Jackler and D.E. Brackmann (Eds.), 1994, p. 971. St. Louis: Mosby. Copyright 1994 by Mosby-Yearbook, Inc. Reprinted with permission.)

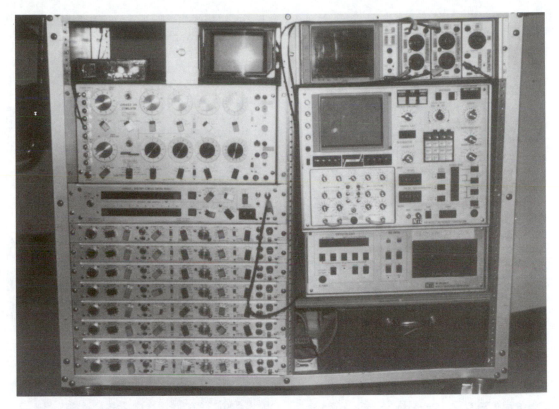

Figure 15–2. The custom-built multichannel EMG and ABR monitoring system used at the University of California at San Francisco (UCSF) for intraoperative cranial nerve monitoring during acoustic neuroma surgery. (Left, top to bottom) Audio and video monitors, dual-channel electrical stimulator, acoustic stimulator, and eight EEG amplifiers. (Right) Multichannel storage oscilloscope, averaging computer, disk drive for averaging computer, and storage drawer. (From *Neurotology* by R. K. Jackler and D.E. Brackmann (Eds.), 1994, p. 971. St. Louis: Mosby. Copyright 1994 by Mosby-Yearbook, Inc. Reprinted with permission.)

liable and easy to use, and, unlike surface electrodes, they are not susceptible to a gradual change in impedance over time (Bankaitis & Keith, 1993). For these reasons, needle electrodes generally have supplanted the use of surface electrodes, which have the disadvantage of being more prone to artifact. For facial nerve monitoring, two channels typically are used, with one pair of electrodes inserted into the orbicularis oculi muscle and a more distantly located pair inserted into the orbicularis oris. Monitoring the motor component of the trigeminal nerve requires insertion of electrodes into the masseter or temporalis muscles. The accessory nerve can be monitored via an electrode inserted in the trapezius muscle or, occasionally, in the sternomastoid muscle, if there is wasting of the trapezius, providing a marker for the location of the jugular foramen complex (see Figure 15–3).

The polarity of a stimulating electrode can be either unipolar or bipolar. Theoretically, a bipolar electrode should offer more specificity and precision but, in practice, this is not the case, because these attributes depend on the orientation of the electrode with respect to the long axis of the nerve when stimulation occurs. A monopolar electrode is less bulky than a bipolar electrode and is the preferred choice in the limited

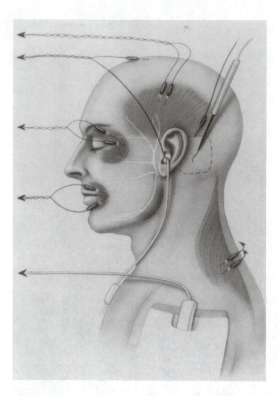

Figure 15–3. A diagrammatic representation of electrode placement for monitoring during acoustic neuroma surgery with attempted hearing preservation. Pairs of electrodes are placed in the following muscles: temporalis (CN V3M), orbicularis oris and orbicularis oculi (VII), and trapezius (XI). Click stimuli from a small transducer on the chest are fed through plastic tubing into the ipsilateral ear through a foil-covered sponge insert. This insert also serves as a recording electrode that is referred to a needle electrode on the forehead or vertex. An electrocautery ground pad is placed on the arm as a signal ground. A flexible-tip probe is used to stimulate cranial motor nerves, with a needle electrode as the stimulator ground placed in the margin of the craniotomy. (Redrawn from "Acoustic Neuroma," by R.K. Jackler and L.K. Pitts, 1990, *Neurosurgical Clinics of North America, 1,* pp. 199–223. Copyright 1990 by W. B. Saunders Company. Adapted with permission.)

Treace), (see Figure 15–4). The end of the probe can be angled and used to probe within dissection planes or on the medial surface of the tumor away from direct vision, thus aiding in the identification of the site of the nerve before it can be seen directly.

Unfortunately, the operating room (OR) is an electronically hostile environment, with many sources of interference. Every effort must be made to reduce 60 Hz interference, as well as electronic noise from the operating room equipment, such as the suc-

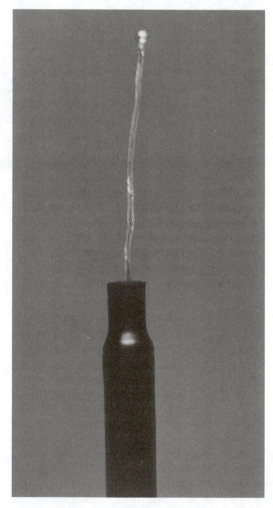

Figure 15–4. Flexible-tip probe used for intracranial stimulation. The entire probe and flexible wire are insulated from the 0.5 mm ball at the distal end. This allows accurate localization of stimulation.

space available during acoustic neuroma surgery. Several types of unipolar electrode are available. The authors use a probe with a flexible platinum-iridium tip that is insulated from a 0.5-mm ball on the end (Xomed-

tion apparatus, electrocautery instrumentation, the anesthesia machines, and the operating table controls. Elimination or at least reduction of interference may be possible by grounding the equipment, rerouting cables, or plugging the cables into a different outlet. It also is important to ensure that the patient is grounded adequately to the recording apparatus. An electrocautery ground pad can be adapted easily to this purpose and is very effective.

Identification and elimination of artifacts that can arise at any time during a case is entrusted best to an experienced neurophysiologist, audiologist, or other professional who is trained specifically in intraoperative monitoring. Successful monitoring cannot be accomplished by simply bringing another piece of equipment into the operating room. Failure to recognize and correct technical problems or identify true EMG activity correctly (which can occur simultaneously with non-EMG artifacts) can lead to a false sense of security, which may be worse than no monitoring at all.

MONITORING TECHNIQUES

Motor Nerves

Monitoring of motor cranial nerve activity includes the following: (a) monitoring of ongoing activity to check for increases that may represent irritation of the nerve due to intraoperative events, such as retraction, cautery, dissection, and so on (Figure 15–5); (b) identification of nerves by evoking activity in the nerve by intracranial stimulation; (c) assessing integrity of a nerve at the end of a procedure using evoked EMG methods. In acoustic neuroma surgery, we routinely monitor the motor division of the trigeminal nerve, two independent channels for the facial nerve, and the accessory nerve. If hearing conservation is being attempted, the cochlear nerve is monitored.

Near the beginning of the procedure, it is important to check the integrity of the system to avoid false-positive and false-negative results. This is done either by stimulating the facial nerve in its vertical segment in the mastoid during translabyrinthine craniotomy or by stimulating the accessory nerve after retrosigmoid craniotomy and confirming an EMG response. Dissection then proceeds, approaching the tumor. In the presence of a small tumor, the facial nerve usually can be identified relatively easily and the threshold established. Subsequent sweeping or probing of the tumor surface then is carried out at approximately three times the threshold value, up to 1 V. In the presence of larger tumors, the facial nerve usually is obscured by the tumor. Electrical stimulation is begun at 0.3 V. If there is no response at this level, the voltage is increased to 0.5 V, then 1 V. If there still is no response, it is assumed that the facial nerve is not in the immediate vicinity, and dissection is continued. When the facial nerve is thought to be identified, its presence can be confirmed. At the end of the surgical procedure, nerve thresholds can be obtained in the internal auditory canal and brainstem to check the integrity of the nerve. Other nerves in the surgical field can be identified and monitored in a similar way.

Cochlear Nerve

During procedures involving hearing conservation, auditory brainstem responses can be used to check the integrity of the cochlear nerve both during and at the end of the procedure. Most clinical ABR systems are easily adaptable for use in the operating room, although standard earphones must be replaced by a tube connected to an earphone located some distance from the ear so as not to compromise the operative field, as previously described. The technique of auditory brainstem response recording for the purpose of intraoperative monitoring of the cochlear nerve is similar to that used in diagnostic testing. However, the stimuli used for eliciting the ABR intraoperatively are delivered at higher rates (20–30/s) in or-

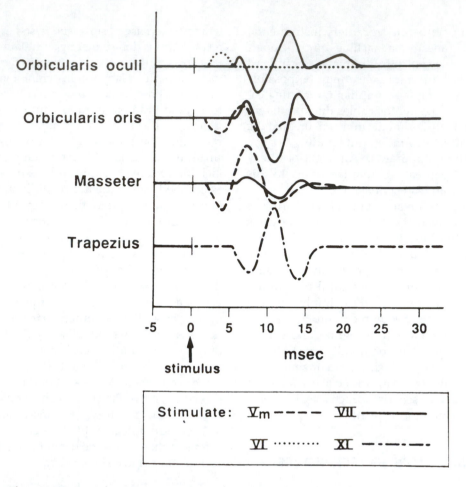

Figure 15–5. Schematic representation of responses obtained using four-channel montage (as depicted in Figures 15–1 and 15–2) with intracranial stimulation of cranial nerves (CN) Vm, VI, VII, and XI. Despite crosstalk between the CN V and VII channels, these nerves can be distinguished clearly by the shorter latency of responses to Vm stimulation. Stimulation of CN VI produces a short-latency response that is localized to the orbicularis oculi channel, due to volume conduction from the nearby lateral rectus. Responses to CN XI stimulation are restricted to the trapezius channel. (From "Acoustic Neuroma," by R.K. Jackler and L.K. Pitts, 1990, *Neurosurgical Clinics of North America, 1*, pp. 199–223. Copyright 1990 by W. B. Saunders Company. Reprinted with permission.)

der to reduce the averaging time and, thus, reduce the lag period between initiating the test and achieving a result. It is important to be aware that the ABR may not be normal in patients with acoustic tumors, but it usually is possible to obtain clear definition of wave I. An alternative to ABR recording is to measure evoked potentials from the cochlear nucleus by inserting an electrode into the lateral recess of the fourth ventricle prior to tumor removal. Because these recordings have larger amplitudes that ABR recordings, fewer stimuli are required, with consequent reduction in the length of time needed to establish whether the nerve is under threat of damage (Møller, Jho, & Jannetta, 1994).

ANESTHETIC CONSIDERATIONS

Motor Nerves

At any time when cranial nerves other than the cochlear nerve are being monitored, it is important that no neuromuscular blocking agents are present, because even low levels will affect the EMG and, in particular, the small amplitude signals associated with mechanical manipulation may be missed (Kartush & Bouchard, 1992). It has been shown that this is particularly true of the chronically injured facial nerve in an animal model (Blair, Teeple, Sutherland, Shih, & Chen, 1994).

If lidocaine injection is used, it must be remembered that it is possible to anesthetize the facial nerve inadvertently at the stylomastoid foramen. This obviously invalidates further attempts at facial nerve monitoring. Because the local anesthetic usually is a vehicle for delivery of epinephrine to aid hemostasis, it has been suggested that epinephrine 1:100,000 alone may be used (Jones & Mellert, 1991).

Cochlear Nerve

The auditory brainstem responses are not known to be affected by pharmacologic influences, but they may be affected by nonspecific influences, such as cerebrospinal fluid drainage and core temperature (Lenarz & Ernst, 1992). Therefore, normal brain temperature must be maintained. Another factor that may affect the ABR is the craniotomy itself, which may allow new pathways for current flow and physical changes in the cochlear nerve (e.g., sequelae, due to the exposure to air). These conditions are not clinically significant, but they can affect the recordings. Thus, it is important to obtain an intraoperative baseline after the craniotomy and placement of retractors, rather than rely on the baseline obtained before the commencement of the procedure.

SURGICAL OUTCOME

Facial Nerve

Acoustic neuroma surgery is now a relatively safe procedure with very few mortalities. We now are at the stage where we can turn our attention to further reduction of the associated morbidity.

Postoperative facial nerve function is of great concern to the patient who undergoes excision of acoustic neuroma. Intraoperative facial nerve monitoring is of great benefit in reducing this particular aspect of morbidity. Several studies have compared facial nerve outcome, with and without facial nerve monitoring. During the infratemporal approach to the skull base, requiring rerouting of the facial nerve, Leonetti, Brackmann, and Prass (1989) compared the results from 20 cases in which facial nerve monitoring was used with the results from 31 cases in which facial nerve monitoring was not used. Immediate postoperative facial function was normal in 93% of the monitored group, compared with only 70% in the unmonitored group. In addition, 48% of the unmonitored group had grade 5 or 6 facial paresis, whereas none of the monitored group fell into this category. Niparko, Kileny, Kemink, Lee, and Graham (1989) compared facial nerve outcome after translabyrinthine removal of acoustic neuroma in 29 monitored cases versus 75 unmonitored cases. For tumors larger than 2 cm, a statistically significant association was found between monitoring and satisfactory long-term facial nerve outcome. For smaller tumors, a nonsignificant trend for improved facial nerve outcome was seen with monitoring. Harner, Daube, Beatty, and Ebersold (1988) compared 91 consecutive acoustic neuroma removals using intraoperative cranial nerve monitoring with an unmonitored control group of 91 patients selected from a pool of 173 cases to match the monitored group in tumor size, most recent year of operation, and age of the patient. The difference in facial nerve preservation rate (92% in the monitored group and 84% in the unmonitored group) was not statistically significant between the two groups. However, at 1 year postoperatively, grade 1 facial function was present in 45% of the monitored cases versus 27% of the unmonitored cases, and this difference was statistically significant. In addition, 6% of the unmonitored group had grade 6 facial function at one year, whereas only 2% of the unmonitored group had facial paralysis as severe. Data presented by Yingling (1994), based on a review of over 1,000 published cases of acoustic neuroma surgery with and without facial nerve monitoring and with at least 6 months follow-up, showed that the incidence of severe facial palsy (House/Brackmann Grades V or VI) dropped from 12% to 4% with the addition of cranial nerve monitoring. Improvements in the outcomes shown in these series may be simply the result of greater experience on the part of the surgeon, because most of the monitored cases were performed subsequent to the unmonitored cases. However, intraoperative monitoring may have contributed to the technical skills necessary for acoustic neuroma removal, while preserving cranial nerves. Lalwani, Butt, Jackler, Pitts, and Yingling, (1994) reported facial nerve outcome after acoustic neuroma removal in a series of 129 patients. They showed that it is possible to predict long-term facial function by using facial nerve stimulation at the end of the removal of acoustic neuromas. They assessed the voltage required to reach facial nerve threshold. Their data suggest that, if the facial EMG can be evoked with a proximal seventh nerve stimulation of 0.2 V or less, prognosis for grade 1 or 2 facial nerve function at 1 year is excellent. However, these results were not predictive of facial nerve function in the immediate postoperative period. This ability for prediction of long-term facial nerve function is useful in preoperative discussions of anticipated results and potential complications.

Cochlear Nerve

It is difficult to provide a consensus opinion on the usefulness of cochlear nerve monitoring in acoustic tumor surgery due to several factors. First, there is a great deal of variation in the definition of useful hearing postoperatively. Some authors have defined hearing preservation as any useful speech discrimination or pure tone thresholds better than 70 dB HL between 0.5 and 2.0 kHz (Nadol, Ojemann, Martuza, Montgomery, & Klevens de Sandoval, 1987) while others require pure tone thresholds better than 50 dB HL and word recognition scores of better than 50% (Kanzaki, Kunihiro, D-Uchi, Shiobara, & Toya, 1991).

Second, it is difficult to compare groups of patients who have differing presurgical hearing status and different tumor size. The studies that have reported hearing conservation after excision of tumors less than 2 cm in size have shown hearing preservation rates of 30% to 45% (Kanzaki, Ogawa, & Toya, 1989; Nadol, et al., 1987). However, it is noteworthy that, in Baldwin, King, and Morrison's 1990 series, in which they described results of posterior fossa approaches to 44 acoustic neuromas of less than 2 cm, there was anatomical preservation of the cochlear nerve in 26 cases, but only 14 of those had mean pure-tone thresholds of 50 dB HL, or word recognition scores better than 50%.

FUTURE TRENDS

It is likely that, in the next few years, we will see significant improvement in equipment for intraoperative cranial nerve monitoring in the form of integrated compact packages. These systems will have better artifact rejection with on-line digital filters and automated control of stimulation and recording parameters.

Large-scale controlled studies will lead to a better understanding of the relationship of intraoperative recording patterns and clinical outcome. These developments ultimately will lead to an improved outcome in terms of morbidity for patients undergoing surgical removal of acoustic neuroma.

REFERENCES

Baldwin, D.L., King, T.T., & Morrison, A.W. (1990). Hearing conservation in acoustic neuroma surgery via the posterior fossa. *Journal of Laryngology and Otology, 104,* 463–467.

Bankaitis, A.E., & Keith, R.W. (1993). Cranial nerve monitoring beyond the facial and auditory nerves. *Seminars in Hearing, 14,* 163–171.

Blair, E.A., Teeple, E., Jr., Sutherland, R.M., Shih, T., & Chen, D. (1994). Effect of neuromuscular blockade on facial nerve monitoring. *American Journal of Otology, 15,* 161–167.

Delgado, T.E., Buchheit, W.A., Rosenholtz, H.R., & Chrissian, S. (1979). Intraoperative monitoring of facial muscle evoked responses obtained by intracranial stimulation of the facial nerve: A more accurate technique for facial nerve dissection. *Neurosurgery, 4,* 418–421.

Frazier, C.H. (1912). Intracranial division of the auditory nerve for persistent aural vertigo. *Surgery, Gynecology and Obstetrics, 15,* 524–529.

Harner, S.G., Daube, J.R., Beatty, C.W., & Ebersold, M.J. (1988). Intraoperative monitoring of the facial nerve *Laryngoscope, 98,* 209–212.

Jellinek, D.A., Tan, L.C., & Symon, L. (1991). The impact of continuous electrophysiological monitoring on preservation of the facial nerve during acoustic tumor surgery. *British Journal of Neurosurgery, 5,* 19–24.

Jones, R., & Mellert, T. (1991). Use of dilute epinephrine as an aid in facial nerve monitoring. *American Journal of Otology, 12,* 446–449.

Kanzaki, J., Kunihiro, T., D-Uchi, T., Shiobara, R., & Toya, S. (1991). Preservation of facial nerve function in acoustic neuroma surgery by the extended middle fossa approach. *Acta Otolaryngologica, 487*(Suppl.) 36–40.

Kartush, J., & Bouchard, K. (1992). Intraoperative facial nerve monitoring. In J. Kartush & K. Bouchard (Eds.), *Neuromonitoring in otology and head and neck surgery* (pp. 99–120). New York: Raven Press.

Krause, F. (1912). *Surgery of the brain and spinal cord.* New York: Rebman.

Lalwani, A.K., Butt, F.Y., Jackler, R.K., Pitts, L.H., & Yingling, C.D. (1994). Facial nerve outcomes after acoustic neuroma surgery study from the era of cranial nerve monitoring. *Otolaryngology—Head and Neck Surgery, 111,* 561–570.

Lenarz, T., & Ernst, A. (1992). Intraoperative monitoring by transtympanic electrocochleography and brainstem electrical response audiometry in acoustic neuroma surgery. *European Archives of Otorhinolaryngology, 249,* 257–262.

Leonetti, J.P., Brackmann, D.E., & Prass, R.L. (1989). Improved preservation of facial nerve function in the infratemporal approach to the skull base. *Archives of Otolaryngology—Head and Neck Surgery, 101,* 74–78.

Møller, A.R., Jho, H.D., & Jannetta, P.J. (1994). Preservation of hearing in operations on acoustic tumors: An alternative to recording brainstem auditory evoked potentials. *Neurosurgery, 34,* 688–693.

Nadol, J.B., Ojemann, R.G., Martuza, R.L., Montgomery, W.W., & Klevens de Sandoval, P. (1987). Preservation of hearing in surgical removal of acoustic neuromas of the internal auditory canal and cerebellar pontine angle. *Laryngoscope, 97,* 1287–1294.

Niparko, J.K., Kileny, P.R., Kemink, J.L., Lee, H.M., & Graham, M.D. (1989). Neurophysiologic intraoperative monitoring. II. Facial nerve function. *American Journal of Otology, 10,* 55–61.

Yingling, C.D. (1994). Intraoperative monitoring of cranial nerves in skull base surgery. In R.K. Jackler & D.E. Brackmann (Eds.), *Neurotology* (pp. 967–1002). St. Louis: C.V. Mosby.

CHAPTER 16

Facial Nerve Result

Rick A. Friedman, M.D., Ph.D.
John W. House, M.D.

HISTORICAL PERSPECTIVE

In the earlier part of this century, many patients with acoustic neuromas presented with facial weakness (Cross, 1981). Olivecrona (1967) reported facial paresis at the time of tumor diagnosis in 54.7% of his patients. This fact combined with the emphasis placed on preservation of life certainly explain Dandy's (1941) statement. "Paralysis of the facial nerve must usually be accepted as a necessary sequel of the operation." (p. 1030). Pennybacker and Cairns (1950), in their review of 130 cases of acoustic neuroma, stated that "complete facial paralysis seems a small price to pay for relief from an acoustic tumour" (p. 276).

Facial nerve preservation in acoustic tumor surgery, like surgical mortality, has undergone tremendous evolution over the past century. With the introduction of the operating microscope and the revival of the translabyrinthine approach by William House in 1961, mortality rates dropped significantly, and the focus of acoustic tumor removal shifted to the preservation of neural function. Most patients undergoing acoustic tumor surgery today expect that they will

survive surgery and are most concerned with preservation of facial function and, when appropriate, auditory function. The importance of facial nerve preservation in modern neurotology is emphasized by the survey conducted by Wiegand and Fickel's (1989) survey of the Acoustic Neuroma Association patients who underwent tumor resection between 1973 and 1983. The survey showed that the majority of patients considered postoperative facial weakness to be their most significant problem.

A critical review of the literature in this area is difficult for a number of reasons. Until the publication of the House-Brackmann facial nerve grading scale in 1985, there were no quantitative measures of facial nerve outcomes. Furthermore, comparisons of outcomes have been hampered by the lack of consistent reporting of tumor size, anatomic versus functional preservation of the facial nerve, operative technique, duration of follow-up, and completeness of tumor resection. Despite these shortcomings, a brief review of the history of facial nerve preservation in acoustic tumor surgery will put the state of the art into perspective.

As alluded to earlier, in the days of Cushing and Dandy, facial nerve paralysis was an expected postoperative outcome. In fact, Dandy's technique involved electrocautery of the dura at the porus acusticus after tumor removal. This hemostatic measure resulted in damage to the facial nerve. The first documented case of an acoustic tumor removal with anatomic preservation of the facial nerve was reported by Cairns (1931).

Between 1922 and 1946, Olivecrona (1967) conducted a series of surgeries in which he completely excised the tumor in 72% of the cases, and reported facial nerve preservation in approximately 30%. Among these patients, 34% demonstrated complete recovery of function, 34% demonstrated partial recovery of function, and 32% demonstrated no recovery. Pool (1966) described immediate postoperative facial nerve function in 76 patients who underwent surgery between 1950 and 1965. Eighty-six percent of the patients with large tumors that were completely excised demonstrated facial palsy. This is in contrast to a 20% incidence of palsy in moderately sized tumors that were completely excised.

McCarty (1975) reported his series of 132 cases of acoustic tumors that were removed through the suboccipital approach between 1967 and 1972. The facial nerve was preserved anatomically in 68 patients and was described as functioning in 66% of this group. Smith, Miller, and Cox (1973) reported outcomes in their series of 15 tumors. Postoperative facial nerve function was normal when the tumors were small (that is, within the internal auditory canal, or IAC) or medium sized (≤2 cm beyond the porus acusticus) and satisfactory in five of eight large tumors (>2 cm). That same year, Montgomery (1973) reported an 18% incidence of total facial paralysis in 75 consecutive cases.

Later in the same decade, Palva and Troupp (1979) reported their results on 104 patients, for which they compared the translabyrinthine and suboccipital approaches to acoustic tumor removal. Unfortunately, tumor size was not specified for the two groups, so meaningful conclusions are difficult to draw. However, permanent facial paralysis occurred in 8% of the translabyrinthine group and 51% of the suboccipital group.

King and Morrison (1980) described their results in 150 cases using a qualitative scale of facial nerve function, and they compared groups with tumors of different sizes. An "excellent" result meant normal facial function, a "good" result meant slight weakness or asymmetry, and a "fair" result meant marked weakness, asymmetry, and synkinesis. Although the length of follow-up was unspecified, the facial nerve was preserved functionally in 54% of the patients. Facial nerve function was preserved and rated "excellent" in 100% of patients with small tumors. Sixty-five percent of patients with medium-sized tumors achieved "excellent" outcomes compared to 50% of the large tumor group. Overall, 63% of the patients were reported to have "excellent" facial nerve function at the final follow-up visit.

Gardner, Robertson, Clark, Bellott, and Hamm (1983) reported on their series of 105 patients whose tumors were removed with the aid of a CO_2 laser. They reported facial nerve outcome qualitatively as the percentage of normal function and compared groups of patients with small (0–1 cm), medium (1.1–3.9 cm), and large (≥4 cm) tumors. Overall, 65% of the patients achieved 90% or better long-term function. Fourteen percent of patients overall had absent function long-term, including 7% of patients with small tumors, 8% of patients with medium tumors, and 42% of patients with large tumors. Devriese, van der Werf, and van der Borden (1984) created a five-point grading scale of facial nerve function by observing the lower eyelid and nasolabial folds. Their scale included the presence or absence of synkinesis as evidence of prior denervation. Utilizing this scale, they reported the facial nerve outcome in patients whose nerves were preserved (66%), with an average follow-up of 31.1 months. While facial nerve function was normal in 18.3%, there was slight paresis in 23.3%, moderate paresis in 31.7%, subtotal loss of function in 20%, and complete loss of function in 6.7%.

In 1985, House and Leutje, utilizing patient questionnaires, reported the long-term facial nerve function of the House Ear Clinic's first 500 patients with acoustic tumors. With 96.6% facial nerve preservation, and 414 respondents with 1 year of follow-up, 13.5% reported complete paralysis. The incidence of postoperative complete facial paralysis was 0% in patients with small tumors, 10.4% in patients with medium tumors, and 21.4% in patients with large tumors.

After the publication of the House and Brackmann (1985) facial nerve grading scale, reports of facial nerve outcome became standardized, allowing for more meaningful comparisons (see Table 16–1). Utilizing this scale, Moffat, Croxson, Baguley, and Hardy (1989) described the outcome for 76 patients who underwent acoustic tumor removal. Their overall anatomic preservation

rate was 82%. Of these patients, 65% had a satisfactory outcome (House Grade I to III), while 35% achieved only a House Grade IV to VI. In a more recent publication, Cerullo, Grutsch, Heiferman, and Osterdock (1993) reported that 86% of 102 patients who were surgically treated for acoustic tumors retained normal facial function (House Grade I or II) postoperatively.

The facial nerve outcomes for patients operated upon by members of the House Ear Clinic between 1982 and 1993, with a minimum of 1 year of follow-up, can be seen in Table 16–2. The results of our most recent cases with follow-up of 1 year or more reveal good postoperative function (House Grade I or II) in 92.1% of patients with tumors less than 2 cm and 67.2% of patients with tumors that are 2 to 4 cm in size. Only 6.2% of the total group displayed poor postoperative function (House Grade V or VI), and the vast majority of these patients had tumors larger than 4 cm.

TABLE 16–1. House-Brackmann facial nerve grading scale.

Degree of Injury	Grade	Definition
Normal	I	Normal symmetric function in all areas
Mild dysfunction	II	Slight weakness noticeable only on close inspection; complete eye closure with minimal effort; slight asymmetry of smile with maximal effort; synkinesis barely noticeable; contracture or spasm absent
Moderate dysfunction	III	Obvious weakness but not disfiguring; may not be able to lift eyebrow; complete eye closure and strong but asymmetric mouth movement with maximal effort; obvious but not disfiguring synkinesis, mass movement, or spasm
Moderately severe dysfunction	IV	Obvious disfiguring weakness; inability to lift brow; incomplete eye closure and asymmetry of mouth with maximal effort; severe synkinesis, mass movement, or spasm
Severe dysfunction	V	Motion barely perceptible; incomplete eye closure, slight movement of corner of mouth; synkinesis, contracture, and spasm usually absent
Total paralysis	VI	No movement; loss of tone; no synkinesis, contracture, or spasm

TABLE 16–2. House Ear Clinic facial nerve outcomes from 1982 to 1993.

	<2 cm	2 to 4 cm	>4 cm	Total
Grade I	75.0	49.3	24.2	61.4
Grade II	11.8	13.7	9.7	12.5
Grade III	7.9	16.8	14.5	12.0
Grade IV	3.0	9.3	19.4	6.6
Grade V	0.5	4.4	12.9	2.9
Grade VI	1.8	6.4	19.4	4.7

FACIAL NERVE MONITORING

Identification of the facial nerve during acoustic tumor dissection has been facilitated by the use of intraoperative facial nerve monitoring. The first published report of electromyographic (EMG) monitoring of the facial nerve during acoustic tumor surgery was by Delgado, Delgado, Bucheit, Rosenholtz, and Chrissian, (1979). Since this publication, a variety of techniques have been described, including constant-current stimulation, constant voltage stimulation, and the use of monopolar versus bipolar stimulator probes.

At the House Ear Clinic, we use EMG facial nerve monitoring for all cases in which acoustic tumors are removed. We currently employ the Nerve Integrity Monitor (NIM-2) (Xomed-Treace, Jacksonville, FL) or the Brackmann EMG monitor (W.R. Medical Electronics, Stillwater, MN). Our technique involves the insertion of (a) Teflon-coated, silver bipolar, hookwire electrodes into the superior and inferior orbicularis oris muscle, (b) a monopolar ground electrode into the forehead, and (c) a monopolar electrode into the ipsilateral shoulder to serve as the anode for the stimulator probe. A flexible flush-tip monopolar stimulating probe is used to identify and map the facial nerve, using a constant-current stimulus. Stimulus intensities vary from 0.05 mA to 3.0 mA, and the monitor screen is calibrated to detect EMG activity up to 1500 mV. EMG activity is monitored continuously both visually and acoustically.

Kwartler, Luxford, Atkins, and Shelton (1991) evaluated the impact of intraoperative facial nerve monitoring on 89 patients who underwent translabyrinthine acoustic tumor removal at the House Ear Clinic and compared the results to a control group of 155 patients who had undergone the same procedure but without facial nerve monitoring. They found that a larger proportion of the monitored patients yielded a satisfactory result (House Grade I or II) when evaluated immediately postoperatively, at the time of discharge, and at 1 year follow-up. The differences between the two groups of patients were statistically significant only for the first two evaluation periods. Long-term outcomes between the groups were not significantly different. When facial nerve outcome was analyzed on the basis of tumor size, there were no significant differences between groups for tumors less than 2.5 cm. For tumors larger than 2.5 cm, the monitored patients showed better function at the immediate and discharge evaluation times, when compared to the unmonitored patients, but the differences were not statistically significant.

In a similar study by Hammerschlag and Cohen (1990), there was no significant difference in outcomes based on monitoring for small- and medium-sized tumors. Furthermore, although the incidence of facial paralysis in the monitored group of patients with tumors greater than 3 cm was lower than in the unmonitored control group, the difference was not significant.

Although, intuitively, facial nerve monitoring would seem to play a greater role in functional preservation, this has not been borne out by either the literature or our own experience at the House Ear Clinic. Further study with larger sample sizes is warranted. Despite these findings, we continue to recommend intraoperative facial EMG for acoustic tumor surgery.

SURGICAL TECHNIQUE

The middle cranial fossa and translabyrinthine approaches allow early and precise identification of the facial nerve at the most lateral aspect of the internal auditory canal, the fundus. In a review of the surgical removal of 164 tumors (≤1.5 cm in size) conducted by the members of the House Ear Clinic. Arriaga, Luxford, and Berliner (1994) examined the impact of approach on immediate, intermediate, and long-term facial nerve function postoperatively. All patients had normal preoperative facial nerve function and were followed up for a minimum of 1 year. In this group of patients, there was no significant difference in facial nerve outcome between the middle fossa group and the translabyrinthine group at any of the three postoperative time intervals.

The translabyrinthine approach is the one most commonly used at the House Ear Clinic. Although the technique is described in detail elsewhere (House, 1994), several important technical and anatomic considerations for identification and preservation of the facial nerve during translabyrinthine craniotomy will be reviewed.

The first surgical consideration is early identification of the facial nerve at a consistent landmark. After completion of the labyrinthectomy and skeletonization of the internal auditory canal, the bone that is superior to the canal and inferior to the middle fossa floor is removed to the level of the anterior wall of the IAC, beginning medially at the sinodural angle and progressing laterally toward the fundus. Removing this bone allows identification of the facial nerve from above rather than behind. Utilizing this technique, Bill's bar (vertical crest) can be identified easily, and the exact location of the facial nerve (where it is not involved with tumor) can be determined.

The next consideration is delivery of the tumor and identification of the proximal facial nerve at its origin from the brainstem. Intracapsular enucleation of large tumors is performed to allow development of dissection planes anteriorly, posteriorly, superiorly, and inferiorly. Enucleation facilitates posterior dissection of large tumors, obviating the need to push forward on the tumor and risk stretching the facial nerve. Development of the tumor capsular plane posteriorly allows identification of the proximal facial nerve at the brainstem, where it lies ventral and caudal to the vestibulocochlear nerve.

Sharp, rather than blunt, dissection of the tumor from the facial nerve is the preferred technique of the members of the House Ear Clinic. The process of tumor growth within the IAC dictates the necessity for sharp dissection. Throughout its length, the tumor is enveloped in an arachnoid sheath. Growth of the tumor pushes the arachnoid out of the canal medially, causing it to double over on itself in the distal part of the meatus and at the porus (Tos, Thomsen, & Harmsen, 1988). This thick layer of the arachnoid surrounding the tumor, in combination with its dense adhesion to the tumor in the region of the porus acusticus, necessitates sharp dissection. We have found that sharp dissection of the tumor from the facial nerve and its dense attachments to the arachnoid at the porus is associated with less EMG evidence of mechanical irritation of the nerve.

In an evaluation of the causes of facial nerve paresis after translabyrinthine surgery, Tos, Thomsen, Youssef, and Turgut (1992) found that suctioning on the nerve was the most important factor for perioperative facial nerve damage, and cauterization was the least important factor. To reduce inadvertent suction injury to the facial nerve, we use the Brackmann fenestrated suction device during tumor dissection.

In the event that the facial nerve cannot be preserved anatomically, the members of the House Ear Clinic advocate immediate repair of the nerve in the cerebellopontine angle (Brackmann, Hitselberger, & Robinson, 1978). This is facilitated by identifying the proximal stump at the brainstem and rerouting the tympanic and mastoid segments with either primary end-to-end anastamosis or interposition grafting with the greater auricular nerve. Primary repair often will result in a satisfactory outcome (House Grade III or IV) and will preserve emotional expression. If the proximal stump cannot be identified, a nerve substitution technique can be utilized.

PREDICTORS OF FACIAL NERVE OUTCOME

Many aspects of acoustic tumor biology and surgical management have been examined in an effort to identify certain intrinsic and extrinsic factors that would allow prediction of facial nerve outcomes after treatment. One aspect of tumor biology that has been examined is the infiltrative nature of vestibular schwannomas. Neely and Neblett (1983) have presented data suggesting tumor infiltration of the cochlear nerve. Although infiltration of the facial nerve by a vestibular schwannoma is exceedingly rare, Luetje, Whittaker, Callaway, and Veraga (1983) reported two cases of histologically inseparable planes between the schwannoma and the facial nerve. Jaaskelainen et al. (1994) examined the tumor-facial nerve interface histologically in 20 cases requiring intraoperative sacrifice of the facial nerve due to tumor adherence. In each case, they found areas that were at least partially devoid of a clear histologic cleavage plane. Frank embedding of tumor within the facial nerve was more frequent in NF-2 cases.

Tumor size has a strong relationship to facial nerve outcome in several large series (Devriese et al., 1984; Moffat et al., 1989; Nutik, 1994; Tos et al., 1988). In an analysis of how tumor size and volume relate to postoperative facial nerve function, Kirkpatrick, Tierney, Gleeson, and Strong (1993) found that patients whose tumors had diameters no larger than 2.5 cm and calculated volumes less than 5 ml constituted the largest proportion achieving a good outcome (House Grade I or II).

Preoperative facial nerve weakness is an unusual finding in patients with acoustic tumors. Neely and Neblett (1983) found preoperative weakness in 6.1% of patients with acoustic tumors, compared to 66.6% of patients with other tumors of the IAC. Furthermore, they found that those patients with acoustic tumors and preoperative weakness universally had permanent loss of facial function postoperatively. Moffat and colleagues (1989) found a 44% satisfactory postoperative outcome (House Grade I or II) in patients with preoperative weakness, compared to a 65% satisfactory outcome overall.

In an attempt to quantify facial nerve dysfunction preoperatively and correlate it with postoperative function, Kartush, Niparko, Graham, and Kemink (1987) performed preoperative electroneurography (ENoG) on 52 patients with acoustic tumors. They found that preoperative ENoG amplitude was reduced more often with large tumors. However, preoperative ENoG amplitude reduction did not accurately predict postoperative facial nerve function.

Several studies in the literature have attempted to correlate intraoperative EMG thresholds to postoperative function. Beck, Atkins, Benecke, and Brackmann (1991) reviewed 56 patients from the House Ear Clinic who underwent acoustic tumor removal with facial nerve monitoring and from whom data on intraoperative thresholds had been obtained. Of the 29 patients who demonstrated less than 500 μV of ongoing intraoperative EMG irritative activity and who yielded a contraction greater than 500 μV to a 0.05 mA constant-current stimulus to the proximal nerve, 97% demonstrated House Grade I function at the time of discharge. The groups with more intraoperative irritation and poorer electrical response to stimulation did not fare as well at the time of discharge. Unfortunately, long-term follow-up data on these patients were not available. Prasad, Hirsch, Kamerer, Durrant, and Sekhar (1993) examined facial nerve outcome in the immediate and late postoperative periods. They found a statistically significant difference between a group of patients who demonstrated intraoperative thresholds to proximal facial nerve stimulation that were no greater than 0.2 V and a group of patients whose thresholds exceeded 0.2 V. For the group with lower thresholds, 93% had early, and 85% had late House Grade I or II function. In contrast, for the group with higher thresholds, 31% demonstrated early, and 44 % demonstrated late postoperative House Grade I or II. In a similar study, Lalwani, Butt, Jackler, Pitts, and Yingling (1994) found intraoperative thresholds less than 0.2 V to be most predictive of long-term function.

Although preoperative and intraoperative factors can aid in prognosticating postoperative facial nerve function, the final answer lies in the postoperative examination. In a review of 515 consecutive acoustic tumor removals at the House Ear Clinic, Arriaga, Luxford, Atkins, and Kwartler (1993), assessed the predictability of long-term facial outcome, based on early postoperative function. Long-term function was significantly different for patients with good, intermediate, or poor function at the immediate and time of discharge time intervals. In general, acceptable function (House Grades I to IV) immediately after surgery predicted long-term acceptable function in 98% of patients. Acceptable function at the time of discharge was associated with acceptable long-term function in 99.7% of patients. Among patients with delayed postoperative paralysis, 88% displayed long-term acceptable function, while 12% had long-term House Grade V or VI results. Finally, of those with immediate postoperative House Grade V or VI function, only 30% remained at this level on long-term follow-up. Therefore, even with a poor early result, if the nerve is preserved, 70% of patients will develop acceptable long-term function. Nutik (1994) found similar results in his recent review of facial nerve outcomes after acoustic tumor removal. Specifically, patients with normal, early, postoperative function remained normal late. Patients with weak, early function generally displayed normal late function. Function that was lost early returned later, although incompletely. Additionally, it was reported that, of 11 patients with some early postoperative function who progressed to paralysis in the first week, only three were normal at the 1-year point.

CONCLUSIONS

Acoustic tumor management has come a long way since the turn of the century. Preservation of life is no longer the sole issue, and now preservation of function is the new frontier. The anatomical and functional preservation of the facial nerve is the norm in acoustic tumor surgery today. The future likely holds improved methods for preservation of auditory function.

REFERENCES

Arriaga, M.A., Luxford, W.M., Atkins, J.S., & Kwartler, J.A. (1993). Predicting long-term facial nerve outcome after acoustic neuroma surgery. *Archives of Otolaryngology—Head and Neck Surgery, 108,* 220–224.

Arriaga, M.A., Luxford, W.M., & Berliner, K.I. (1994). Facial nerve function following middle fossa and translabyrinthine acoustic tumor surgery: A comparison. *The American Journal of Otology, 15,* 620–624.

Beck, D.L., Atkins, J.S., Benecke, J.E., & Brackmann, D.E. (1991). Intraoperative facial nerve monitoring: Prognostic aspects during acoustic tumor removal. Archives of *Otolaryngology—Head and Neck Surgery, 104,* 780–782.

Brackmann, D.E., Hitselberger, W.E., & Robinson, J.V. (1978). Facial nerve repair in cerebellopontine angle surgery. *Annals of Otology, Rhinology, and Laryngology, 87*, 772–777.

Cairns, H. (1931). Acoustic neurinoma of the right cerebellopontine angle. Complete removal. Spontaneous recovery from postoperative facial palsy. *Proceedings of the Royal Society of Medicine, 25*, 7–12.

Cerullo, L.J., Grutsch, J.F., Heiferman, K., & Osterdock, R. (1993). The preservation of hearing and facial nerve function in a consecutive series of unilateral vestibular nerve schwannoma surgical patients (acoustic neuroma). *Surgical Neurology, 39*, 485–493.

Cross, J.P. (1981). Unilateral neurilemmomas of the eighth cranial nerve: Then and now. *The American Journal of Otology, 3*, 28–34.

Dandy, W.E. (1941). Results of removal of acoustic tumors by the unilateral approach. *Archives of Surgery, 42*, 1026–1033.

Delgado, T.E., Buchheit, W.A., Rosenholtz, H.R., & Chrissans, S. (1990). Intraoperative monitoring of facial muscle evoked responses obtained by stimulation of the facial nerve: A more accurate technique for facial nerve dissection. *Neurosurgery, 4*, 418–421.

Devriese, P.P., van der Werf, A.J.M., & van der Borden, J. (1984). Facial nerve function after suboccipital removal of acoustic neurinoma. *Archives of Otorhinolaryngology, 240*, 193–206.

Gardner, G., Robertson, J.H., Clark, W.C., Bellott, A.L., & Hamm, C.W. (1983). Acoustic tumor management—combined approach surgery with CO_2 laser. *The American Journal of Otology, 5*, 87–108.

Hammerschlag, P.E., & Cohen, N.L. (1990). Intraoperative monitoring of facial nerve function in cerebellopontine angle surgery. *Archives of Otolaryngology—Head and Neck Surgery, 103*, 681–684.

House, J.W., & Brackmann, D.E. (1985). Facial nerve grading system. *Archives of Otolaryngology—Head and Neck Surgery, 93*, 146–147.

House, J.W. (1994). Translabyrinthine approach. In D.E. Brackmann, C. Shelton, & M.A. Arriaga (Eds.), *Otologic surgery* (pp. 605–616). Philadelphia: W.B. Saunders.

Jaaskelainen, J., Paetau, A., Pyykko, I., Blomstedt, G., Palva, T., & Troupp, H. (1994). Interface between the facial nerve and large acoustic neurinomas. *Journal of Neurosurgery, 80*, 541–547.

Kartush, J.M., Niparko, J.K., Graham, M.D., & Kemink, J.L. (1987). Electroneurography: Preoperative facial nerve assessment for tumors of the temporal bone. *Archives of Otolaryngology—Head and Neck Surgery, 97*, 257–261.

King, T.T., & Morrison, A.W. (1980). Translabyrinthine and transtentorial removal of acoustic nerve tumors. Results in 150 cases. *Journal of Neurosurgery, 52*, 210–216.

Kirkpatrick, P.J., Tierney, P., Gleeson, M.J., & Strong, A.J. (1993). Acoustic tumour volume and the prediction of facial nerve functional outcome from intraoperative monitoring. *British Journal of Neurosurgery, 7*, 657–664.

Kwartler, J.A., Luxford, W.M., Atkins, J., & Shelton, C. (1991). Facial nerve monitoring in acoustic tumor surgery. *Archives of Otolaryngology—Head and Neck Surgery, 104*, 814–817.

Lalwani, A.K., Butt, F. Y.-S., Jackler, R.K., Pitts, L.H., & Yingling, C.D. (1994). Facial nerve outcome after acoustic neuroma surgery: A study from the era of cranial nerve monitoring. *Archives of Otolaryngology—Head and Neck Surgery, 111*, 561–570.

Luetje, C.M., Whittaker, C.K., Callaway, L.A., & Veraga, G. (1983). Histological acoustic tumor involvement of the VIIth nerve and multicentric origin in the VIIIth nerve. *Laryngoscope, 93*, 1133–1138.

McCarty, C.S. (1975). Acoustic neuroma and the suboccipital approach (1967–1972). *Mayo Clinic Proceedings, 50*, 15–16.

Moffat, D.A., Croxson, G.R., Baguley, D.M., & Hardy, D.G. (1989). Facial nerve recovery after acoustic neuroma removal. *Journal of Laryngology and Otology, 103*, 169–172.

Montgomery, W.W. (1973). Surgery for acoustic neurinoma. *Annals of Otology, Rhinology, and Laryngology, 82*, 428–424.

Neely, J.G., & Neblett, C.R. (1983). Differential facial nerve function in tumors of the internal auditory meatus. *Annals of Otology, Rhinology, and Laryngology, 92*, 39–41.

Nutik, S.L. (1994). Facial nerve outcome after acoustic neuroma surgery. *Surgical Neurology, 41*, 28–33.

Olivecrona, H. (1967). Acoustic tumors. *Journal of Neurosurgery, 26*, 6–13.

Palva, T., & Troupp, H. (1979). Recent experience in the surgery of acoustic neurinomas. *Acta Otolaryngologica, 360*(Suppl.) 48–50.

Pennybacker, J.B., & Cairns, H. (1950). Results in 130 cases of acoustic neurinoma. *Journal of Neurology, Neurosurgery, and Psychiatry, 13*, 272–277.

Pool, J.L. (1966). Suboccipital surgery for acoustic neurinomas: Advantages and disadvantages. *Journal of Neurosurgery, 24*, 483–492.

Prasad, S., Hirsch, B.E., Kamerer, D.B., Durrant, J., & Sekhar, L.N. (1993). Facial nerve function following cerebellopontine angle surgery: Prognostic value of intraoperative thresholds. *American Journal of Otology, 14*, 330–333.

Smith, M.F.W., Miller, R.N., & Cox, D.J. (1973). Suboccipital microsurgical removal of acoustic neurinomas of all sizes. *Annals of Otology, Rhinology, and Laryngology, 82*, 407–414.

Tos, M., Thomsen, J., & Harmsen, A. (1988). Results of translabyrinthine removal of 300 acoustic neuromas related to tumour size. *Acta Otolaryngologica, 452*(Suppl.), 38–51.

Tos, M., Thomsen, J., Youssef, M., & Turgut, S. (1992). Causes of facial nerve paresis after translabyrinthine surgery for acoustic neuroma. *Annals of Otology, Rhinology, and Laryngology, 101*, 821–825.

Wiegand, D.A., & Fickel, V. (1989). Acoustic neuromas, the patient's perspective. Subjective assessment of symptoms, diagnosis, therapy, and outcome in 541 patients. *Laryngoscope, 99*, 179–187.

CHAPTER 17

Surgical Treatment of Facial Paralysis

William H. Slattery, III, M.D.
Robert E. Levine, M.D.

FACIAL REANIMATION

Today, facial nerve paralysis is the most feared outcome for patients who undergo acoustic neuroma surgery. Fortunately, facial nerve results have improved over the years as a result of improvements in microsurgical techniques and the introduction of facial nerve monitoring.

The selection of surgical rehabilitation is dependent on the status of the injured nerve, the degree of facial nerve paralysis, and the time from onset of the paralysis. Surgical treatment typically is directed toward restoring resting muscle tone to allow facial symmetry at rest, providing volitional and emotional facial movement to allow more natural facial expression, and providing protection of the eye to prevent corneal complications. There are several surgical techniques that accomplish these goals, including nerve grafts, nerve transpositions, muscle transpositions, and surgical implants for the eye.

Nerve Grafts

There is a negative relationship between the size of an acoustic neuroma and the facial nerve results, which are always best when the facial nerve is preserved. The facial nerve usually can be separated from the tumor. In 98.7% of acoustic neuroma surgeries performed at the House Ear Clinic, surgeons were able to preserve the nerve anatomically intact (Arriaga, Luxford, Atkins, & Kwartler, 1993). Facial nerve paralysis still may occur, even with nerve preservation. Acoustic tumors may invade the facial nerve itself, thus requiring the surgeon to sever it. In a large tumor, the facial nerve may be stretched and, therefore, the proximal and distal stumps can be reapproximated.

Direct facial nerve end-to-end anastomosis is performed most easily when using the translabyrinthine approach. The intracranial portion of the facial nerve is devoid of perineurium and covered with only a thin layer of glia. This makes neurorraphy much more difficult than peripheral nerve neurorrhaphy, where a thick perineurial layer exists for the suturing. In the cerebellopontine angle, a portion of the nerve must be incorporated in the suture ties to allow adequate tissue to support the neurorraphy.

In many cases, the facial nerve cannot be reapproximated after tumor excision due to either a missing segment or severe thinning of the nerve that does not allow adequate length for reapproximation. The distal segment of the facial nerve may be rerouted to allow good approximation without tension across the suture line. During neurorraphy, it is extremely important that there is no tension across the suture line, because results are affected by the amount of tension. This is extremely important in the cerebellopontine angle, where neurorraphy is quite tenuous, and usually only one or two sutures can be completed. Rerouting requires bone to be removed around the labyrinthine and horizontal segments of the facial nerve. The superficial petrosal nerve must be cut as it exits from the geniculate ganglion. The bone is thinned carefully around the nerve to create an eggshell layer. This is removed carefully, and the facial nerve is released from the fallopian canal. Rerouting of the nerve usually will provide an adequate length to allow end-to-end anastomosis within the cerebellopontine angle. This, of course, requires that the proximal stump at the brainstem be of sufficient length for suturing. When this is not the case, other reanimation procedures must be considered postoperatively.

Hypoglossal Anastomosis

The hypoglossal nerve anastomosis technique is preferred when direct nerve reanastomosis cannot be performed. When there is facial nerve discontinuity, the procedure should be performed as soon as possible following acoustic neuroma surgery. Muscle atrophy and degeneration may occur quickly following denervation, and early repair limits the amount of muscle degeneration.

This technique also may be used in individuals following acoustic neuroma surgery in which the facial nerve is anatomically preserved, but nonfunctional. Facial nerve paralysis tends to improve over the first year following surgery. Therefore, this technique usually is not performed until 1 year following surgery in patients who have no recovery of facial nerve function. If the patient has no clinically defined recovery at 1 year, then hypoglossal anastomosis is considered. Confirmation of denervation may be determined using evoked electromyography. This test can determine if there are functional motor endplates. A patient in whom there is minimum function and very poor clinical function still may be considered a candidate for nerve anastomosis, because there may be a few surviving fibers, and the reanastomosis may provide a greater number of fibers to the muscles of the face.

The spinal accessory, phrenic, and ansa hypoglossal nerves also have been proposed for facial reanimation, although the use of these nerves results in greater morbidity and fewer functional axons, and the clinical results have not been consistent. Therefore, the hypoglossal nerve still is recommended as the nerve of choice for facial reanimation. The hypoglossal nerve is in close anatomical proximity to the facial nerve in the neck. The disadvantage of the hypoglossal nerve transfer is the loss of motion to the ipsilateral side of the tongue.

Surgical Technique

The procedure is performed through a typical parotid incision extended anteriorly approximately 2 cm under the mandible. The parotid gland is separated from the sternocleidomastoid muscle and the external auditory canal. The facial nerve is identified at the level of the digastric muscle and dissected from the parotid gland to the pes anserinus, thereby exposing approximately 2 cm of the facial nerve. The hypoglossal nerve is dissected from the undersurface of the posterior belly of the digastric muscle. The hypoglossal nerve then is transected as far distally as possible prior to its branching into the tongue. The facial nerve is transected at the stylomastoid foramen. The hypoglossal nerve then is rotated superiorly deep to the posterior belly of the digastric muscle. The nerve ends should lie together without tension. The ends should be severed with a sharp knife to ensure a sharp cut that allows a flush anastomosis. Three-to-four 9–0 nylon sutures approximate the perineurium together. Care must be taken not to damage the neural tissue.

A modification of the classic facial hypoglossal anastomosis technique was recently introduced by May (May, Sobol, & Mester, 1991). This technique involves splitting the hypoglossal nerve in half and using a jump graft to attach the proximal segment of the partially severed hypoglossal nerve to the distal stump of the facial nerve. The hypoglossal nerve is divided in half, and two or three 9–0 nylon sutures are used to attach the jump graft to the proximal side of the cut hypoglossal nerve. The jump graft may come from the greater auricular nerve found in the same vicinity. The advantage is that it allows tongue function to be preserved. The disadvantage of this technique is that it does not provide as many potential axons for reinnervation.

Results

Results from facial hypoglossal anastomosis are not seen until approximately 4 to 6 months following surgery. Axonal growth begins at the brainstem and occurs at the rate of 1 mm per day. An increase in muscle tone and resting symmetry usually is the first sign of reinnervation. Volitional movement may become possible as reinnervation occurs. Maximal results typically are seen 1 year following the procedure, although small improvement may be seen past that time. Rehabilitation training can improve the functional results following nerve transposition. The patient is taught to use the

tongue to elicit different facial movements, depending on the muscles that are reinnervated. Some patients are able to obtain significant control of facial movements with rehabilitation. Anastomosis also may be helpful to individuals during eating, because the normal movement of the tongue increases oral muscular tone. Electromyographic feedback can enhance a rehabilitation training program and is used intermittently to assess patient improvement.

Synkinesis

Synkinesis results from misdirected reinnervation. This may occur in patients who have facial paralysis with an intact facial nerve, following either direct nerve anastomosis or XII–VII nerve anastomosis. This problem typically involves eye closure with movement of the lower face; however, other muscle groups may be similarly affected. Puckering of the mouth usually will demonstrate the synkinesis. Synkinesis may be reduced with biofeedback therapy or, in severe cases, botulism toxin can be injected selectively into muscle groups and may provide adequate temporary control. Botulism toxin usually requires reinjection every 4 to 6 months to control the symptoms.

Muscle Transpositions

Muscle transposition techniques may be employed in individuals who have poor facial function. Patients with long-standing facial nerve paralysis may not be candidates for nerve grafting or facial hypoglossal grafting due to fibrosis that occurs in the distal facial nerve over time. Temporalis muscle transposition is the most common muscle transfer technique used to reanimate the lower face (Baker & Conley, 1979). This technique may be used in combination with the nerve grafting techniques described previously to augment the results of facial nerve repair.

Ideally, postoperative acoustic neuroma patients must have an intact ipsilateral trigeminal nerve to be considered a candidate for a muscle transposition. A lack of innervation leads to temporalis muscle atrophy that may be detected preoperatively by palpating the temporalis muscle superior to the zygomatic arch. The purpose of temporalis muscle transfer is to allow movement to the lower aspect of the face by contracting the temporalis muscle.

The patient must have realistic expectations about the results of muscle transposition surgery. While purposeful movement may be obtained in some patients, the overall objective is to improve facial symmetry.

Surgical Technique

Temporal muscle transfer is performed under general anesthesia with contralateral nasotracheal intubation. This allows full exposure of the mouth area. Preoperative intravenous antibiotics are required. A vertical incision that extends from the preauricular area superiorly is created and carried down to the temporalis fascia. An incision is created in the ipsilateral vermilion border. An alternative is to make an incision in what should be the nasolabial crease or fold. The skin is elevated to expose the orbicularis oris muscle and perioral musculature.

A tunnel at least two finger breadths wide is then made under the skin and superficial to the musculoaponeurotic system (SMAS), connecting the two operative fields. Remaining just under the skin will protect any facial nerve fibers that may be partially functioning or have the potential for recovery.

The slips of temporalis muscle and fascia will be sewn to the orbicularis oris muscle near the corner of the mouth. The length between this area and the zygomatic arch is measured, and the appropriate length of temporalis muscle is approximated. A 4-cm-wide segment is obtained from the midportion of the muscle. The muscle flap then is rotated through the previously created pocket to reach the area of the orbicularis oris muscle. The muscle is divided near the corner of the mouth so that one slip of muscle may be attached to the upper area of the mouth and another extended to support the inferior corner of the mouth. Sutures (2–0 Prolene) are used to connect temporalis muscle with the underlying facial musculature. Overcorrection of the smile is obtained, as some stretching of muscle and fascia will occur. An attempt is made to overcorrect the smile such that the second molar can be seen. The temporalis donor site then is drained, and the wound is closed in layers.

Results

After the initial swelling of surgery resolves, improved symmetry is noted almost immediately. Movement is noted several weeks following surgery. However, the patient is instructed not to attempt movement, because it creates tension on the suture lines. At approximately 6 to 8 weeks following the procedure, the patient is instructed to bite down on the ipsilateral side, causing the temporalis muscle to contract. The patient is instructed not to bite severely, because dental problems can arise. Biofeedback therapy can be very helpful in allowing the patient to learn purposeful movement with the muscle transfer. Some patients are able to develop symmetry of smiling with extensive rehabilitation.

MANAGEMENT OF THE EYE

Many patients will experience eye discomfort following acoustic neuroma surgery. The sequelae may range from minimum to severe, and the aggressive management and rehabilitation of eye disorders are important.

Factors that determine the extent to which the patient is at risk of developing ocular complications should be emphasized in the examination. The position and degree of functional impairment of either or both eyelids and the brow should be noted. Corneal sensitivity, corneal injury, if any, and tear function should be evaluated. The extent to which the globe rolls upward with attempted lid closure (Bell's phenomenon) also should be noted, because it is a major factor in determining how well the cornea is protected during sleep. Patients who have a fifth nerve deficit, a poor Bell's phenomenon coexistent with a seventh nerve defect, or both, are prone to serious corneal complications.

Additional observations provide a baseline for gauging changes in the patient's ocular and neurological status. Visual acuity is a sensitive indicator of corneal change and, therefore, should be noted. The optic disc should be examined for edema. Any ocular motility deficit, especially a lateral rectus deficit resulting from sixth nerve involvement, should be measured.

The persistence of a coexistent sixth nerve paresis, causing diplopia in the primary position of gaze, influences the management of seventh nerve impairment. Even if lid function were to be restored, the patient would have to occlude one eye to prevent diplopia.

The progression of the return of function of the fifth, sixth, and seventh cranial nerves should help determine the mode of therapy. Bandage contact lenses, temporary methods of lid closure, or both, are best for patients in whom fifth nerve function, seventh nerve function, or both, is expected to improve within 2 or 3 months. On the other hand, definitive procedures to improve lid closure and function, possibly combined with bandage contact lenses, must be considered for patients who are expected to have poor function of the fifth nerve, the seventh nerve, or both for longer periods.

The patient's occupation and social environment must be integrated carefully with therapy. For example, taping an eye shut for months may be acceptable for someone at home, but unacceptable for one who deals with the public. Similarly, a patient who is reliable, has interested helpful family members, and has easy access to medical care at regular intervals may be managed conservatively, whereas the same problem occurring in an unreliable patient living alone in a remote area may warrant an early definitive surgical procedure.

Although occasionally we have seen neurotrophic keratitis (arising from fifth nerve involvement) as the sole eye problem in patients with acoustic tumors, the usual eye problems are those due to facial nerve weakness. Instances in which the seventh nerve defect is complicated by coexistent fifth nerve involvement are the most difficult cases to manage. Therefore, the therapy of eye problems secondary to both fifth and seventh nerve deficits is discussed concurrently.

Medical Management

Use of Eye Drops and Ointments

The simplest therapeutic regimen consists of protecting the cornea with artificial tears, such as methylcellulose 0.5% or 1.0%, carboxymethylcellulose 0.5% (Refresh Plus), or 1.0% (Celluvisc), or polyvinyl alcohol 1.5% (Liquifilm) or 3.0% (Liquifilm Forte). Drops remain in the conjunctival sac only briefly, thus requiring instillations as frequently as hourly. Some patients benefit from the addition of wetting agents, such as polyvinylpyrrolidone (Adapt). The wetting agent is instilled first and, a minute or two later, the artificial tear drop is instilled. In our experience, patients who benefit from the use of wetting agents seem to do better with sequential drops than with combination drops that contain both wetting agents and artificial tears.

If drops are not successful in relieving symptoms or in eliminating corneal staining, ointment may be added at bedtime. Ointment stays on the surface of the eye for hours, but it has the disadvantage of blurring vision. When used at bedtime, it is generally cleared from the eye by morning.

When used liberally, it helps keep the eye closed during sleep by sticking the lashes together. A bland ophthalmic ointment may be used, for example, 5% boric acid ointment or sterile white petrolatum (Lacrilube, Duolube, Refresh PM). Antimicrobial preparations have the added advantage of protecting against infection. Sulfa-containing ointments are preferred to preparations with neomycin or tetracycline, which are associated with a high incidence of allergy. If the use of drops during the day is insufficient to protect the eye adequately, supplementary daytime use of ointment may be employed. The visual blurring caused by using ointment may be acceptable in cases in which surgical management is better postponed.

Injuries to denervated corneas often are complicated by vascular ingrowth and marked uveitis. To prevent these sequelae, early therapy, including the judicious use of topical steroids and cycloplegics, is important. Such drops generally are used in conjunction with therapy (e.g., a lid suture) to prevent further corneal injury.

Use of Tape

Patients in whom adequate ocular protection cannot be achieved with instillations of ointment may benefit by having the lids taped shut. Clear plastic tape, for example, Transpore, is satisfactory for this purpose. Lid taping should be utilized in situations in which it can be supervised. Special care must be taken with patients with hypesthetic or anesthetic corneas, because they may not be able to determine when their lids have been closed adequately. In this regard, it is helpful to ask the patient whether light can be seen after the lids have been taped shut.

Droop of the lower lid can be benefitted by taping. This is accomplished best by using a one-quarter to one-half inch wide strip of clear plastic or paper tape or surgical skin closure tape, such as Steri-Strips. The end of the tape is applied at the center of the lower lid, with the upper edge about one quarter of an inch below the lashes. The tape is used like a pull tab, with the tension directed up and laterally, and is secured lateral to the orbital rim. Trial and error will demonstrate the best way of eliminating lid droop in a given patient. Some of our female patients even have applied makeup over the tape to make its use in public cosmetically less objectionable.

A crescentic piece of tape can be placed overriding the lid fold in the upper lid. It functions as a splint to limit the ability of the lid to open excessively. Alternatively, a strip of tape analogous to that used for the lower lid can be placed across the lid fold and pulled downward and laterally to help the lid close. The combination of the two pieces of tape is referred to as "X-taping" of the lid.

Protective Glasses and Moisture Chambers

Protective lenses, such as wrap-around sunglasses or goggles, may be used to decrease the normal evaporation from the eye. These devices are useful especially in patients with limited tearing, limited lid function, or both who are comfortable indoors but who cannot compensate for the additional corneal drying induced by exposure to wind. A simple and inexpensive moisture chamber is available that can be attached to ordinary spectacles or secured with an elastic band around the head.

Room Humidifiers

Evaporation of tears is accelerated by low humidity. Therefore, maintaining high room humidity may be of significant benefit.

Avoiding Ocular Irritants

Eyes with impaired fifth and seventh nerve functions are much more subject to injury by irritants such as fumes, aerosols, cosmetics, chlorinated pool water, and drying air currents. Patients should be alerted to the hazards of such irritants and urged to guard against them.

Lid Sutures

When the eye is difficult to tape shut, placing a lid suture may be preferable. A simple and effective means of lid closure is to place a 5–0 nonresorbable suture through the skin of the upper lid, then tape it to the cheek. Such a suture should be used whenever temporary lid closure is indicated and when tape is inadequate to keep the lids shut. The eye still may be opened easily to check pupillary reflexes as often as necessary. Should the surgeon choose to leave the lid open at intervals, the ends of the suture may be taped loosely to the forehead. Generally, such a suture can be left in place for 4 to 6 weeks; thereafter, it tends to extrude. The lid suture is a satisfactory technique for managing difficult cases after surgery until a more definitive solution can be achieved.

Bandage Contact Lenses

It is difficult to keep bandage contact lenses (disposable soft lenses) in place in patients who have marked lower lid droop or marked impairment of lid closure. Soft contact lenses may be helpful if the degree of functional lid deficit is mild, or if the lenses are used in conjunction with some of the measures available to improve lid position and closure. We have found the greatest utility of soft contact lenses to be in managing the neurotrophic component in patients whose lid problems already have been solved by definitive surgical procedures.

Soft lenses also can be used in cases of upper lid entropion to protect the cornea until surgery is performed. Whenever hydrophilic lenses are used, only drops compatible with such lenses should be instilled in the eye.

Surgical Management

Tarsorrhaphy

Tarsorrhaphy has been long advocated as a method of managing neurotrophic and ex-posure keratitis. Even when the cornea is protected adequately by a two-pillar tarsorrhaphy, it is cosmetically objectionable and restricts vision. Lateral tarsorrhaphy is successful in cases of mild lagophthalmos. Frequently, however, stretching and fibrosis of the tarsus adjacent to the adhesion may leave a wedge-shaped area of cornea unprotected. In addition, after opening the tarsorrhaphy, there may be irregularity of the lid margins and trichiasis. Further, tarsorrhaphies are disfiguring and add to the psychological load the patient is already facing.

The objections to tarsorrhaphy, especially in younger patients, have led to the suggestion of alternative methods of improving lid position and function. With the availability of the alternatives discussed below, we rarely find an indication to perform tarsorrhaphy.

Procedures to Correct Lower Lid Droop or Ectropion

Technique of Medial Canthoplasty. In patients who have marked lower lid droop, pulling the lid laterally without first anchoring it medially, may bring the lacrimal punctum to a point almost tangential to the limbus. Medial canthoplasty avoids both excising tarsus and displacing the punctum centrally. The technique we employ currently (Beard, 1964) is as follows.

With the globe protected with scleral shell and the lacrimal canaliculi protected with probes, infiltration anesthesia is placed at the medial canthus. A 4-mm square of skin-muscle is reflected below, with its lateral extent 2 mm medial to the lacrimal punctum and its palpebral extent at the mucocutaneous junction. A double-armed 5–0 Polyester suture is placed at the insertion of the medial canthal tendon in the lower lid and then directed superonasally into the origin of the medial canthal tendon and tied. To obtain greater correction, a similar skin flap is formed in the upper lid, and a second double-armed suture is placed between the arms of the tendon. The skin is closed with running 6–0 plain gut suture.

We have found the medial canthoplasty to be of great value as a temporary or permanent means of correcting mild degrees of lower lid droop, and we perform it almost routinely to correct lower lid problems when we need to place a palpebral spring in the upper lid or when we need to anchor the lower lid prior to performing a lateral canthoplasty.

Technique of Lateral Canthoplasty. For this technique (Tenzel, 1969; Tenzel, Buffam, & Miller, 1977), the lateral canthus is clamped, and a canthotomy is performed. The inferior canthal tendon is cut, and the lower lid is mobilized. A tarsal tongue is created laterally by excising 3 mm of the skin-muscle lamina. Both arms of a 5–0 Polyester suture are sewn through the tarsal tongue. A tunnel then is made under the superior arm of the lateral tendon. The tarsal tongue is drawn into the tunnel and secured by the two arms of the Polyester suture to periosteum at the inner aspect of the lateral orbital rim, placing the sutures superior to the lateral raphe and as posterior as possible. Lid position is checked with the patient in both the supine and seated positions, and final knots are tied. Skin is closed with 6-0 plain gut suture.

Procedures to Reanimate the Upper Lid: Palpebral Spring and Gold Weight

Patients who require these devices can be divided into two groups. The first group includes patients who are not medically manageable and who will have return of nerve function in 6 to 12 months (either by spontaneous recovery or following nerve anastomosis). Implantation of the prosthetic device improves the patient functionally, psychologically, and cosmetically until the return of orbicularis function permits removal of the device.

The second group includes patients with permanent defects in lid position or function that cannot be adequately managed by medical means or lesser surgical proce-dures. The prosthetic device may be placed in such a patient's eyelid with the understanding that repositioning, resuturing, or replacement of the device might be required in the months or years that follow. In our experience, extrusion has not been a frequent problem with either device, but patients who submit to an implantation procedure must be made clearly aware of the risk of extrusion. Implantation should not be performed in any patient who cannot make provisions for medical follow-up. Patients should be made aware preoperatively that neither device can ensure perfect symmetry of the affected eye, compared to the normal eye.

Technique of Palpebral Spring Implantation (Levine, 1979, 1980, 1982a, 1982b, 1985, 1986, 1989, 1992, 1994; Levine, House, & Hitselberger, 1972; Morel-Fatio & Lalardrie, 1964, 1965). For this technique, the spring is prepared prior to surgery; minor adjustments may be made at the time of surgery. The spring is fashioned by making a loop in a piece of stainless steel orthodontic wire measuring 0.011 in. in diameter. It is important that the loop at the fulcrum of the spring measure about 5 mm in diameter and be as flat as possible. The posterior extension of the loop is the upper arm of the spring, which rests on the periosteum of the orbital rim. The anterior extension of the loop is the lower arm, which will be positioned in the lid overlying the tarsal plate.

Two curves are placed in each arm of the spring to make it conform properly on the contour of the lid. One curve is made in the frontal plane to allow the upper arm of the spring to conform to the curvature of the orbital rim and to allow the lower arm to conform to the contour of the upper lid. A second curve is made anteroposteriorly to allow the spring to accommodate the orbital rim above and the meridional curvature of the globe below.

When the lids are closed, separation of the arms of the spring should measure one-and-a-half times the separation when the lids are open. In cases of severe lagophthalmos, this factor should be increased to double the separation. Because it is easier subsequently to lessen the tension of the spring than to increase the tension, it is preferable that the arms initially be too far apart than too close together.

The surgical technique is depicted in Figure 17–1 and is conducted as follows. A lid fold incision is made, starting at the medial limbus and continuing across the orbital rim. Dissection is carried down medially to expose the anterior surface of the tarsus. Laterally, the dissection is carried to expose the periosteum of the lateral orbital rim. Hemostasis is achieved with bipolar cautery.

While protecting the eye with a scleral shell, a blunted 22-gauge spinal needle, with its stylet in place, is passed from the medial aspect of the incision, beginning mid-tarsus along the plane between the anterior surface of the tarsus and the orbicularis oculi, projecting in a slightly inferior direction. The undersurface of the lid should be checked to ensure that the tarsus has not been perforated inadvertently. The end of the previously prepared spring is passed into the needle and, as the needle is withdrawn, the spring is brought into position.

A 4–0 Mersilene suture is placed through the fulcrum of the spring to secure it to orbital rim periosteum, taking an extra bit of periosteum in the stitch before tying it. Four additional 4–0 Mersilene sutures are placed to secure the fulcrum, taking an additional bit of periosteum with each stitch.

Loops then are fashioned at the upper and lower ends of the wire with special orthodontic pliers designed for that purpose. The superior loop should be made at the upper end of the lateral incision, and the inferior loop should be made at the center of the upper lid. The inferior loop should be placed superior to the lower arm of the spring. If the loop is formed inferiorly, the lower arm loses its smooth contour on its palpebral aspect. The wire is cut, and each loop is closed carefully so that there are no sharp free ends that may perforate adjacent tissues.

It is imperative that the spring be placed precisely so that pressure exerted on the adjacent tissues is minimal. Any point of pressure on the tissues could lead potentially to migration or extrusion of the spring. Therefore, the lower loop position should be checked with the eyes open and closed and with the scleral shell removed.

The lower loop of the spring is not sutured. Rather, it is secured in its position by encasing it in a folded piece of 0.2-mm thick Dacron patch material. The crease in the patch is accomplished best by folding the material in a Gelfoam press that subsequently is put through the normal steam autoclave cycle. A piece of folded Dacron, approximately 5 mm wide and 10 mm long, is cut and converted to a tiny sack by closing the long, open side and one short, open side with 8–0 nylon sutures. The Dacron is placed around the wire, with the crease directed toward the lid margin, and the remaining open side is closed with 8-0 nylon. The Dacron is held in position in the upper lid by fixing it to the tarsus with the same suture material and by closing overlying tissue meticulously with 6–0 plain gut suture. In time, granulation tissue will invade the Dacron and fix it solidly to its surrounding tissues. The tension on the spring is adjusted with the patient in both the seated and supine positions. Deeper tissues overlying the spring then are closed with 5–0 plain gut suture to assure that the spring and the Mersilene sutures are well covered. Skin and muscle are closed with running 6–0 plain gut, fast-absorbing suture.

Technique of Enhanced Palpebral Spring Implantation. In recent years, we have been enhancing the effect of the palpebral spring by tightening the levator at the same time (Levine, 1994). This allows for increased tension on the spring, with better blinking and less pseudoptosis. The technique is used for those patients who will require a permanent spring and for those for whom it is felt that the optimal functional result, even for a shorter term, is worth the extra procedure.

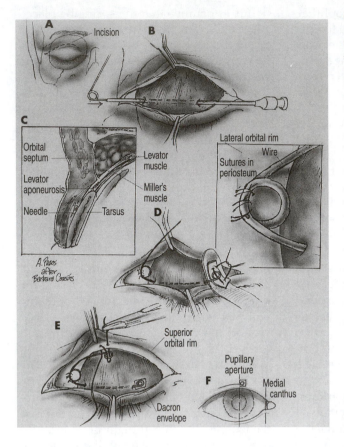

Figure 17-1. The palpebral spring implantation technique. **A.** With a protective scleral shell in place, an incision is made along the lateral two-thirds of the lid crease and carried across the orbital rim laterally. Dissection is carried downward at the medial end of the incision to expose the tarsal plate. Dissection also is carried upward and laterally to expose the orbital rim. **B.** A 22-gauge blunted spinal needle with the stylet in place is passed from the medial end of the dissection to emerge laterally in the plane between orbicularis and tarsus. The passage should be carried out overlying mid-tarsus. The needle is angulated slightly downward at its lateral extent. The exit of the needle tract should be close to lateral orbital rim periosteum. The lid is everted to confirm that the needle has not inadvertently perforated the tarsus. The previously prepared wire spring (which has been autoclaved) is passed through the needle, and the needle is withdrawn. **C.** A cross-section of the lid illustrates placement of the needle over the mid-tarsus in the plane between the tarsus and orbicularis. The wire spring should be resting on the epitarsal surface. **D.** The scleral shell is removed, and the fulcrum of the spring is brought into the desired position along the orbital rim. The spring should be placed in a position where its curves conform perfectly to the eyelid con-

tour. (*Inset:* The fulcrum of the spring is secured to lateral orbital rim periosteum with five 4–0 Mersilene sutures, taking an extra bite of the periosteum with each stitch.) Loops are fashioned at each end, and the spring is cut to size. The loops should be flat and tightly closed to leave no sharp edges. The medial loop is enveloped in 0.2-mm thick Dacron patch material, to which it is secured by means of three 8–0 nylon sutures tied internally. The Dacron patch material is creased in a Gelfoam press before surgery and autoclaved with the other instruments. The folded Dacron envelope is cut to size at surgery. The crease in the patch material should be directed downward so that the spring and patch together provide a smooth inferior surface. The loop at the end of the inferior arm is directed upward for the same reason. Suturing of the loop to the Dacron is facilitated by resting the Dacron on a retractor. **E.** The end of the spring, with its Dacron envelope, is reposited into the lid between tarsus and orbicularis. In time, the end of the spring will become fixed to the tarsus by granulation tissue integrating into the Dacron patch. It is helpful to secure the patch to the tarsus directly with an additional running 8–0 nylon suture to provide fixation until connective tissue grows into the Dacron. The tension on the spring is checked, with the patient in both the upright and supine positions. The tension can be adjusted by grasping the upper end of the spring with forceps and changing its position. When the correct tension has been determined, the upper loop of the spring is secured to the orbital rim periosteum with a 4–0 Mersilene suture. An extra bite of the periosteum may be taken in the stitch before tying. When placing sutures to secure either the fulcrum or the upper loop of the spring to the orbital rim periosteum, it is safer to sew in the direction away from the globe. Spring tension again is checked with the patient both seated and supine. Additional adjustments can be made by bending the wire or repositioning the loop. When the adjustments are completed, four additional 4–0 Mersilene sutures are placed through the upper loop in a manner similar to the initial suture. Deeper tissues overlying the spring then are closed with 5–0 plain gut suture to assure that the spring and the Mersilene sutures are well covered. Skin and muscle are closed with running 6–0 plain gut fast-absorbing suture. **F.** The end of the spring should be between the pupillary axis and the medial limbus, with the eyes in the primary position of gaze. (From *Oculoplastic Surgery* (p. 723), by D. Tse and K.W. Wright (Eds.), 1992, Philadelphia: J.B. Lippincott. Copyright 1992 by J.B. Lippincott. Artwork by Barbara Coustus. Reprinted with permission.)

The technique, as shown in Figure 17–2, is the same as described above, except that dissection is carried upward to expose the levator. Two horizontal mattress sutures of 5–0 Mersilene are placed from the tarsus through the levator to tighten it. Technically, it is easier to place these sutures prior to placing the spring. They should be placed in tarsus above the level where the spring will be located. The more medial suture is not completed until after the spring is placed, so it can be passed through the Dacron envelope and tied before completing its passage through the levator, thus helping to fixate the spring. The tension on the levator sutures and on the spring is adjusted with the patient in both the seated and supine positions.

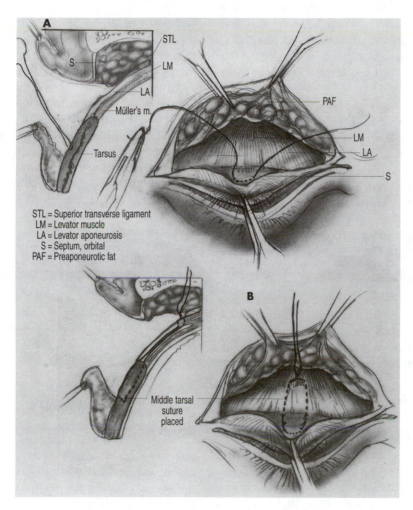

STL = Superior transverse ligament
LM = Levator muscle
LA = Levator aponeurosis
S = Septum, orbital
PAF = Preaponeurotic fat

Figure 17–2. The enhanced palpebral spring implantation technique. **A.** The levator aponeurosis and the inferior aspect of the muscular portion of the levator are exposed. Centrally, the superior portion of the tarsus also is exposed. A double-armed 5–0 Mersilene suture then is placed through mid-tarsus. **B.** Each arm of the suture is brought superiorly through the levator to emerge just above the point where the aponeurosis meets the levator muscle. Temporary knots are tied. If necessary, an additional lateral suture and, possibly, an additional medial suture are placed in a similar manner. (*Inset:* The course of the suture is illustrated in cross section. Check to be sure that the suture has not perforated either tarsus or conjunctiva). (From *Otologic Surgery*, by D.E. Brackmann, C. Shelton, and M.A. Arriaga (Eds.), 1994, p. 724. Philadelphia: W.B. Saunders. Copyright 1994 by W.B. Saunders. Reprinted with permission.)

Technique of Gold Weight Implantation. This technique (Jobe, 1974; May, 1985) is conducted as follows. Preoperatively, with the patient seated, a gold weight that is estimated to be suitable for the degree of lagophthalmos is selected and secured to the patient's upper lid either with cyanoacrylate glue or with a temporary lid suture. The patient then is asked to open and close the eye, and it is determined if the weight is correct or if a heavier or lighter weight should be used. The evaluation is repeated with the patient is the supine position. Weights in the range of 1.2 to 1.6 g seem suitable in most cases.

A scleral shell is placed. An incision is made in the lid fold, and dissection is carried upward to expose orbital septum. The pre-aponeurotic fat can be seen through the septum. The septum is opened, and the weight is secured to the levator with a single 5–0 Dacron suture placed through the holes in the weight. The knot is buried.

The weight may be fixated either supratarsally or tarsally. Fixating it supra-tarsally is preferable, unless the weight is so large that is not practical. The function of the weight then is tested with the patient in the seated and supine positions. If the desired effect is not obtained, a different size weight may be tried. Overlying skin muscle is closed with running 6–0 plain gut suture.

Procedures to Correct Upper Lid Entropion and Brow Droop

The cornea can be protected against the upper lid lashes or brow hair by a soft lens until surgical correction can be undertaken. We frequently have combined entropion correction, brow elevation, or both with spring implantation.

Technique of Correction of Upper Lid Entropion. This technique (Levine, 1994) is carried out as follows. After infiltration of local anesthesia in the upper lid, an incision is made across the lid several millimeters below the upper border of the tarsus and parallel to it.

If entropion correction is combined with spring implantation, the usual upper lid incision is merely extended medially. A series of 6–0 Vicryl sutures is placed from subcuticular tissue at the lower aspect of the wound to levator muscle. These sutures will evert the lid and correct the entropion. The skin incision is closed with interrupted 6-0 plain gut suture.

Technique of Brow Lift. For this technique (Beard, 1964), local infiltration anesthesia is placed. The brow is placed at a position symmetrical to the opposite brow, and a skin incision is made just above the upper border of the brow and parallel to it. Dissection is carried to periosteum and slightly upwards. A double-armed, Prolene 4–0 suture is placed through the deeper tissues at the lower edge of the wound, and both arms are brought through periosteum several millimeters above the brow incision. The suture is tied with adequate tension to elevate the brow centrally to the desired height. This is checked with the patient in the supine and upright positions. In a similar manner, two additional sutures are placed medially and laterally to obtain the desired brow elevation and curvature. Wound closure is achieved with deep 5–0 Vicryl sutures, 6–0 plain gut sutures, and a Steri-Strip for the skin.

COMMENTS

Facial nerve paralysis remains a risk for all patients who have treatment of an acoustic neuroma. Therefore, the physician caring for the acoustic neuroma patient must understand the indications, benefits, and limitations of current facial rehabilitation techniques.

Future techniques for facial paralysis associated with acoustic neuroma surgery may include medications that will prevent or decrease the degree of facial nerve paralysis. The development of more effective nerve muscle transfers allowing animated facial expression and implantable facial nerve stimulators are areas of active research and may be clinically utilized in the future.

REFERENCES

Arriaga, M.A., Luxford, W.M., Atkins, J.S., Jr., & Kwartler J.A. (1993). Predicting long-term facial nerve outcome after acoustic neuroma surgery. *Archives of Otolaryngology—Head and Neck Surgery, 108*(3), 220–224.

Beard, C. (1964). Canthoplasty and brow elevation for facial palsy. *Archives of Ophthalmology, 71*, 386–388.

Baker, D.C., & Conley, J., (1979). Regional muscle transposition for rehabilitation of the paralyzed face. *Clinical Plastic Surgery, 6*(3), 317–331.

Jobe, R.P., (1974). A technique for lid-loading in the management of lagophthalmos in facial paralysis. *Plastic and Reconstructive Surgery, 53*, 29–31.

Levine, R.E. (1979). Management of the eye after acoustic tumor surgery. In W.F. House & C.M. Luetje (Eds.), *Acoustic tumors* (Vol. 2), (pp. 105–149). Baltimore: University Park Press.

Levine, R.E. (1980) Management of the ophthalmologic complications of facial paralysis. *Trans. Pacific Coast Oto-Opthalmologic Soc., 61*, 85–93.

Levine, R.E. (1982a). Protection of the exposed eye. In D. E. Brackmann (Ed.), *Neurological surgery of the ear and skull base* (pp. 81–87). New York: Raven Press.

Levine, R.E. (1982b). Protection of the exposed eye in facial paralysis. In M.D. Graham & W.F. House (Eds.), *Disorders of the facial nerve* (pp. 336–375). New York: Raven Press.

Levine, R.E. (1985). Eyelid reanimation surgery. In M. May (Ed.), *The facial nerve* (pp. 681–694). New York : Thieme-Stratton.

Levine, R.E. (1986). Palpebral spring for lagophthalmos due to facial nerve palsy. In R.E.

Wesley (Ed.,) *Techniques in ophthalmic plastic surgery* (pp. 424–427). New York: John Wiley & Sons.

Levine, R.E. (1989). Management of lagophthalmos with palpebral spring and silastic elastic prosthesis. In A. Hornblass (Ed.), *Ophthalmic and orbital plastic reconstructive surgery* (Vol. 1) (pp. 384–392). Baltimore: Williams & Wilkins.

Levine, R.E. (1992). Lid reanimation with the palpebral spring. In K. Wright and D. Tse (Eds.), *Color atlas of ophthalmic surgery* (pp. 231–238). Philadelphia: J. B. Lippincott.

Levine, R.E. (1994) Eyelid reanimation, In D. E. Brackmann, C. Shelton, & A. Arriaga (Eds.), *Otologic surgery* (pp. 717–740). Philadelphia: W. B. Saunders.

Levine, R.E., House, W.F., & Hitselberger, W.E. (1972). Ocular complications of seventh nerve paralysis and management with the palpebral spring. *American Journal of Ophthalmology, 73*, 219–228.

May, M. (1985). Surgical rehabilitation of facial palsy. In M. May (Ed.), *The facial nerve* (pp. 695–777). New York: Thieme-Stratton.

May, M., Sobol, S.M., & Mester, S.J. (1991). Hypoglossal-facial nerve interpositional-jump graft for facial reanimation without tongue atrophy. *Archives of Otolaryngology—Head and Neck Surgery, 104*, 818–825.

Morel-Fatio, D. & Lalardrie, J.P. (1964). Palliative surgical treatment of facial paralysis: The palpebral spring. *Plastic and Reconstructive Surgery, 33*, 446–456.

Morel-Fatio, D., & Lalardrie, J.P. (1965). Le ressort palpebral: Contribution a l'etude de la chirurgie plastique de la paralysie faciale. *Neurochirurgie, 11*, 303–310.

Tenzel, R.R. (1969). Treatment of lagophthalmos of the lower lid. *Archives of Ophthalmology, 88*, 366–368.

Tenzel, R.R., Buffam, F.V., & Miller, G.R. (1977). The use of the lateral canthal sling in ectropion repair. *Canadian Journal of Ophthalmology, 12*, 199–202.

Preoperative and Postoperative Care of Patients with Acoustic Tumors

Patricia Gentner, R.N.
Charles M. Luetje, M.D.

An increased comprehension of the requirements for the care of patients with acoustic tumors has evolved, inspired by surgical refinement, improved surgical results, and a concept of "centers of excellence" (Lunsford, 1995), the definition of which remains to be clarified. Clearly, the beneficial and significant influence on patient awareness in general by the Acoustic Neuroma Association[1] has been a major factor in focusing on patient care. Any team involved in caring for patients with acoustic tumors must be prepared to provide for the needs of these patients in an expert and professionally appropriate manner.

We define the preoperative to postoperative period as that span of time from diagnosis to incision and all that occurs after placement of the dressing. This chapter addresses important issues within these time frames. The detail presented may differ from others, but it is a method that has evolved for the authors. Further, it may seem elementary to some readers but, nevertheless it details important steps in preoperative preparation and postoperative care that are felt to be in the patient's best interest. It provides guidelines for those who are interested.

PREOPERATIVE PREPARATION

Moment of Impact

The most common symptoms of acoustic tumors are unilateral hearing loss, tinnitus, and balance disturbance, the latter of which may be slight and even unnoticeable, unless attention is directed toward it. Eventually, radiographic evaluation leads to diagnosis, the moment of impact. The ensuing explanation by the physician and nurse re-

[1]P.O. Box 12402, Atlanta, GA 30355.

garding the findings and proposed treatment never will be forgotten by the patient. It is at this stage that a caring and competent team approach must be established firmly.

Initial Team Contact

Referral patterns usually are otolaryngologic in origin because of the nature of the symptomatology. However, more imaging scans that are obtained by various physician practices for unrelated complaints occasionally do identify small, or even large, acoustic tumors. The resultant referral may either be neurosurgical, neurotologic, or a combination. However it occurs, an unhurried, careful, detailed, and educational analysis of all aspects of the treatment alternatives is mandatory. Confidence must be instilled at this visit.

Radiographic Analysis

The appropriateness of the imaging detail of soft tissue and bone, either by magnetic resonance imaging (MRI) or computerized tomography (CT), must be determined. Usually, MRI is the study in hand for review. This affords the essentials of tumor size and configuration. Particular information regarding tumor displacement of the brainstem, the fourth ventricle, hydrocephalus, extension into Meckel's cave and the tentorial notch, cystic degeneration, and blood vessel flow voids should be recorded as seen on T1, T1 enhanced, and T2 weighted images. If a CT is the only study available, MRI is indicated. An idea of the temporal bone air cell system can be gleaned from air cell void on MRI, but is more accurate with CT bone windows.

Patient Examination

The time-honored neurologic evaluation of these patients usually is not revealing, except to document the presence or absence of cranial nerve deficits and cerebellar func-

tion. However, careful historical documentation may disclose other related neurologic abnormalities and, to some extent, afford the opportunity to assess the cognitive abilities of the patient.

Patient Discussion

This is the meat of the preoperative preparation. At no other time is it more important to explain in full detail the risks, complications, and alternatives to the patient. Subsequent reinforcement of these factors may be called upon, because patients forget information. They receive the opinions of friends and family, and other influences may enter into the decision making process. There must be no waffling by the surgeon; rather, a genuine willingness to consider questions generated by the patient about alternatives must be displayed and, if indicated, the surgeon must make changes.

The authors have enjoyed the advantages of a team approach by the same individuals within each specialty who have been together for almost 20 years. This includes the neurotologic surgeon, the registered nurse in the neurotologic office (who, in addition, scrubs the case), and the neurosurgeon. The initial visit usually begins with the neurotologist. Surgical evaluation and discussion occur first. The nurse, using a patient information letter she has prepared previously, discusses in great detail the step-by-step events that happen to the patient. A final wrap-up is conducted by the neurotologist, and other professional literature reprints are given to the patient. Arrangements are made to see the neurosurgeon. For patients who travel long distances, appointments are coordinated ahead of time.

Neurosurgical and neurotologic opinions may differ at times because of an insight gained by the neurosurgeon at the subsequent evaluation, or an identified and unrecognized risk factor seen by one and not the other. By the time the patient is seen by the neurosurgeon, there has been time to think about the issues involved and ask pertinent questions. In general, the neurotologist and neurosurgeon should have similar surgical philosophies that develop only through a mutual respect for each others' skills by working together over time. This solidifies the team approach.

The authors' team has learned that alternative treatments are based on patient age and health, tumor size, ventricular size and cerebrospinal fluid (CSF) flow dynamics, brainstem compression, and the patient's own wishes. Three distinct alternatives have evolved: interval imaging follow-up without surgery, surgery, and stereotactic radiation.

Informed Consent

Once the decision has been made by the patient for surgical removal of the tumor, the standard informed consent protocol is accomplished. The authors have the patient sign a form explaining the risks and complications involved and an office form securing permission to operate, separate from the hospital operative permit. By this time, the patient has read all the information provided, perhaps talked to another patient whose name has been provided, and has had all questions answered.

There is no place for scare tactics or other unethical methods to hustle a patient to the operating room to remove this benign tumor, the surgery for which, though refined, carries the risks of injury to the cranial nerves, brainstem, and cerebellum, as well as death. We agree with Lunsford (1995) that the decision must be the patient's. An orderly progression of events leading to the operating room is mandatory. In this way, the patient, though naturally frightened, can approach surgery with confidence that the team is doing all that is possible. Surgical complications, though not desired by the patient or the treating team, are understood based on thorough preparation.

Medical Preparation

The onerous task of insurance preauthorization and precertification falls upon the shoulders of the office nurse. No one better understands the conversations that must occur with reimbursement personnel, with whom the initial and sustaining contacts are conducted. Unless there are circumstances of special needs based on physiologic abnormalities or tumor size, we have been forced by reimbursing agencies and their medical directors to admit patients the morning of surgery. Most preoperative medical assessments are managed under outpatient care. These all are arranged well in advance of surgery.

A unit of autologous blood is obtained and prepared for transfer to the hospital for the day of surgery. This usually is two weeks in advance, and the patient is started on iron. Individuals who have gastrointestinal problems may need prescription types of iron preparations, rather than off-the-shelf elemental iron. We rarely need the blood, but we feel that it is in the patient's best interest that one has one's own blood, if needed. Indeed, this usually is the patient's own preference, as well.

Since 1980, all patients, regardless of tumor size, are given dexamethasone preoperatively. If the tumor is very large, the dosage is begun 4 to 5 days preoperatively. If the tumor is smaller, it is given intramuscularly at midnight and 6:00 a.m., preceding surgery. Dexamethasone will be mentioned again in more detail in the postoperative section.

The patient is seen in the neurotology office the day before surgery, where a preoperative audiological evaluation, electronystagmography (ENG), and possibly an auditory brainstem response test are conducted. The ENG has no diagnostic importance, but it is helpful in our discussion of postoperative vestibular dysfunction with each patient. We have found that the reduction of the preoperative ENG response usually means less postoperative vertigo and compensation. It is helpful to patients to counsel them in this regard.

At the preoperative visit, the risks and complications sheets and operative permit are signed and witnessed by the nurse. A financial responsibility sheet, previously given, also is signed. There are no financial surprises for the patient. Final overview of surgery again is outlined to the patient, and it is here that the finishing touches of confidence are solidified. The patient is made to feel that nothing will be on the minds of the surgical team other than providing the very best in tumor removal and postoperative care.

Orders and copies of appropriate documents from the neurotologist's office (office notes, test results, etc.) are given to the patient to carry to the admissions desk of the hospital. MRI films are taken to the operating room by the neurotologist, and the chart goes with the nurse. If the neurosurgical visit is subsequent to the neurotologist preoperative visit, the patient takes the X-ray films to the hospital and is given strict instructions to keep them "under the pillow" and to give them to no one. The patient carries the films to the hospital surgical holding area, where they are given personally to the surgeon during preparation for surgery.

If surgery is on the day of admission, laboratory studies, chest X-rays, and electrocardiography are conducted the day prior. Anesthesia consultation is obtained. In some instances in which it appears advisable for optimal patient care, hospitalization occurs the day prior to surgery. There are no set criteria for hospital admission the day prior to surgery, and it always means a lengthy discussion with the patient's managed care personnel. The factors that are considered important in making this determination for early admission are the patient's physical and mental health, the necessity of inpatient medication, and hospital consultation. Preferably, the patient is sedated and rests well the night before surgery. The hair is shampooed with an antiseptic soap at bedtime and again at 5:00 a.m., and steroids are given at midnight and 6:00 A.M.

It is the opinion of the authors that patients do better when they are hospitalized and sedated and when their environment is controlled during the 12 hours preceding surgery. This opinion is not shared by third party medical directors for reimbursement companies. The emotional energy intensity level at home usually is high, and unknown factors often interfere with the orderly progression of patient to the holding area in preparation for surgery the morning of admission. These intangibles are not accepted by administrators for third party reimbursement companies. Often, the surgeon must be persuasive in making sure that the patient arrives in the operating room area properly prepared for a craniotomy.

Adequate hair removal is completed, an intravenous (IV) is started, and a final chart check is conducted in the surgical holding area. The nurse sees the patient in the holding area prior to returning to the operating room. The hospital operative permit, nurse's notes, surgeon's history and physical, neurosurgeon's consultative report, laboratory results, chest X-ray, and EKG all are reviewed by the operating surgeons. The status of ordered blood is confirmed, ready for use. The side for surgery clearly is delineated once again.

In the operating room, the gowned and masked surgical nurse greets the patient. A wedge is placed under the popliteal fossae to provide a bend in the knees. The patient is intubated, and a nasogastric tube is placed to prevent accumulation of gastric juice in the stomach. The first dose of prophylactic antibiotics, usually Rocephin, is given. A core body temperature Foley catheter is inserted. The patient is positioned on the operating table according to the surgeon's preference. For the translabyrinthine approach, a sheepskin is placed under the head to prevent sheet burn skin irritation and localized alopecia. Facial nerve monitoring electrodes are inserted, and if hearing preservation measures are to be undertaken, appropriate electrodes are placed. An arterial line is established. Surgical skin preparation is 10 min and, for the translabyrinthine approach, abdominal skin is prepped simultaneously.

POSTOPERATIVE MANAGEMENT

Postoperative care begins the moment the dressing is applied. Immediate assessments are made of pupillary size, extremity movement, swallowing, spontaneous respiration and other signs of activity indicative of brainstem function. Nasal flaring is the first indication of facial function. Often, definitive assessment is difficult if anesthesia has been deep and prolonged. However, careful observation is the word. The microscope is left draped until there is assurance that all is satisfactory. The surgeons stay with the patient from operating room to recovery room.

Recovery Room

The surgeons continue to observe the patient in the recovery room until there is assurance that breathing is satisfactory and oxygen saturations are normal, extremity movement can be assessed, facial function is noted, and the surgeons feel that a complete but preliminary report can be given to the family. Zofran (32 mg) is given intravenously to help reduce retching, nausea, and vomiting.

The family is notified when the patient is ready to leave the recovery room for the intensive care unit. The surgeons have talked with the family, dictated their operative reports, and revisited the patient for final assessments. At this point, all neurologic signs are stable, other recovery parameters have been satisfied, and safe transportation is anticipated. This transfer occurs without physician accompaniment.

Intensive Care Unit

The patient's stay in the intensive care (ICU) includes the night of surgery, and the patient is discharged to the floor the following morning. Glasgow coma scale measurements are made hourly with vital sign checks, deep breathing is initiated, and care-

ful continuous assessment is made of neurological function. After initial assessments have been made and all is stable, the family is allowed in the room. The nasogastric tube that was placed at intubation usually is removed within a few hours, and ice chips and liquids are given when the patient is alert. Nasal oxygen (via a nasal cannula) is given continuously at 2–3 L/min until the morning following surgery, when the patient is discharged from the ICU. Arterial oxygen saturation measurements are not used as a criterion, nasal oxygen simply is given empirically. A microscope is available for immediate reopening of the wound and tumor bed clot evacuation should a sudden hemorrhage and rapid, neurological deterioration occur. Fortunately, the authors have not had this experience.

The biggest problems are nausea and vertigo. It is of the patient's best interest to control these as much as possible. The smaller the tumor and the more vestibular function that is present preoperatively, the worse the problem. The authors' experience with Zofran has been favorable, although a prospective study has not been accomplished. This medication is used by the oncologists for the nausea and vomiting produced from chemotherapy, and it usually is effective for 8–12 hr. The literature suggests that 8 mg be used for postsurgical nausea (Higgins, Kilpatric, Bruce, Jones, & Tyers, 1989), but the authors feel that the full 32 mg oncologic dose is better. It does not impair neurological function or level of consciousness. The dose may be repeated in 12 hr, but it is rare to give further doses. Dramamine (100 mg) also is used routinely for nausea, vomiting, and vertigo.

Narcotics are avoided, with the exception of codeine, which is given liberally (45–60 mg at 2-hr intervals, as needed). The switch to oral acetaminophen (with or without codeine) is encouraged early. Phenothiazaines are not given because of unpredictable extrapyramidal reactions. Rocephin (1 g) is given for three successive IV doses at 12-hr intervals. Dexamethasone (4 mg) is given at

6-hr intervals, with a rapid taper over 3–4 days for patients with smaller tumors, and a slower taper for patients with larger tumors who have been taking the drug preoperatively for 4–5 days. Procardia (10 mg) is given sublingually as needed to keep systolic blood pressure below 160 mm.

The morning following surgery, careful neurological assessment is made, and the arterial line and nasal oxygen are discontinued. The Foley catheter is left in place, depending upon the gender and anticipated activity of the patient. The patient is helped to the sitting position on the side of the bed, then to the standing position. If tolerated, the patient may sit in a chair beside the bed or even take a few steps. This occurs after surgeon rounds, during which time the amount of nystagmus is noted. With third-degree nystagmus, direction-fixed nystagmus in all directions of gaze, there usually is considerable nausea and vertigo. In these instances, the approach generally is not as cavalier, and a more conservative patient movement approach is taken.

Nursing Floor

Transfer occurs the morning after surgery, when the surgeons are satisfied with neurological recovery. A private room directly across from the nurse's station is ordered so that intensive neurosurgical nursing care can be continued. Vital sign checks are reduced to 2-hr intervals until evening, and the dietitians are instructed to give the patient whatever he or she selects to eat, not a "routine" dietary progression. The same medicines and IV fluids are given unless necessity dictates differently. Activity level is modest, depending upon the disequilibrium. The first day usually is a quiet one.

Dressing removal occurs on the second postoperative day. Usually, the Foley catheter is removed on this day and, toward evening, the IV is discontinued. Activity then includes going to the bathroom with help and sitting in a chair, then back to bed. Early ambulation is the goal as soon as possible, even the first day, if tolerated. The thromboembolic deterrent (TED) hose that was placed preoperatively may be removed at this point, although some patients like to keep them on.

The tapering off of steroids usually begins on the second day and is fairly rapid over 3–4 days. There have been two or three cases of steroid psychosis, the main symptom of which is hallucination. This problem can be controlled within 24–36 hr via steroid elimination and the administration of Haldol. The authors feel this small risk of psychosis is worth the benefits from steroids. The problem of low-grade fever on the second or third postoperative day has been eliminated since the institution of prophylactic antibiotics and steroids in all patients, regardless of tumor size, in 1980. Before 1980, low-grade fever used to be a problem because of uncertainty as to etiology. Frequently, lumbar puncture and equivocal interpretations regarding meningitis were entertained. Terms such as "chemical" meningitis were mentioned. Criteria for the institution of antibiotics were loose and confusing. Hospital stays were prolonged and, in some cases, dependent upon further spinal fluid analysis. This no longer occurs with the use of antibiotics and steroids.

Since 1980, the authors have obliterated the eustachian tube via the facial recess with periosteum and fascia (Glasscock, Hays, & Murphy, 1975; Pulec, 1974), filled the middle ear with muscle, reconstituted the dura of the craniotomy defect with abdominal fascia, which is tamponaded with abdominal fat (translabyrinthine cases), and used prophylactic antibiotics and steroids. The incidence of CSF leak has dropped to less than 1–2% and meningitis to less than 1% (Luetje & Whittaker, 1994). Nevertheless, these are the complications of concern on the nursing floor. The hospital team nurses are constantly on the lookout for signs of CSF leak and temperature elevation. In addition, attention is paid to the gradual activity progression, dependency on medications, and general recovery pattern. By the third and fourth postoperative days, the expectation is self-ambulation in the hallway. Discharge usually is on the fourth postoperative day, occasionally on the fifth day and, sometimes, later.

The role of vestibular rehabilitation remains to be defined clearly. Although it is becoming more popular to initiate this early and during hospitalization, the benefits seem doubtful. Patients seem to learn what they can and cannot do, they are motivated to progress at a satisfactory level, and they rarely need anything beyond the surgeon's encouragement and clarification of activities. There are no major activity limitations for a surgical point. The limiting factor to a patient's activity is simply the inability due to disequilibrium, fatigue, or headache.

Rarely do the patients go home with any medication other than the last few tapered steroids or acetaminophen. Occasionally, codeine or other similar oral analgesics are used. Dramamine seems to be helpful in many patients for disequilibrium, but increasing activity seems equally as helpful. Out-of-city patients remove steri strip wound coverage themselves and usually return for a postoperative visit in 2–4 weeks, depending on geographic location.

The most common and distressing postoperative problem is facial paralysis and ipsilateral eye care. It is the worst cosmetic, neurological complication and should never be taken lightly. The potential for loss of vision is very real because of poor eye care. It is easy for the surgeon and the patient to forget about aggressive eye care until too late. Eye protection begins in the hospital with artificial tears during the day, then taping the eye closed over lubrication at night. The patient and family are taught proper techniques for taping the eyelid closed. Additionally, the technique of applying the ipsilateral index finger knuckle to the eyelid for forced lid closure is taught.

Appropriate ophthalmological care must be obtained for the patient. It is the operating surgeon's responsibility to make sure that the ophthalmologist is interested not only in seeing the patient but also possesses a high degree of intellectual and surgical skill. Eye care cannot be stressed enough for patients who have facial paralysis.

Home

There are no restrictions on physical activity, unless some special problem exists. Patients are limited by their own disequilibrium, fatigue, or headache. It is usual to tire quickly and take naps. Imbalance is expected for the first few weeks to months. Thus, patient activity seeks its own level. The craniotomy defect is sealed within a few days. Natural limitation due to how the patient feels is sufficient to reduce activity. Patients are told that they can do anything they feel like doing, but to avoid heavy lifting or straining for a couple of weeks. Most can resume office work within a month. Laborers may take 2 or 3 months before they can return to work.

Occasionally, prolonged disequilibrium is a problem and, for these patients, vestibular rehabilitation seems to be helpful. Headache is not a major problem and is usually controlled with acetaminophen or ibuprophen. It takes 3 to 4 months for individuals to develop stamina as they had preoperatively. They are told this. Most will persevere and, gradually, will overcome their short-term disability through compensation. A few patients will not succeed in this regard, and will become dependency problem patients. These few will require patience, understanding, and as little medication as possible.

CONCLUSION

A total team approach for patients with acoustic tumors has been established well. The future dictates that "centers of excellence" be identified for referral for surgical removal of these tumors. There always will be a place for surgical removal of acoustic tumors. Irradiation may reduce the number of smaller tumors for surgical excision. Thus, the surgical team must be skilled at removal of larger tumors, as well as those that may grow after irradiation.

In these centers, the team involved must instill confidence in the patient. Well-prepared teams will have evolved a method of caring for these patients. This chapter details some of the more important aspects of patient care that have been found to be effective over the last 20 years. These guidelines are meant to be a reference for others in search of a methodology that may be modified for a particular patient care setting.

REFERENCES

Glasscock, M.E., Hays, J.W., & Murphy, J.P. (1975). Complications in acoustic neuroma surgery. *Annals of Otology, Rhinology, and Laryngology, 84,* 530–540

Higgins, G.A., Kilpatric, G.J., Bruce, K.T., Jones, B.J., & Tyers, M.B. (1989). 5-HTZ receptor antagonists injected into the area postrema inhibit cisplatin-induced emesis in the ferret. *British Journal of Pharmacology, 97,* 247–255.

Luetje, C.M., & Whittaker, C.K. (1994, January). *Factors and surgical techniques in preventing postoperative complications in acoustic tumor surgery.* Paper presented at the Middle Section Meeting of the American Laryngological, Rhinological and Otological Society, Rochester, MN.

Lunsford, L.D. (1995). Commentary on the article Results of surgery following sterostactic irradiation for acoustic tumors. *American Journal of Otology, 16,* 319–321.

Pulec, J.L. (1994). Technique to avoid cerebrospinal fluid otorhinorrhea with translabyrinthine removal of acoustic neuroma. *Laryngoscope, 104,* 382–386.

CHAPTER 19

Complications After Acoustic Neuroma Surgery

C. Y. Joseph Chang, M.D.
Steven W. Cheung, M.D.

The morbidity and mortality rates associated with the surgical treatment of acoustic neuromas have undergone evolutionary changes during the past century. Prior to the early 1900's, mortality rates of surgery approached 80%. Subsequently, Harvey Cushing developed techniques to reduce the mortality rate of surgery to 20% by 1917 with an even lower mortality rate by 1931. However, preservation of hearing and facial nerve function was thought to be futile, and tumor resection was usually subtotal. Most patients who survived surgery eventually succumbed to complications of tumor growth.

Since then, major advances in anesthesia, pharmacology, and surgical technique have been developed. The occurrence of serious complications after acoustic tumor surgery has become uncommon (Table 19–1), and posterior fossa surgery has become almost routine. Anatomic preservation of cranial nerves, including the facial nerve, is now largely expected, with excellent functional outcome in a large majority of cases. Only the preservation of serviceable hearing re-

TABLE 19–1. Rates of complications after acoustic neuroma surgery.

Complication	Incidence (%)
Cerebrospinal leak	2.6–15.0
Severe headache	0.4–14.3
Bacterial meningitis	0.7– 7.0
Pulmonary complications	0.6– 2.7
Lower cranial nerve palsy	0.0– 3.1
Ataxia	1.7– 1.9
Urinary tract infection	0.0– 1.9
Hydrocephalus	0.7– 1.7
Death	0.6– 1.7
Trigeminal dysfunction	0.0– 1.4
Cerebrovascular accident	0.0– 1.7
Sixth nerve palsy	1.2– 1.6
Cardiac complications	0.0– 0.4
Intracranial bleed	0.4– 0.6
Deep venous thrombosis	0.4– 0.6
Wound complication	0.0– 0.7

Note: Data compiled from Cohen et al., 1993; Ebersold et al., 1992; Mangham, 1988; Wiet, Teixido, & Liang, 1986.

mains problematic, although hearing preservation rates have been improving steadily over the past decade.

Despite the almost routine nature of posterior fossa surgery today, serious complications do occur occasionally, and the surgeon must take all necessary precautions to avoid adverse outcomes. When a significant complication does occur, the surgeon must be able to recognize it early and treat it expeditiously in order to maximize the patient's chances of a full recovery. The goals of this chapter are to discuss both minor and major complications associated with acoustic tumor surgery, to elucidate ways to prevent these complications, and to explore the ways in which problems can be identified quickly so that appropriate treatment can be instituted in a timely fashion.

INTRAOPERATIVE COMPLICATIONS

Many of the problems that the surgeon can encounter intraoperatively are potentially catastrophic and require immediate recognition and corrective action. The majority of these complications are vascular in nature and include both venous and arterial systems.

Venous Hemorrhage

The most common sources of venous bleeding during acoustic tumor surgery are the sigmoid sinus, jugular bulb, and superior petrosal sinus. In the translabyrinthine approach, the sigmoid and superior petrosal sinuses can be injured during venous decompression, and the jugular bulb can be injured when dissecting the internal auditory canal (IAC), especially if the bulb is high-riding. In the retrosigmoid approach, the sigmoid and transverse sinuses can be injured while performing the craniectomy, and the jugular bulb can be lacerated when opening the posterior lip of the IAC. In the middle fossa approach, the superior petrosal sinus is vulnerable to injury during dural elevation off the petrous ridge. In general,

violation of dural venous sinuses occurs infrequently when careful surgical technique utilizing the diamond burr to decompress venous structures is used. When bleeding is encountered, proper management is required to control hemorrhage and to proceed expeditiously with the remainder of the procedure.

If the dural sinus laceration occurs prior to bony decompression, the bleeding is best managed using bone wax. An island of bone around the waxed area can be maintained for the remainder of the procedure. If the dural sinus puncture occurs after bony decompression, the bleeding can be controlled with bipolar cautery, placement of hemostatic agents such as oxidized cellulose (Surgicel™) or microfibrillary collagen (Avitene™), or repair using 6-O or 7-O monofilament suture. Bleeding from the superior petrosal sinus that is refractory to control with bipolar cautery can be managed by creating dural incisions on both sides of the sinus to allow application of hemoclips. For large sigmoid sinus rents that do not respond to topical hemostatic agents, extraluminal or intraluminal packing may be used. Extraluminal packing can only be used if there is adequate bone around the venous structure against which to pack, both proximal and distal to the bleeding site. When extraluminal packing is not possible, intraluminal packing is used. The hemostatic material utilized should be large enough so that a portion remains outside the venous opening. The danger of placing small pieces of Surgicel™ into the venous lumen is embolization to the heart and lungs. With either intraluminal or extraluminal packing of the sigmoid sinus, care must be taken not to pack into the region of the vein of Labbe.

Air embolism is a potential complication if the venous sinus opening is significant, especially when the patient is in the sitting position (Raskin, Benjamin, & Iberti, 1985). Signs of this complication include intravascular crepitation, hypotension, tachycardia, and a decline in end-expiratory pCO_2. The classic sign of air embolus is a mechanical sounding heart murmur. When this complication is detected, inhalational anesthetic agents are stopped, and 100% oxygen is administered while the bleeding site is controlled with direct pressure. In order to reduce air flow into the venous lumen, the local venous pressure should be increased by placing the patient in the Trendelenberg position. The table should be rotated to the patient's left in order to trap the intravascular air within the right ventricle. The air then can be aspirated through a central venous catheter (Kletzker, Smith, Backer, & Leonetti, 1994).

Venous Infarction

A significant injury to the vein of Labbe or another structure providing temporal lobe venous drainage can lead to temporal lobe infarction with subsequent recurrent seizures. Additionally a temporal lobe infarction on the dominant side can cause language dysfunction, with expressive and receptive aphasia. The temporal lobe venous system is most at risk in acoustic tumor surgery during the middle fossa approach when temporal lobe retraction occasionally can impede venous outflow. These temporal lobe vessels also are at risk at their drainage points into the transverse sinus during manipulation of the sigmoid and transverse sinuses.

Injury to the temporal lobe venous system is quite unusual in acoustic tumor surgery. Such venous complications can be avoided by gentle use of temporal lobe retraction and preservation of venous outflow from the vein of Labbe while manipulating the sigmoid and transverse sinuses. Patients who develop seizures due to temporal lobe infarction should be treated with anti-seizure medications, and language deficits should be treated with speech and language rehabilitation.

Arterial Complications

Major arterial bleeding is an uncommon complication in posterior fossa surgery, unless the tumor is so large that the basilar artery is involved. In contrast, the anterior inferior cerebellar artery (AICA), which supplies the lateral pontomedullary region of the brainstem, is frequently within the surgical field and often requires dissection during acoustic tumor surgery. This vessel usually forms a loop within the cerebellopontine angle (CPA), may be intermingled between cranial nerves VII and VIII, and may even form a loop within the IAC. Tumor dissection in this area must be performed with care in order to preserve the main loop of the AICA and its distal tributaries. If vasospasm occurs, papaverine should be administered to the vessel topically. The structures at risk following injury to AICA include the vestibulocochlear nerve, the labyrinth, the nuclei of the facial and trigeminal nerves, the medial lemniscus, the lateral lemniscus, the central tegmental tract, the spinothalamic tract, and the cerebellar peduncles. The clinical symptoms can vary due to variations in blood flow patterns from the ipsilateral AICA within the regions at risk, and they include ipsilateral trigeminal nerve dysfunction, hearing loss, Horner's syndrome, vertigo, cerebellar ataxia, and myoclonus of the uvula and pharynx (Atkinson, 1949). Contralateral decrease in pain and temperature sensation as well as hemiparesis can also occur (Perneczky, Parneczky, Tschabitscher, & Samec, 1981). In recent surgical experience, deficits resulting from brainstem infarction have been limited to cerebellar dysfunction due to wedge infarcts involving the cerebellar peduncle; major deficits, such as the full AICA and posterior inferior cerebellar artery (PICA) syndromes, rarely have been seen (Rigby, Cheung, Sim, & Jackler, 1996).

Brainstem infarction is a serious complication and, in addition to the symptoms described above, also can lead to increased intracranial pressure, autonomic dysfunction, and possible death. Only supportive treatment is available at this stage, including administration of corticosteroids, pharmacologic agents to support blood pressure, mechanical ventilation, and placement of a ventriculostomy for cerebrospinal fluid (CSF) pressure control.

POSTOPERATIVE COMPLICATIONS

Adverse postoperative events that require emergent treatment include cerebral edema, intracranial hemorrhage, pneumocephalus, and bacterial meningitis. Other complications include CSF leak, cerebrovascular accident, dysfunction of trigeminal and lower cranial nerves, vertigo and dysequilibrium, headache, contralateral hearing loss, and various medical complications. Management of acute, transient facial nerve paralysis is also discussed.

Cerebral Edema

Postoperative cerebral edema is most likely to occur after the removal of large CPA tumors, during which a significant amount of cerebral or cerebellar retraction has been necessary. Cerebral edema also can result from ischemia or infarction. Since prevention is always preferable to treatment of the complication, the minimal amount of brain retraction should be used to achieve the surgical objective. The retrosigmoid approach is thought to require a larger amount of cerebellar retraction than the translabyrinthine or middle fossa approaches, but modern techniques have minimized this problem. The intraoperative use of agents that reduce CSF volume, such as mannitol and furosemide, as well as anesthetic techniques including hyperventilation, have been useful. An important surgical maneuver during the retrosigmoid approach is early decompression of the medullary cistern. In many cases, use of a retractor is unnecessary, because relaxation of the cerebellum with gradual evacuation of CSF during the posterior fossa approach provides ample exposure. A few minutes of patience at this stage can prevent major cerebellar morbidity.

The middle fossa approach can cause temporal lobe swelling due to retraction of this structure. Since the retraction is extradural in most of these cases, the occurrence of significant temporal lobe trauma during the middle fossa approach is unusual. Intraoperative somatosensory evoked potential monitoring can be used to follow the functional status of the temporal lobe so that the retraction can be relaxed, should any changes in cerebral function be detected.

The symptoms of an acute increase in intracranial pressure include decreased patient alertness or level of consciousness followed by progressive development of focal neurological deficits, such as aphasia and extremity weakness. The differential diagnosis includes intracranial hemorrhage, acute hydrocephalus, and meningitis. Unless a rapid and fulminant deterioration of the patient's neurological and hemodynamic status occurs that is consistent with an acute intracranial bleed, a non-contrast computerized tomography (CT) scan of the head should be obtained to rule out hemorrhage and acute hydrocephalus.

The goal of treatment is to reduce the intracranial pressure using pharmacologic, ventilatory, and surgical means. Acutely, hyperventilation to reduce the serum pCO_2 level to 25 to 30 mmHg can be used, if the patient has been intubated. This modality is effective only for approximately 36 hrs. Hyperosmolar agents, such as mannitol, are administered intravenously (IV) in doses of 0.5 to 2.0 mg/kg every 6 to 12 hr, and furosemide is given 20 to 60 mg IV every 4 to 6 hr to reduce CSF volume acutely. If these measures prove inadequate, a ventriculostomy can be placed to drain CSF and control intracranial pressure more directly. A lumbar drain also can be used to drain CSF to reduce intracranial pressure but, if the aqueduct and fourth ventricle are obstructed, as is often the case with posterior fossa pathology, there is a significant risk of downward brainstem herniation. Therefore, placement of a lumbar drain is contraindicated in these situations.

Steroid therapy is thought to be an effective treatment for reduction of cerebral edema, but its onset of action is not immediate. It is given often intraoperatively, especially if the posterior fossa tumor is large. The loading dose for dexamethasone is 6 to 12 mg IV, while maintenance therapy is given in doses of 4 to 6 mg every 6 hr. Steroid therapy is tapered once the cerebral edema has subsided. Short-term steroid administration can be associated with gastric distress, mood changes, and alterations in glucose control, especially in diabetic patients. The occurrence of other long-term sequelae with short-term use of steroids is uncommon.

Severe cerebral edema may place the patient at risk for cerebral ischemic complications, so consideration should be given to providing cerebral protection utilizing induced hypertension, hypothermia (30° to 32°C), and barbiturate coma. In a dire emergency, a subtotal resection of the cerebellum or temporal lobe can be undertaken as a life-saving measure.

Hemorrhage

Posterior fossa hemorrhage after acoustic neuroma surgery can be catastrophic and, fortunately, occurs only rarely. Again, prevention is preferable to management of the complication itself. Any history of bleeding problems or laboratory abnormalities in platelet or coagulation function should be evaluated and treated prior to surgery. All aspirin, nonsteroidal anti-inflammatory agents, and other medications that can compromise clot formation and maintenance of a hemostatic plug should be discontinued well in advance of surgery to allow adequate recovery of the coagulation system. During surgery, all vessels feeding the tumor should be controlled with bipolar cautery or hemoclips. Bleeding at the dural edge should be controlled similarly. Prior to closure, a Valsalva maneuver should be performed to identify residual bleeding sites.

The posterior fossa should be irrigated, and the irrigant should remain clear. Dural sinus bleeding usually is controlled adequately with local packing or suture closure, as described previously. Postoperatively, the patient should be kept at bedrest for 24 hr, and systolic blood pressure should be maintained within 20 mmHg of the patient's baseline pressure. Patients who are at risk for seizures should be treated prophylactically with phenytoin or phenobarbital.

The signs of acute intracranial bleed consist of the signs of increased intracranial pressure. The patient develops an altered level of consciousness, followed by acute neurological deficits. Classically, the patient has hemiparalysis with obtundation, a fixed and dilated pupil, respiratory distress, bradycardia, and systolic hypertension, but the presentation can be quite variable. A CT scan of the head should be performed immediately to identify the pathology but, if the patient deteriorates too rapidly, immediate intracranial re-exploration in the operating room is necessary. The clot may be epidural, subdural, or intracranial, but the goal of surgical therapy remains the same. The wound is opened, the blood clot is evacuated using copious irrigation, and the bleeding source is controlled. In the meantime, efforts to reduce the intracranial pressure, including use of a ventriculostomy, should be made. If the patient fails to improve neurologically after drainage of the hematoma, a repeat CT scan should be performed to rule out recurrent hemorrhage.

Pneumocephalus

Although intracranial air often is present after acoustic tumor surgery, it should resolve within 7 to 10 days. The volume of intracranial air should not enlarge to the point of hampering brain function. Symptomatic pneumocephalus occurs rarely after posterior fossa surgery. It is most often associated with an intracranial procedure performed in anatomic continuity with the aerodigestive tract, as in a craniofacial resection. A dural defect allowing communication between the subarachnoid and aerodigestive spaces allows air to enter the intracranial space. If a ball-valve effect occurs, the volume and pressure of intracranial air can become significant, leading to acute elevation of intracranial pressure. A CT scan of the head usually will lead to the proper diagnosis and exclude other complications.

Treatment of symptomatic pneumocephalus usually is conservative. The patient is administered 100% oxygen, and a search for the site of air leak is made and sealed, if found. Often, a concurrent CSF leak exists, and this requires treatment, as well. If the patient's neurological status is unstable, the intracranial air should be removed, either percutaneously with or without CT guidance or with wound re-exploration.

Cerebrovascular Accident

The incidence of stroke after acoustic neuroma surgery is very low. Immediate infarction can be the result of intraoperative events, such as excessive brain retraction or injury to key arteries or veins, as discussed previously. Postoperative etiologies include emboli, vascular thrombosis, arterial spasm, or intimal dissection. The clinical findings can vary, depending on the size and location of the territories affected.

Treatment is largely supportive. The acute sequelae of stroke can include cerebral edema, spread of infarction, and hemorrhage, so efforts should be made to control the intracranial pressure and limit the damage to the brain by maintaining normal blood pressure. Aspirin can be given, but care must be taken to monitor for a change to a hemorrhagic infarct, indicated by an acute deterioration in the patient's neurological status. Anticoagulation therapy with heparin is controversial and is not advised.

Cerebrospinal Fluid Leak

Perhaps the most common complication following acoustic tumor surgery is CSF leak. The incidence of this complication after the translabyrinthine and retrosigmoid approaches is approximately 12% in the literature (Hoffman, 1994). The leak can occur through the nose, wound, or ear canal. The path of CSF leakage consists of a dural defect that connects the subarachnoid compartment to the mastoid and perilabyrinthine air cells. These air cells communicate widely and variably, allowing CSF to flow to the wound, middle ear, and eustachian tube. In general, CSF otorrhea after any approach is rare, unless the external auditory canal skin or tympanic membrane has been violated. CSF leakage through the wound occurs more frequently, but proper wound closure prevents most potential leaks. CSF otorrhea and wound leak therefore should be rare, and one must suspect inadequate surgical technique if they occur with any regularity. In contrast, CSF rhinorrhea is more difficult to prevent, since dural closure after any approach for acoustic tumor surgery is rarely watertight, and routine obliteration of the eustachian tube is not practical, except perhaps with the translabyrinthine approach.

Prevention

Anatomic barriers to undesirable CSF flow in acoustic tumor surgery include watertight dural closure, blockage of air cells adjacent to dural defects, obliteration of potential routes of CSF flow within the middle ear and mastoid, and watertight closure of the skin incision, ear canal skin, and eustachian tube. Methods to block CSF flow at each of these sites are available, but the particular sets of barriers that are implemented depend on the approach being used.

There are two main routes of CSF leakage in the retrosigmoid approach: through the dural defect at the craniectomy, and through exposed IAC air cells (Figure 19–1). CSF

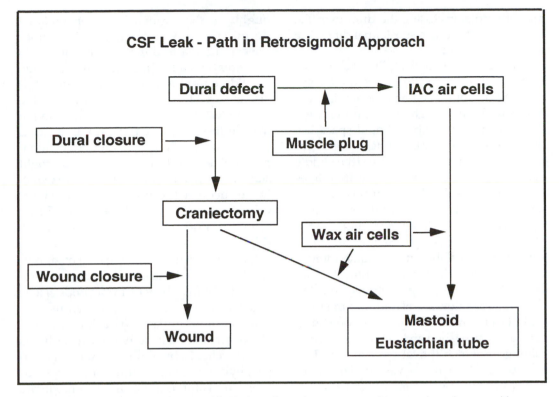

Figure 19–1. Paths of cerebrospinal fluid (CSF) flow after retrosigmoid approach and potential barriers to CSF leak. IAC = Internal Auditory Canal

flowing through the dural defect at the craniectomy can flow through the posterior neck musculature and through any defect in the skin closure. Alternatively, the CSF can escape through any open mastoid air cells within the craniectomy into the mastoid cavity, middle ear space, and eustachian tube to cause CSF rhinorrhea. Since the retrosigmoid approach does not expose the mastoid cavity and middle ear routinely, obliteration of the mastoid and eustachian tube is not a viable option. The first barrier to CSF leak is the dural closure, which potentially can be made watertight. Although the dural incision can be shaped in many different ways, it can be categorized into cruciate and curvilinear types. Either type of incision can be difficult to close primarily because of dural shrinkage during the procedure. Even though the cruciate incision may provide somewhat better access to the surgical site, it is more difficult to repair, compared to the curvilinear incision. Primary closure is attempted using 4-O Surgilon™ or silk, and any areas that will not approximate well can be reinforced with a piece of fascia or muscle plug. The posterior neck musculature and skin should be closed well enough so that a CSF leak through the wound will not occur, even if the dural closure is not watertight. In addition, any mastoid air cells in the craniectomy defect should be waxed to prevent CSF flow into the mastoid cavity.

The dural defect in the IAC usually cannot be closed primarily, so CSF flow through open air cells of the IAC should be blocked by wax. Waxing these air cells alone is likely as effective as any technique, since the use of fibrin glue, muscle or fascia plugs, and attempts at closing the dura over the IAC have not made a substantial difference in CSF leakage rates.

The routes of potential CSF leakage in the translabyrinthine approach are quite complex. Waxing of specific air cells in this situation is futile. Watertight dural closure is not possible, and the subarachnoid space has wide access to the air cell system of the temporal bone. CSF also can leak into the middle ear through the oval window if the stapes footplate has been subluxed during incus removal and there is significant communication between the vestibule and fundus of the IAC. The first barrier to CSF leakage in closure of the translabyrinthine craniectomy is formed within the mastoid cavity (Figure 19–2). Autologous, free fat grafts from the abdomen or thigh are placed into the mastoid defect. Partial dural closure sometimes can be accomplished and can provide a scaffolding on which the fat graft can lay. It is also possible to use a vascularized flap, such as the temporalis muscle or temporoparietal fascia flap based on the superficial temporal artery, but the use of such flaps has not been accepted widely. The wound closure must be watertight after the translabyrinthine approach, since CSF is expected to percolate through the fat to some degree.

The barrier to CSF leakage into the eustachian tube in translabyrinthine surgery is most commonly formed at the aditus ad antrum. A piece of fascia or muscle plug is placed into the mastoid antrum with or without removal of the incus. Additionally some surgeons obliterate the eustachian tube through the facial recess using fascia, muscle plugs, bone wax, bone dust, incus, and other materials. The use of fibrin glue has not been shown to reduce the incidence of CSF leakage (Hoffman, 1994).

The most common path of CSF leakage after the middle cranial fossa approach is through the dural defect in the IAC to the exposed suprameatal air cells and into the mastoid and middle ear, exiting through the eustachian tube (Figure 19–3). These open IAC air cells should be waxed thor-oughly. If the tegmen has been violated during surgery, CSF can flow into the middle ear and mastoid through this defect. In this situation, a fascia graft or muscle plug should be used to close the bony defect. It also is possible for CSF to leak through the wound, but this occurs infrequently. In the middle fossa approach, the dural defect is small and usually is in a more dependent position relative to the wound. Watertight skin and subcutaneous tissue closure usually are adequate for prevention of incisional CSF leakage. The overall rate of CSF leak after the middle fossa approach is 7% (Hoffman, 1994).

Finally, patients with evidence of significantly increased intracranial pressure preoperatively may benefit from prophylactic placement of a CSF shunt, which usually consists of a lumbar subarachnoid drain. However, the obstructive hydrocephalus often is relieved by removal of the tumor, so prophylactic use of a shunt for acoustic tumor removal in cases of mild to moderate degrees of hydrocephalus is not accepted universally.

Treatment

CSF leakage through the wound after any surgical approach for acoustic tumor surgery can be treated with the placement of Nylon™ or Surgilon™ sutures to augment the wound closure and the placement of a pressure dressing. The patient should remain at bedrest as much as possible, and the head should remain elevated to at least 30°. If these conservative measures fail after 24 hr, a lumbar drain should be placed to remove CSF at a rate of approximately 10 cc per hr. If the CSF leak persists after continuous lumbar drainage for three days, revision surgery may be necessary.

After any surgical approach, CSF rhinorrhea initially should be treated conservatively with head elevation and bedrest. A pressure dressing also can be applied. If the CSF leak does not cease after 24 hr, a lumbar drain should be placed. If the CSF leak-

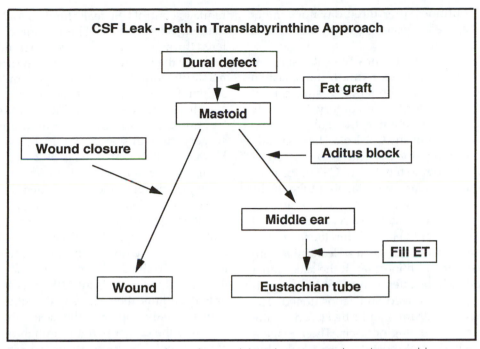

Figure 19–2. Paths of CSF flow after translabyrinthine approach and potential barriers to CSF leak. ET = Eustachian Tube

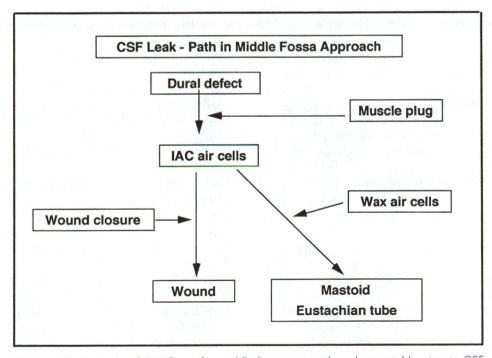

Figure 19–3. Paths of CSF flow after middle fossa approach and potential barriers to CSF leak. IAC = Internal Auditory Canal.

age continues after three days of lumbar drainage, a surgical wound revision should be considered.

Revision surgery for CSF leak usually is performed by an extradural, transmastoid procedure, regardless of the surgical approach used for tumor surgery. It is rarely necessary to re-enter the subarachnoid space to control any CSF leak. The goal of revision surgery for CSF leak is to form an effective barrier to the flow of CSF in the mastoid, middle ear, or eustachian tube. If the CSF leak occurred after a translabyrinthine approach, the same incision is utilized, and the location of the leak within the fat graft is sought. If found, the area of leakage is reinforced with additional fat. If the leak cannot be located, the lateral layers of the fat graft should be removed and repositioned. The aditus ad antrum should be closed tightly with a muscle plug or fascia. These maneuvers will control most persistent leaks, but more extensive procedures are required in some cases.

The next barrier to CSF flow can be formed at the eustachian tube, which must be sealed for cases in which there is an obvious flow of CSF from air cells anterior to the aditus ad antrum. The facial recess is opened to provide access to the middle ear and protympanum. The incus is removed, the mucosa of the eustachian tube is scarified, and the eustachian tube is plugged with bone wax, bone dust, ossicles, fascia, muscle, or a combination of materials. The middle ear and mastoid also are filled with fat. If this intervention fails to control the leak, the middle ear and mastoid can be obliterated by taking down the bony canal wall, removing the mucosa from the middle ear and protympanum, making certain that the eustachian tube has been sealed adequately, filling the entire cavity with fat, and closing the external auditory canal.

For CSF leaks after middle fossa and retrosigmoid approaches that persist after conservative measures, a transmastoid procedure is used. Since some of the patients may have useful residual hearing, the tech-

nique to control CSF leak should avoid permanent hearing loss. The mastoid is entered through an incision separate from that used for the initial surgery. Once the simple mastoidectomy has been performed, a search for the area of leakage is made. Usually, the leak will be visible from a retrolabyrinthine air cell tract after retrosigmoid surgery, and this area should be waxed. However, all potential areas of leakage, including spaces anterior to the ossicles, hypotympanic air cells, and any tegmen defects, must be considered. If there is no apparent leakage anterior to the aditus ad antrum, the aditus is blocked with a piece of muscle or fascia without removing the incus. The mastoid cavity is filled with autologous fat, and the wound is closed. If the leakage is anterior to the aditus, then access to this site is obtained by either opening the facial recess or exposing the epitympanum through the zygomatic root. The incudostapedial joint can be separated and the incus removed, if necessary. An ossicular reconstruction can be performed at a later time if the patient has useful residual sensorineural hearing. Attempts to control the CSF leak with bone wax should be made after adequate access has been obtained, and the eustachian tube and middle ear should be packed with fascia and muscle. These materials have been shown to resorb over time, thereby reconstituting a pneumatized middle ear space (Bryce, Nedzelski, Rowed, & Rappaport, 1991). The mastoid cavity is filled with autologous fat prior to skin closure.

Although there are some conflicting data (Mangham, 1988; Rodgers & Luxford, 1993), there is compelling evidence that patients with CSF leak are at a significantly increased risk of developing bacterial meningitis (Bryce et al., 1991; Hardy, Macfarlane, Baguley, & Moffat, 1989; Hoffman, 1994; Tos & Thomsen, 1982). The prophylactic use of antibiotics for CSF leaks is controversial. Some believe that the use of prophylactic antibiotics reduces the incidence of meningitis in the setting of CSF leak, but others believe that there is no such benefit and, in fact, those who eventually develop meningitis may have a higher chance of harboring a resistant organism. We believe that prophylactic antibiotics in the setting of CSF leak after acoustic neuroma surgery is not beneficial, and we reserve the use of antibiotics until after a presumptive diagnosis of bacterial meningitis has been made. The best prophylaxis against the development of meningitis in the setting of CSF leakage is to control the fistula promptly.

Meningitis

The risk of bacterial meningitis after acoustic tumor surgery is relatively low, ranging from 0.7% to 7% (Cohen, Lewis, & Ransohoff, 1993; Ebersold, Harner, Beatty, Harper, & Quest, 1992; Mangham, 1988; Rodgers & Luxford, 1993; Wiet, Kazan, Raslan, & Herzon, 1986). Meningitis often is a sequela of CSF leakage and, therefore prompt treatment of the leak should limit the risk of meningitis. Although the incidence of meningitis after acoustic tumor surgery is low, the potential morbidity and mortality are high. Without prompt treatment, fulminant bacterial meningitis has a high mortality rate, and those who survive can have major sequelae, including permanent brain damage with symptoms of cognitive dysfunction, seizure disorders, motor and coordination abnormalities, and hearing loss.

The signs and symptoms of meningitis include fever, headache, neck stiffness, photophobia, lethargy, and mental status changes. There may be Kernig's or Brudzinski's signs and focal neurological deficits, although the absence of these signs does not rule out meningitis. If clinical evidence of significantly increased intracranial pressure exists, a CT of the head should be performed to rule out obstructive hydrocephalus, intracranial hematoma, or other pathology that may increase the risk of cerebral herniation during lumbar puncture. In these cases, it is more appropriate to perform a ventriculostomy to obtain a CSF sample. Otherwise, the diagnosis of meningitis is confirmed by performing a lumbar puncture to obtain CSF for chemistries, cell counts, and cultures. Since the morbidity and mortality of bacterial meningitis increase significantly with delay in therapy, antibiotics are administered immediately after a CSF sample has been obtained. Antibiotic coverage should include gram positive organisms, such as Staphylococcus and Streptococcus, and gram negative organisms, such as Klebsiella and Hemophilus. We use a combination of vancomycin and ceftizoxime as initial therapy, and we direct treatment according to the culture results.

Differentiating cases of bacterial meningitis from cases of aseptic meningitis, which are best treated with steroids, presents a diagnostic dilemma. A significant percentage of patients without bacterial meningitis develop CSF changes consistent with meningitis after posterior fossa surgery. Carmel, Fraser, and Bennett (1974) noted that 70% of such patients exhibited these CSF changes without clinical evidence of bacterial meningitis. Although patients with bacterial meningitis tend to have higher fevers, greater incidence of neurological deficits, higher systemic white cell counts, higher CSF white cell counts, and higher incidence of CSF leak (Table 19–2), there is a large overlap in these parameters among cases of bacterial and aseptic meningitis, and no clinical or laboratory criteria can be used to differentiate the two conditions (Ross, Rosegay, & Pons, 1988). The diagnosis of bacterial meningitis can be confirmed only by the presence of organisms on the CSF smear, which occurs rarely, or with positive bacterial cultures, which are not available until two days later. In the absence of CSF leak and implantation of intracranial hardware, the continuation of antibiotics in patients with negative cultures after 2 days has not been found to be beneficial (Blomsted, 1987). Therefore, we continue antibiotic coverage for 2 days until the culture results are available. If the cultures are positive, the patient is treated with culture-directed antibiotics for 2 weeks. If the cultures are negative and the patient continues to have symptoms, steroids, such as dexamethasone (4 mg IV or po q 6 hr), are given over the course of 1 week tapered subsequently. Antibiotics are not continued in these cases unless there is a high suspicion of bacterial meningitis, as in the setting of CSF leak.

Facial Nerve

The preservation of facial nerve function has become almost routine in modern neurotology. The factors that are thought to be impor-

tant in facial nerve preservation include the use of the operating microscope, the use of intraoperative facial nerve monitoring, and the surgeon's experience. The proportion of overall, long-term House-Brackmann grade I to II facial nerve function reported in recent surgical series is 90% (Lalwani, Butt, Jackler, Pitts, & Vingling, 1993; Silverstein, Rosenberg, Flanzer, & Seidman, 1993; Uziel, Benezech, & Frerebeau, 1993).

Acutely after surgery, however, there is a significant incidence of transient facial nerve dysfunction that may last a few weeks to several months. In these patients, the eye should be protected against corneal dessica-

TABLE 19–2. Clinical and laboratory findings in patients with bacterial or aseptic meningitis.

Feature	Aseptic Meningitis	Bacterial Meningitis
Highest oral temperature (¡C)	38.3 ± 0.2	38.9 ± 0.2
Headache	74%	78%
Neck stiffness	74%	72%
Nausea/vomiting	46%	33%
Altered mental status	26%	39%
CSF leak	0%	56%
New focal deficit	0%	11%
Peripheral WBC ($\times\ 10^3$/mm^3)	10.5 ± 0.7	14.9 ± 1.6
Range ($\times\ 10^3$/mm^3)	4.9–18.2	2.5–27.5
CSF WBC (/mm^3)	1012 ± 257	6178 ± 2291
Range (/mm^3)	2–5150	23–40400
CSF PMN	61% ± 6.9%	81% ± 4.5%
Range	1%–98%	25%–98%
CSF lymphocytes	25% ± 6%	7% ± 3%
Range	1%–95%	0%–42%
CSF glucose (mg/dl)	44 ± 4	32 ± 6
Range (mg/dl)	9–100	0–82
CSF protein (mg/dl)	187 ± 35	279 ± 82
Range (mg/dl)	29–760	74–1230

Note. CSF = Cerebrospinal Fluid. WBC = White Blood Cell. PMN = Polymorphonuclear leukocytes. Values reported are mean ± standard error of the mean. From "Differentiation of Aseptic and Bacterial Meningitis in Postoperative Neurosurgical Patients, "by D. Ross, H. Rosegay, and V. Pons, 1988, *Journal of Neurosurgery, 69,* pp. 669–674. Copyright 1991 by American Association of Neurological Surgeons. Reprinted/Adapted with permission of the author.

tion and injury due to inadvertent abrasion, especially if the fifth cranial nerve function also has been affected. Eye lubrication, consisting of tear substitutes, such as hydroxypropylcellulose (Tearisol™), during the day and ophthalmic ointment, such as LacriLube™, at night should be used. The use of a protective shield over the eye also has been found to be useful. If facial nerve function does not recover after 4 to 6 weeks or is not expected to recover for several months, additional measures should be considered. These include an upper eyelid loading procedure, such as the insertion of a gold weight or spring, and a lower eyelid suspension procedure, such as the lateral tarsal strip or wedge resection for those with paralytic ectropion or those at high risk of developing ectropion. Elderly patients, whose soft tissue support of the lower eyelid tends to be lax, are more likely to require a lower lid procedure. When adequate facial nerve function returns, the gold weight or spring can be removed. Lower lid suspension procedures in general do not require a subsequent procedure for reversal. If the facial nerve function fails to return after several months, or is not expected to return due to its transection at the root entry zone, a XII to VII anastamosis is performed.

Should a corneal complication, such as an abrasion, occur, the ophthalmologist is consulted to perform a full eye examination, specifically looking for the extent of corneal damage. Such eye complications are most common in patients who have facial nerve dysfunction together with corneal anesthesia and reduced tearing. Treatment of corneal pathology should be coordinated with the consulting ophthalmologist.

Other Cranial Nerves

Trigeminal Nerve

The incidence of facial numbness after acoustic tumor surgery is thought to be low. In re-cent series, 0% to 1.4% of patients were affected (Ebersold et al., 1992; Harner, Beatty, & Ebersold, 1990; Wiet et al., 1986). Trigeminal dysfunction usually is associated with the surgical excision of large tumors, especially if a significant amount of dissection is required to separate the tumor from the trigeminal nerve. The main morbidity associated with facial numbness is anesthesia of the eye. Transient dysfunction of the trigeminal nerve occurs frequently with transient facial nerve dysfunction, since both are associated with the resection of large tumors. Appropriate eye care should be given in these cases, as discussed previously.

Abducens Nerve

Injury to the sixth cranial nerve is rare but can occur during the resection of large acoustic tumors that penetrate medially. While dissecting medially along the brain stem, one must be cognizant of the presence of the abducens nerve, which may be found in an unexpected location due to anatomic distortion by the tumor. If the nerve is divided, an attempt should be made to repair it primarily. A sixth nerve palsy results in the patient's inability to abduct the ipsilateral eye, and the main complaint will be horizontal diplopia on lateral gaze toward the surgical side. An eye patch can be worn on the paretic side if the diplopia is bothersome. Once the patient has recovered sufficiently from the initial surgery and the abducens palsy is confirmed to be permanent, the ophthalmologist can proceed with extraocular muscle surgery to help alleviate the patient's diplopia.

Dysphagia

There are two etiologies of swallowing dysfunction after acoustic tumor surgery. The first is an acute lower cranial nerve dysfunction, and the second is a combined facial and trigeminal nerve dysfunction. Injury to the lower cranial nerves during acoustic tumor surgery can occur in the setting of a large tumor that extends to the jugular foramen and is adherent to cranial nerves IX, X, and XI. Permanent injury to these nerves is infrequent when they are identified and dissected off the tumor using microsurgical techniques. Injury to cranial nerves IX and X results in abnormalities of both motor and sensory function of the pharynx and larynx. Acute lower cranial nerve deficits can result in dysphagia and aspiration. Initial treatment should include an evaluation of swallowing function, followed by rehabilitation by the speech pathologist. Nutrition should be provided through a small-caliber nasogastric tube or gastric tube until adequate swallowing function returns. If the return of glottic competence is poor and results in persistent aspiration, a Teflon injection or thyroplasty can be performed to medialize the denervated vocal cord.

Oral-facial dysphagia due to facial nerve and trigeminal nerve dysfunction results from abnormalities in the oral phase of swallowing. Oral commissure weakness can lead to oral sphincter incompetence with drooling, and poor buccal tone can result in the undesirable collection of food in the oral gutter. Poor oral sensation and any tongue dysfunction (cranial nerve XII) can compromise further oral function. Treatment again should include swallowing evaluation and therapy by the speech pathologist. For prolonged facial nerve dysfunction, facial function can be augmented by a XII to VII anastamosis. However, disruption of hypoglossal nerve function in the setting of cranial nerves IX and X dysfunction can result in further progression of dysphagia. There is a relative contraindication to performing a XII to VII anastamosis in these cases. Oral commissure rehabilitation utilizing a fascial sling procedure is more appropriate in this setting, although recently developed techniques of XII to VII anastamosis with preservation of hypoglossal function may be used.

Vertigo and Dysequilibrium

Patients can experience vertigo and dysequilibrium caused by the acute loss of residual ipsilateral vestibular function after acoustic tumor surgery. The magnitude of the patient's acute symptoms is related directly to the amount of residual vestibular function present prior to surgery. In patients whose vestibular end-organ or nerve function has been completely obliterated over time by tumor, postoperative vestibular symptoms are relatively mild. In contrast, patients with a significant amount of residual vestibular function prior to surgery experience significant vertigo in the early postoperative period. Symptomatic patients usually recover their balance function over a period of days to weeks as central compensation takes place. Some patients benefit from a short course of physical and vestibular therapy during this period of compensation.

There are some patients who continue to experience balance disturbances beyond the initial compensatory period. These symptoms can be caused by injury to the cerebellum or brainstem, either by the tumor itself or as a result of surgery. Elderly patients appear to be the most susceptible to this type of problem due to their overall reduced ability to compensate for vestibular deficits. Fortunately, reported incidences of vertigo and dysequilibrium at long term follow-up after acoustic neuroma surgery have decreased over the past two decades, and the incidence of persistent cerebellar ataxia after surgery is now only 1% to 2% (Ebersold et al., 1992; Harner et al. 1990). This low incidence likely relates to improved surgical technique, especially with the retrosigmoid approach in which retraction may have been more extensive in the past. Cerebellar retraction is minimal with today's technique of decompressing the CSF cisternal spaces early, allowing nontraumatic relaxation of the cerebellum. In addition, much of the vascular supply to the brainstem is better preserved with contemporary microsurgical dissection techniques for tumor removal.

Chronic dysequilibrium and ataxia due to cerebellar or brainstem contusion are treated with a long course of physical and vestibular rehabilitation therapy. Since many of these patients continue to experience residual deficits, proper surgical technique remains critical in avoiding brainstem and cerebellar injury.

Headache

Chronic headache after acoustic tumor surgery has been reported, but the incidence has been quite variable among different reports, ranging from 0.4% (Ebersold et al., 1992) to 15% (Cohen et al., 1993). Survey data from Wiegand and Fickel (1989) showed a 34% incidence, while Parving, Tos, Thomsen, Moller, and Buchwald (1992) reported a 29% incidence in their survey. The difficulty in interpreting these studies is that it is unknown how significant a problem these headaches were and at what point postoperatively the patients were evaluated for headache. Harner, Beatty, and Ebersold (1993) presented a more comprehensive report on headache after retrosigmoid surgery and found significant headache in 16% of patients at 1 year and in 9% of patients at 2 years but, again, the degree of disability was difficult to ascertain.

The occurrence of bothersome headache has been attributed mainly to the retrosigmoid approach, although this relation has never been proven. The etiology of these headaches has been postulated to be contact between the dura and posterior neck musculature in patients whose craniectomy was not reconstructed. Proponents of this theory advocate filling the craniectomy defect with bone chips, abdominal fat, or methylmethacrylate. In the future, this reconstruction may be accomplished utilizing hydroxyapatite cement (Kamerer, Hirsch, Snyderman, Constantino, & Friedman, 1994).

Headaches usually are managed adequately with the use of oral agents, such as acetaminophen, aspirin, and nonsteroidal anti-inflammatory agents. Narcotics are needed only in a few cases at long-term follow-up. Refractory cases may require referral to a chronic pain consultant or neurologist, who, for treatment, may use other pharmacologic agents, such as antidepressants and anti-migraine medications, as well as biofeedback and transcutaneous electrical nerve stimulation.

Contralateral Hearing Loss

Contralateral hearing loss with acute onset is an unusual condition that has been reported in patients who have undergone acoustic tumor surgery. To date, seven such cases have been reported, including the original three by Clemis, Matricola, and Schuler-Vogler (1982). No satisfactory explanation for this phenomenon has been elucidated so far, and all proposed etiologies remain speculative. These include thromboembolic disease in the labyrinthine artery, immune-mediated inner ear disease secondary to exposure of inner ear antigens during surgery, toxicity related to anesthesia or drugs, postoperative meningitis, allergic inner ear disease, acoustic trauma due to drill noise, and endolymphatic hydrops related to changes in CSF pressure during and after surgery. Clinically, many, but not all, of the patients with this sequela had large tumors. In most cases, the time of onset ranged from the immediate postoperative period to a week and a half after surgery, although cases with a more delayed presentation of 4 months (Lustig, Jackler, & Chen, 1995) to several years (Clemis et al., 1982) have been reported. The surgery and postoperative course for most of these patients were otherwise fairly routine. There were several patients with CSF leak, but further information is needed to ascertain whether this is an important risk factor.

Steroids, carbogen, and other agents have been administered for treatment, but it is unclear if any of these interventions alters the natural course of the hearing loss. A large number of these patients, especially those who do not lose all their hearing early, recover some or all of their hearing function over time, starting as late as a year after surgery. For this reason, some have recommended that cochlear implantation be delayed for at least 18 months in such patients who otherwise are good candidates for this procedure (Walsh, Murty, Punt, & Donoghue, 1994).

Medical Complications

Although posterior fossa surgery for removal of acoustic tumors has become somewhat routine, it still is a major operation with the potential for medical complications. A relatively long duration of anesthesia typically is required, and significant blood loss, fluid shifts, and intracranial manipulations can occur. Postoperative stresses include fluid and electrolyte abnormalities, pulmonary and cardiac stresses, coagulation abnormalities, and the possibility of aspiration pneumonia. Prior to surgery, the patient should be in the best possible medical condition, and significant pre-existing conditions, such as coronary artery disease, chronic obstructive pulmonary disease, diabetes mellitus, bleeding disorders, and malnutrition should be treated to optimize the patient's chances of avoiding a major medical complication.

Pulmonary complications represent the most common, potentially serious medical sequelae, and they include atelectasis, pneumonia, and pulmonary embolus from deep venous thrombosis (DVT). Prophylaxis against DVT, consisting of sequential compression stockings, should be instituted prior to surgery and continued until the patient is no longer bedridden. Ambulation is encouraged as soon as the patient is able, and incentive spirometry is begun. Patients with acute lower cranial nerve palsies who are at risk for aspiration should be suctioned vigorously, and those who cannot handle their secretions adequately should undergo tracheotomy for pulmonary toilet and be fed through a nasogastric or gastric tube. Any impending medical problem should be detected and treated as early as possible.

Cardiac complications, including congestive heart failure and coronary ischemia, usually occur in the setting of known coronary artery disease. These patients should be monitored closely after surgery with the maintenance of adequate cardiac and diuretic medications in consultation with the medical specialist. Fluid intake and output should be monitored and controlled closely to avoid fluid overload.

CONCLUSION

Although acoustic tumor surgery has become relatively safe and routine in the past decade, one must keep in mind that it is still major surgery involving manipulation of intracranial structures. Overall rates of morbidity are very low, but a serious complication can still cause significant morbidity and potential mortality. Good surgical results occur with regularity only when there is close cooperation of the entire team, which includes not only the surgical team but also the anesthesia, nursing, and other support staff. All members of the team must work in concert first to eliminate factors that can lead to complications and, second, to detect and treat any complication that does occur early in its course, so as to minimize its impact on the patient.

Acknowledgments. This work was supported in part by NINDS grant F32 NS09708-02 to SWC.

REFERENCES

Atkinson, W. J. (1949). The anterior inferior cerebellar artery: Its variations, pontine distribution, and significance in the surgery of cerebello-pontine angle tumours. *Journal of Neurology, Neurosurgery, and Psychiatry, 12*, 137–151.

Blomstedt, G. C. (1987). Post-operative aseptic meningitis. *Acta Neurochirgica, 89*, 112–116.

Bryce, G. E., Nedzelski, J. M., Rowed, D. W., & Rappaport, J. M. (1991) Cerebrospinal fluid leaks and meningitis in acoustic neuroma surgery. *Archive of Otolaryngology—Head and Neck Surgery, 104*, 81–87.

Carmel, P. W., Fraser, A. R., & Bennett, M. S. (1974). Aseptic meningitis following posterior fossa surgery in children. *Journal of Neurosurgery, 41*, 44–48.

Clemis, J. D., Matricola, P. G., & Schuler-Vogler, M. (1982). Sudden hearing loss in the contralateral ear in postoperative acoustic tumor: Three case reports. *Laryngoscope, 92*, 76–79.

Cohen, N. L., Lewis, W. S., & Ransohoff, J. (1993). Hearing preservation in cerebellopontine angle tumor surgery: The NYU experience, 1974–1991. *American Journal of Otology, 14*, 423–433.

Ebersold, M. J., Harner, S. G., Beatty, C. W., Harper, C. M., & Quast, L. M. (1992). Current results of the retrosigmoid approach to acoustic neurinoma. *Journal of Neurosurgery, 76*, 901–909.

Hardy, D. G., Macfarlane, R., Baguley, D., & Moffat, D. A. (1989). Surgery for acoustic neuromas. *Journal of Neurosurgery, 71*, 799–804.

Harner, S. G., Beatty, C. W., & Ebersold, M. J. (1990). Retrosigmoid removal of acoustic neuroma: Experience 1978–1988. *Archives of Otolaryngology—Head and Neck Surgery, 103*, 40–45.

Harner, S. G., Beatty, C. W., & Ebersold, M. J. (1993). Headache after acoustic neuroma excision. *American Journal of Otology, 14*, 552–555.

Hoffman, R. A. (1994). Cerebrospinal leak following acoustic neuroma removal. *Laryngoscope, 104*, 40–58.

Kamerer, D. B., Hirsch, B. E., Snyderman, C. H., Constantino, P., & Friedman, C. D. (1994). Hydroxyapatite cement: A new method for achieving watertight closure in transtemporal surgery. *American Journal of Otology, 15*, 47–49.

Kletzker, G. R., Smith, P. G., Backer, R. J., Leonetti, J. G. (1994) Complications in neurotologic surgery. In R. K. Jackler & D. E. Brackmann (Eds.), *Neurotology* (pp. 713–727). St Louis: Mosby.

Lalwani, A. K., Butt, F. Y. S., Jackler, R. K., Pitts, L. H., & Yingling, C. D. (1994). Facial nerve outcome after acoustic neuroma surgery: A study from the era of cranial nerve monitoring. *Archives of Otolaryngology—Head and Neck Surgery, 111*, 561–570.

Lustig, L. R., Jackler, R.K., & Chen, D. A. (1995). Contralateral hearing loss after neurotologic surgery. *Archives of Otolaryngology—Head and Neck Surgery, 113*, 276–282.

Mangham, C. A. (1988). Complications of translabyrinthine vs. suboccipital approach for acoustic tumor surgery. *Archives of Otolaryngology—Head and Neck Surgery, 99*, 396–400.

Parving, A., Tos, M., Thomsen, J., Moller, H., & Buchwald, C. (1992). Some aspects of life quality after surgery for acoustic neuroma. *Archives of Otolaryngology—Head and Neck Surgery, 118*, 1061–1064.

Perneczky, A., Perneczky, G., Tschabitscher, M., & Samec, P. (1981). The relationship between the caudolateral pontine syndrome and the anterior inferior cerebellar artery. *Acta Neurochirgica, 58*, 245–257.

Raskin, J. M., Benjamin, E., & Iberti, T. J. (1985). Venous air embolism: Case report and review. *Mount Sinai Journal of Medicine, 52*, 367–370.

Rigby, P., Cheung, S. W., Sim, D., & Jackler, R. K. (1996, May). *Focal infarction of the cerebellar peduncle as a cause of persistent cerebellar dysfunction following acoustic neuroma surgery: A report of 8 cases.* Paper presented at the Annual Meeting of the American Otological Society, Orlando, FL.

Rodgers, G. K., & Luxford, W. M. (1993). Factors affecting the development of cerebrospinal fluid leak and meningitis after translabyrinthine acoustic tumor surgery. *Laryngoscope, 103*, 959–962.

Ross, D., Rosegay, H., & Pons, V. (1988). Differentiation of aseptic and bacterial meningitis in postoperative neurosurgical patients. *Journal of Neurosurgery, 69*, 669–674.

Silverstein, H., Rosenberg, S. I., Flanzer, J., & Seidman, M. D. (1993). Intraoperative facial nerve monitoring in acoustic neuroma surgery. *American Journal of Otology, 14*(6), 524–532.

Tos, M., & Thomsen, J. (1982). The price of preservation of hearing in acoustic neuroma surgery. *Annals of Otology Rhinology and Laryngology, 91,* 240–245.

Uziel, A., Benezech, J., & Frerebeau, P. (1993). Intraoperative facial nerve monitoring in posterior fossa acoustic neuroma surgery. *Archives of Otolaryngology—Head and Neck Surgery, 108,* 126–134.

Walsh, R. M., Murty, G. E., Punt, J. A. G., & Donoghue, G. M. (1994). Sudden contralater-al deafness following cerebellopontine angle tumor surgery. *American Journal of Otology, 15,* 244–246.

Wiegand, D. A., & Fickel, V. (1989). Acoustic neuroma—The patient's perspective: Subjective assessment of symptoms, diagnosis, therapy, and outcome in 541 patients. *Laryngoscope, 99,* 179–187.

Wiet, R. J., Kazan, R. P., Raslan, W., & Herzon, G. D. (1986). Complications in the approach to acoustic tumor surgery. *Annals of Otology, Rhinology, and Laryngology, 95,* 28–31.

Wiet, R. J., Teixido, M., & Liang, J.-G. (1992). Complications in acoustic neuroma surgery. *Otolaryngological Clinics of North America, 25,* 389–412.

CHAPTER 20

Bilateral Acoustic Neuromas (Neurofibromatosis 2)

Karen Jo Doyle, M.D., Ph.D.
Ralph A. Nelson, M.D.

Although bilateral acoustic neuromas had been described 60 years earlier, Fredrich von Recklinghausen (1882) recounted the syndrome of peripheral neurofibromas that became known as von Recklinghausen's disease. Moyes (1968) later discovered that 14 individuals with bilateral acoustic neuromas did not have the café-au-lait spots and subcutaneous neurofibromas characteristic of von Recklinghausen's disease. Today we know that neurofibromatosis-2 (NF-2) is an entity distinct from von Recklinghausen's disease (NF-1). At the 1987 NIH Consensus Development Conference on Neurofibromatosis, the diagnostic criteria for NF-2 were outlined. One criterion includes bilateral eighth nerve masses on magnetic resonance imaging (MRI) or computed tomography (CT). Additional criteria include a first-degree relative with NF-2 and either a unilateral eighth nerve tumor or two of the following: neurofibroma, meningioma, glioma, schwannoma, or posterior subcapsular lenticular opacity. The tumors of NF-2 affect the brain and the spinal cord. NF-2 affects 1 in 35,000–40,000 individuals and, unlike NF-1, which is usually diagnosed in infancy, usually does not become apparent clinically until early adulthood or, in some cases, later.

GENETICS

NF-2 is known to be transmitted in an autosomal dominant manner, with the genetic defect being a deletion on the long arm of chromosome 22 (Rouleau et al., 1987). The NF-2 gene appears to be a tumor suppressor gene that is inactivated in NF-2 tumors (Rouleau et al., 1993.) The DNA sequence and protein product on which it acts have been determined. Penetrance is 100%, but expression is variable. About half of all new cases of NF-2 are new mutations.

The clinical expression of NF-2 is heterogeneous between families (Evans et al., 1992). Two clinical subtypes of NF-2 have been described: a mild form, known as the Gardner subtype, and a severe form, known as the Wishart subtype. The Gardner subtype is characterized by a late onset of symptoms, usually as a result of vestibular schwannomas (hearing loss) and few other associated brain or spinal tumors. In the Wishart subtype, multiple intracranial and spinal tumors develop at an early age, with rapid progression of signs and symptoms. A third subtype, the Lee/Abbott subtype, is characterized by childhood cataracts and early death due to cranial and spinal meningiomas and schwannomas. In a recent study of 63 individuals with NF-2, the mean age of onset of symptoms in individuals of the Gardner subtype was 27 years, and only 12% had meningiomas (Parry et al., 1994). In contrast, patients with the Wishart and Lee/Abbott subtypes presented at 17.4 years and 14.0 years, respectively, and had a greater than 70% incidence of meningiomas. In general, the clinical expression is less heterogeneous within families (Eldridge & Parry, 1992).

MacCollin et al. (1994) described molecular testing of peripheral blood samples obtained from patients with NF-2 that would enable presymptomatic diagnosis in about two thirds of NF-2 families. Harsh et al. (1995) recommend that at-risk families test their children ages 8 to 15 years. For younger children, they recommend that molecular testing be offered to children under age 8 years. Glasscock, Woods, Jackson, and Welling (1989) advocate screening all young family members of patients with NF-2 using contrast-enhanced MRI and following negative MRI with either yearly auditory brainstem response testing or repeat imaging.

DIAGNOSIS

In the past, bilateral acoustic neuromas frequently were not detected until they were large. In the late 1980s, gadolinium-enhanced MRI enabled detection of small tumors before they became symptomatic. With 3-mm cuts overlapping by 1.5 mm through the posterior fossa, MRI with gadolinium can detect acoustic neuromas as small as 2 mm. The diagnosis of NF-2 usually is made on the basis of gadolinium-enhanced MRI obtained in response to patient complaints of hearing loss and tinnitus.

The detection and management of NF-2 should be performed early for family members of individuals already identified with NF-2. In families having two or more affected generations, genetic linkage analysis is possible to identify gene carriers. Currently however, it is rare to genetically diagnose NF-2. About half of NF-2 patients have new mutation and, therefore, will not be identified genetically, and many other patients do not have two affected generations available for genetic testing. Once identified, gene carriers may be screened yearly with gadolinium-enhanced MRI to detect tumors as they appear. MRI of the spine is a necessary part of the evaluation in patients diagnosed with NF-2, because spinal nerve tumors are common.

AUDIOLOGIC FINDINGS

The audiologic test battery in NF-2 consists of pure tone and speech audiometry and auditory brainstem response (ABR) assessment. Linthicum (1972) was the first to observe that hearing and speech discrimination in patients with bilateral acoustic neuromas often are normal or near-normal in the presence of relatively large lesions. These findings were verfied by Bess, Josey, Glasscook, and Wilson (1984), who found that more than half of NF-2 ears exhibited normal hearing or mild hearing loss. More remarkably, 61% of these patients with good hearing had lesions larger than 1.5 cm, and 26% had tumors 4 cm or larger. These findings differ from those pertaining to unilateral acoustic neuroma, which produces a hearing loss early in its development. Linthicum's explanation was that, for NF-2, the lesion invades the cochlear nerve, separating its fibers but not interrupting them.

Standard ABR, formerly the primary diagnostic method for acoustic neuroma before modern cross-sectional imaging techniques were developed, loses sensitivity for lesions less than 1 cm, and a false-negative rate of up to 30% has been seen. Derived-band ABR, on the other hand, relies on amplitude assessment and exhibits a greater sensitivity than standard ABR. Also, derived-band ABR is based on absolute amplitude in each ear, not on interaural latency, making it valuable in bilateral lesions, for which standard ABR fails.

Given that hearing is normal or near-normal more often than not in NF-2, hearing preservation surgery usually is indicated. When hearing preservation surgery is undertaken, ABR or cochlear nerve whole nerve action potentials are monitored intraoperatively. A preoperative ABR is helpful as a baseline and may be useful in the prognosis of whether hearing preservation will be successful.

TREATMENT STRATEGY

Miyamoto, Roos, Campbell, and Worth (1991) point out that the growth pattern of acoustic neuromas in NF-2 patients is unpredictable. Although growth usually is slowly progressive, tumors may progress rapidly, leading to deafness, cerebellar ataxia, visual disturbances, or even death due to brainstem compression. Sequential gadolinium-enhanced MRI of the brain and internal auditory canals can detect the growth patterns of tumors, assisting in treatment planning. Surgery is the mainstay of treatment of NF-2, but radiation therapy and even chemotherapy have been used. The primary goal of treatment for NF-2 is the removal of tumors with preservation of function.

The role of stereotactic radiosurgery in the treatment of acoustic neuroma is discussed in Chapter 21. Most authors would not recommend stereotactic radiosurgery in patients with NF-2, because tumor control rate is significantly poorer in this population than in patients with unilateral acoustic neuromas.

Bilateral acoustic neuromas and their sequelae can present in a variety of ways, including (a) bilateral small tumors (<2.0 cm), with normal hearing; (b) one large and one small tumor, with normal hearing in the ear with the smaller tumor; (c) two large tumors, with bilateral hearing loss; (d) the appearance of a second tumor after a unilateral acoustic neuroma has been removed with loss of hearing; and (e) multiple tumors invading multiple cranial nerves. In the following paragraphs, we will discuss treatment strategies used for the aforementioned scenarios.

Bilateral Small Tumors with Normal Hearing

In the past, small tumors were observed or removed via the translabyrinthine approach, because the rate of hearing preservation was thought to be poorer in NF-2 than in unilateral acoustic tumors (Linthicum & Brackmann, 1980.) The current recommendation for patients with bilateral small tumors (<2 cm) and for whom hearing is normal or near-normal is total removal of either the larger tumor or the tumor in the ear with the worst hearing via the middle cranial fossa surgical approach. If hearing is preserved successfully, the second tumor also is removed via the middle fossa approach. If the hearing is lost at the first excision, the second tumor is observed until hearing begins to deteriorate. At that point, observation may continue, or a middle cranial fossa internal auditory canal decompression may be performed to temporarily preserve hearing (Gadre, Kwartler, Brackmann, House, & Hitselberger, 1990.) In the few cases in which hearing is lost in the first ear, but the cochlear nerve is left intact, cochlear implantation is an option if promontory stimulation testing yields auditory responses (Hoffman, Kohan, & Cohen, 1992). Kemink, Langman, Niparko, and Graham (1991) advocated incomplete resection of some tumors to preserve function of cranial nerves. We feel that subtotal resection is inappropriate in NF-2 patients who already face multiple surgical procedures, particularly since re-operation carries increased rate of cranial nerve palsies, spinal fluid leaks, and infection.

One Large and One Small Tumor

If one tumor is significantly larger than the other (≥ 3 cm), we advocate total removal of the larger tumor via the translabyrinthine approach and placement of an auditory brainstem implant (ABI). If the ABI is unsuccessful or does not produce significant speech understanding, the second tumor may be observed until hearing is lost, at which time the tumor is removed, with placement of another ABI. If the ABI stimulates successfully on the first side, several options are possible for the smaller tumor, including hearing preservation surgery, observation and translabyrinthine removal when the hearing is lost, or middle fossa decompression to delay hearing loss.

In the unusual case in which hearing is worse, and not remediable, on the side with the smaller tumor, we recommend successive, translabyrinthine-approach removals, first of the smaller tumor, with subsequent ABI placement, then of the larger tumor, timed to preserve hearing as long as possible without producing significant brainstem compression.

Two Large Tumors.

In the situation in which there is no residual hearing in either ear, we recommend complete, bilateral, translabyrinthine removal of the tumors, with ABI placement following the first removal. If serviceable hearing is present in one ear in a patient with large tumors (>3 cm), we recommend successive, translabyrinthine-approach removals, first in the poorer-hearing ear, with subsequent ABI placement.

Development of a Second Tumor After First Tumor Has Been Removed with Subsequent Loss of Hearing

This scenario usually is found in older individuals previously treated for unilateral acoustic neuroma in the pre-gadolinium era. Because the tumor occurs in an only-hearing ear, the treatment depends on the size of the tumor. For large tumors (>3 cm), surgical removal via the translabyrinthine approach, with subsequent placement of the auditory brainstem implant, is appropriate. For patients with small- and medium-sized tumors, in which hearing is still good, surgery should be delayed until hearing is no longer usable or when the tumor is large, at which time translabyrinthine surgery and placement of the ABI are recommended. Observation should be performed at 6- to 12-month intervals and should consist of physical examination, audiologic testing, and MRI.

Tumors Invading Multiple Cranial Nerves

When NF-2 occurs in the severe (Wishart) form, spinal tumors, large meningiomas, and schwannomas that invade multiple cranial nerves develop in childhood or early adulthood. It is difficult to generalize about such cases. Sometimes, the number and location of tumors permit successive surgical removal with a minimum of morbidity. In the most severe cases, early mortality is common as a result of spinal or lower cranial nerve tumors.

SURGICAL APPROACHES

Middle Fossa

The middle fossa craniotomy approach has been used successfully to remove bilateral acoustic neuromas completely and preserve hearing. It is suitable for tumors that lie within the internal auditory canal (IAC) and are up to 1 cm in size in the cerebello-pontine angle. The advantage of this approach is the full exposure of the internal auditory canal so as to enable complete tumor excision. Briggs, Brackmann, Baser, and Hitselberger (1994) described several cases of hearing preservation in NF-2 using this approach. The technique is described in Chapter 11.

Translabyrinthine

This approach is suitable only for large tumors or tumors without usable hearing in NF-2. The advantages are excellent visualization of the facial nerve and access to the entire intracanalicular portion of the tumor for complete removal. The translabyrinthine approach permits access to the lateral recess of the fourth ventricle for ABI placement. The technique is described in Chapter 9.

Suboccipital (Retrosigmoid)

For large tumors in ears with serviceable hearing, the suboccipital approach permits debulking or removal without violating the labyrinth. There have been some cases reported in which hearing was preserved in large acoustic tumors, and some authors recommend incomplete tumor removal for NF-2 if intraoperative brainstem auditory evoked potentials are lost. If the cochlear nerve is left intact via the suboccipital approach, it is sometimes possible to perform a cochlear implant at a later date (Hoffman et al., 1992). The suboccipital technique is described in Chapter 12.

Middle Fossa Decompression of the Internal Auditory Canal

Although total tumor removal is the goal in acoustic neuroma surgery, there may be instances in which decompression of the in-ternal auditory canal may be necessary to preserve hearing. Gadre et al. (1990) described a middle fossa decompression procedure during which bone was removed from the superior aspect of the internal auditory canal, followed by a slit in the IAC dura. In five patients with NF-2, the decompression was performed on one side for tumors measuring 1–2 cm. In three patients, speech discrimination improved in the operated ear 6 months after surgery; the other two patients had no change in their preoperatively excellent speech discrimination. Although hearing preservation rates have improved for NF-2 patients undergoing middle fossa tumor removal, there still may be a role for decompression in certain patients, because this procedure appears to delay the progression of hearing loss.

HEARING PRESERVATION

Glasscock et al. (1989) outlined several factors that may have prognostic value in deciding whether to attempt to preserve hearing in NF-2. Although for unilateral acoustic tumors, "serviceable hearing" is defined by a 50 dB speech reception threshold (SRT) and 50% speech discrimination, any amount of hearing in NF-2 should be considered useful. They did not advocate attempting to preserve hearing in only-hearing ears. Previous reports indicated that hearing preservation may be more difficult in NF-2 than in unilateral tumors, but more recent reports, such as that by Doyle and Shelton (1993), found no difference in the hearing preservation rate using the middle fossa approach (67%) compared to that obtained in unilateral acoustic neuromas. Tumors located more medially within the internal auditory canal may be favorable for hearing preservation, because they may be less adherent to the cochlear nerve. Significantly reduced caloric responses with a tumor less than 1.5 cm may reflect involvement of the superior vestibular nerve, with less compression of the cochlear nerve, which may be favorable for hearing preservation, unlike inferior vestibular nerve tumors. Good preoperative morphology of the auditory brainstem response (ABR) may predict a favorable hearing preservation outcome.

With the advent of real-time intraoperative monitoring of the cochlear nerve action potential (Nedzelski, Chiong, Cashman, Stanton, & Rowed, 1994), the surgeon may decide to abandon tumor removal in the only-hearing ear of NF-2 patients in cases in which cochlear function appears compromised during tumor removal.

AUDITORY PROSTHESES

Cochlear Implants

For deafened patients in whom an attempt to preserve hearing has yielded the anatomic preservation of the cochlear nerve, cochlear implantation is a possible alternative for hearing restoration. Cueva, Thedinger, Harris, and Glasscock (1992) performed promontory stimulation on six patients with deafness and intact cochlear nerves. Only one patient noted subjective auditory perception with promontory stimulation, and this patient theoretically would benefit from a cochlear implant. Hoffman et al. (1992) reported a patient with NF-2 who had lost hearing with the first acoustic neuroma removal and who had failed a suboccipital attempt at hearing preservation on the second side. The cochlear nerve was anatomically preserved, and brainstem evoked potentials were lost intraoperatively. One month following surgery, promontory stimulation yielded no response. However, good thresholds were obtained when testing was repeated at 8 weeks, and he underwent successful cochlear implantation. This case demonstrates the feasibility of implant surgery. Hughes, Sismanis, Glasscock, Hays, and Jackson (1982) pointed out that, in some cases, NF-2 tumor invades the cochlea. They theorized that, in such pa-

tients, cochlear implantation could be performed, because the tumor within the cochlea was unlikely to grow. No such cases have been reported in the literature.

One disadvantage of cochlear implantation for patients with NF-2 is that MRI scanning cannot be performed after its insertion. For some patients with NF-2 and multiple tumors, the need for yearly MRI scanning may preclude cochlear implantation. Therefore, before cochlear implantation is undertaken, long-term planning should be undertaken.

Auditory Brainstem Implant

In 1979, William House and William Hitselberger performed the first auditory brainstem implant in a patient with NF-2. She had undergone an earlier translabyrinthine tumor removal in 1964 and subsequently had becomed completely deaf in her other ear due to a large acoustic neuroma. A platinum wire electrode with ball terminals was inserted into the ventral cochlear nucleus. Three years later, the surgeons reported that the patient was able to receive sound through a single-channel stimulator unit and that she scored above chance on closed-set speech tests, similarly to patients with single-channel cochlear implants (Edgerton, House, & Hitselberger, 1982). Since that time, more than 45 patients have received auditory brainstem implants, and many improvements have been introduced into the device (Brackmann et al., 1993). The current device consists of eight disc electrodes mounted on a Dacron mesh carrier. Following tumor removal, the device is placed through the foramen of Luschka into the lateral recess, via the translabyrinthine approach. Monitoring of the electrically evoked auditory brainstem responses is used to determine correct positioning of the electrode array. A transcutaneous electromagnetic coil has replaced the original percutaneous plug used to couple the internal device to the externally worn stimulator.

Most patients show improvement in closed-set speech perception and use the device as an aid to lipreading. A few ABI patients implanted with the eight-electrode array have limited open-set speech understanding.

The ABI currently is not an FDA-approved device, but FDA-monitored clinical trials are in progress at several co-investigator centers. Patient selection criteria currently include the presence of bilateral eighth nerve tumors, age 15 years or older, competence in the English language, psychological suitability, realistic expectations, and willingness to comply with the research protocol. Candidates may wait until removal of the second tumor to receive the ABI but, in some cases, the ABI has been placed at the time of the first tumor removal. It is thought that earlier implantation and experience with the device will enhance performance. In addition, removal of the second tumor often is delayed until the tumor is very large, and the landmarks to identify the cochlear nucleus may become distorted.

OTHER CONSIDERATIONS

As Glasscock et al. (1989) emphasized, NF-2 does not render only deafness. Rather, other central nervous system tumors secondary to NF-2 may result in other morbidities, such as motor deficits and paralysis, blindness, and increased mortality. The potential for permanent disability is great, both psychological and physical. Therefore, other professionals should be involved in the care of patients afflicted with this disorder, such as primary care physicians, psychiatrists, psychologists, occupational therapists, physical therapists, speech pathologists, and genetic counselors.

REFERENCES

Bess, F.H., Josey, A.F., Glasscock, M.E., & Wilson, L.K. (1984). Audiologic manifestations in bilateral acoustic tumors (von Recklinghausen's disease). *Journal of Speech and Hearing Disorders, 49,* 177–182.

Brackmann, D.E., Hitselberger, W.E., Nelson, R.A., Moore, J., Waring, M.D., Portillo, F., Shannon, R.V., & Telischi, F. (1993). Auditory brainstem implant: I. Issues in surgical implantation. *Archives of Otolaryngology—Head and Neck Surgery, 108,* 624–633.

Briggs, R.J.S., Brackmann, D.E., Baser, M.E., & Hitselberger, W.E. (1994). Comprehensive management of bilateral acoustic neuromas. *Archives of Otolaryngology—Head and Neck Surgery, 120,* 1307–1314.

Cueva, R.A., Thedinger, B.A., Harris, J.P., & Glasscock, M.E. (1992). Electrical promontory stimulation in patients with intact cochlear nerve and anacusis following acoustic neuroma surgery. *Laryngoscope, 102,* 1220–1224.

Doyle, K.J., & Shelton, C. (1993). Hearing preservation in bilateral acoustic neuroma surgery. *American Journal of Otology, 14,* 562–565.

Edgerton, B.J., House, W.F., & Hitselberger, W.E. (1982). Hearing by cochlear nucleus stimulation in humans. *Annals of Otology, Rhinology, and Laryngology, 91*(Suppl. 91), 117–124.

Eldredge, R., & Parry, D.M., (1992). Neurofibromatosis 2: Evidence for clinical heterogeneity based on 54 affected individuals studied by MRI with gadolinium, 1987–1991. In M. Tos & J. Thomsen, (Eds.), *Proceedings of the First International Acoustic Neuroma Conference, Copenhagen, Denmark* (pp. 801–804). New York: Kugler.

Evans, D.G., Huson, S.M., Donnai, D., Neary, W., Blair, V., Tears, D., Newton, V., Strachan, T., Ramsden, R., & Harris, R. (1992). A genetic study of type 2 neurofibromatosis in the United Kingdom. I. Prevalence, mutation rate, fitness, and confirmation of maternal transmission effect on severity. *Journal of Medical Genetics, 29,* 841–846.

Gadre, A.K., Kwartler, J.A., Brackmann, D.E., House, W.F., & Hitselberger, W.E. (1990). Middle fossa decompression of the internal auditory canal in acoustic neuroma surgery: A therapeutic alternative. *Laryngoscope, 100,* 948–952.

Glasscock, M.E., Woods, C.I., Jackson, C.G., & Welling, B. (1989). Management of bilateral acoustic tumors. *Laryngoscope, 99,* 475–484.

Harsh, G.R., MacCollin, M., McKenna, M.J., Nadol, J.B., Ojemann, R., & Short, M.P. (1995). Molecular genetic screening for children at risk of neurofibromatosis 2. *Archives of Otolaryngology—Head and Neck Surgery, 121,* 590–591.

Hoffman, R.A., Kohan, D., & Cohen, N.L. (1992). Cochlear implants in the management of bilateral acoustic neuromas. *Archives of Otolaryngology—Head and Neck Surgery, 13,* 525–528.

Hughes, G.B., Sismanis, A., Glasscock, M.E., Hays, J.W., & Jackson C.G. (1982). Management of bilateral acoustic tumors. *Laryngoscope, 92,* 1351–1359.

Kemink, J.L., Langman, A.W., Niparko, J.K., & Graham, M.D. (1991). Operative management of acoustic neuromas: The priority of neurologic function over complete resection. *Archives of Otolaryngology—Head and Neck Surgery, 104,* 96–99.

Linthicum, F.H. (1972). Unusual audiometric and histologic findings in bilateral acoustic neuromas. *Annals of Otolaryngology, 81,* 433–437.

Linthicum, F. H., & Brackmann, D.E. (1980). Bilateral acoustic tumors: A diagnostic and surgical challenge. *Archives of Otolaryngology—Head and Neck Surgery, 106,* 729–733.

MacCollin, M., Ramesh, V., Jacoby, L., Louis, D., Rubio M., Pulaski, K., Trofatter, J., Short, M., Bove, C., Eldridge, R., Parry, D., & Gusella, J. (1994). Mutational analysis of patients with neurofibromatosis 2. *American Journal of Human Genetics, 55,* 314–320.

Miyamoto, R.T., Roos, K.L., Campbell, R.L., & Worth, R.M. (1991). Contemporary management of neurofibromatosis. *Annals of Otology, Rhinology, and Laryngology, 100,* 38–43.

Moyes, P.D. (1968). Familial bilateral acoustic neuroma affecting 14 members from four generations. *Journal of Neurosurgery, 29,* 78–79.

Nedzelski, J.M., Chiong, C.M., Cashman, M.Z., Stanton, S.G., & Rowed D.W. (1994). Hearing preservation in acoustic neuroma surgery: Value of monitoring cochlear nerve action potentials. *Archives of Otolaryngology—Head and Neck Surgery, 111,* 703–709.

Parry, D.M., Eldridge, R., Kaiser-Kipfer, M.I., Bouzas, E.A., Pikus, A., & Patronas, N. (1994). Neurofibromatosis 2 (NF2): Clinical characteristics of 63 affected individuals and clinical evidence for heterogeneity. *American Journal of Medical Genetics, 52,* 450–461.

Rouleau, G.A., Wertelecki, W., Haines, J.L., Hobbs, W.J., Trofatter, J.A., Seizinger, B.R., Martuza, R.L., Superneau, D.W., Conneally, P.M. & Gusella, J.F. (1987). Genetic linkage of bilateral acoustic neurofibromatosis to a DNA marker on chromosome 22. *Nature, 329,* 246–248.

Rouleau, G.A., Merel, P., Lutchman, M., Sanson, M., Zucman, J., Marineau, C., Hoang-Xuan, K., Demczuk, S., Desmaze, C., & Plougastel, B. (1993). Alteration in a new gene encoding a putative membrane-organizing protein causes neurofibromatosis type 2. *Nature, 363,* 515–521.

von Recklinghausen, F. (1882). *Über die Multiplen Fibrone der Haut und Ihre Beziehung zu den Multiplen Neuromen* [About Multiple Fibromas of the Skin and Their Relevance to Multiple Neuromas]. Berlin: A. Hirschwald.

CHAPTER 21

Stereotactic Radiosurgery for Acoustic Neuromas

C. Y. Joseph Chang, M.D.
Donald B. Kamerer, M.D.

The surgical treatment of acoustic neuromas was revolutionized when William House (1964) reported use of the translabyrinthine approach. Prior to this, acoustic neuroma surgery was associated with a high morbidity. The mortality rate was unacceptably high, tumor resection was usually subtotal, and there was no significant chance of preserving hearing or facial nerve function. The recent developments in anesthesia techniques for neurosurgical cases, as well as improved operative techniques, have made surgical resection of acoustic tumors almost routine. The mortality rate for acoustic neuroma surgery is now very low, and the likelihood of normal facial nerve function on long-term follow-up after surgical excision is very high. In addition, the tumor recurrence rate after surgical excision is thought to be extremely low. On the other hand, surgical excision, which can be approached by the middle fossa, translabyrinthine, and retrosigmoid routes, still entails an open intracranial procedure with its attendant risks of possible cerebrovascular accident, cerebral contusion, wound infec-

tion, meningitis, and intracranial bleed. Hearing preservation rates after acoustic neuroma surgery have not been high, although they have been improving. Surgical treatment also requires costly inpatient care. Until recently, the only option available to patients who were poor candidates for major surgery due to pre-existing medical conditions was observation alone.

Lars Leksell (1971), at the Karolinska Institute in Stockholm, Sweden, first reported the use of gamma radiation ports administered stereotactically during a single sitting to halt the growth of acoustic tumors. The lesion was localized precisely for targeting using available imaging modalities, and the radiation ports were designed to maximize the radiation dose to the lesion while minimizing exposure to the normal surrounding structures. The term "stereotactic radiosurgery" was coined to describe this technique, and the particular technology used by Leksell was called the "gamma knife." Since Leksell's early reports, a relatively large experience has been attained in treating benign tumors, vascular anomalies, and malignant neoplasms, either as primary therapy or as adjunctive therapy after subtotal tumor resection.

Since the first gamma knife unit was installed in Stockholm, numerous other sites in Europe acquired this technology. The first gamma knife unit in North America was installed at the University of Pittsburgh in 1987, and over 90 stereotactic radiosurgery units since have become operational in this country (Lunsford & Linskey, 1992). The purpose of this chapter is to familiarize the reader with the basic concepts relating to stereotactic radiosurgery as a treatment modality for acoustic neuromas and discuss the available data regarding morbidities and outcomes.

INTRODUCTION TO STEREOTACTIC RADIOSURGERY

Definition

Stereotactic radiosurgery is characterized by the closed-skull treatment of an intracranial lesion with the use of multiple, precisely directed beams of ionizing radiation delivered during a single treatment session. The radiation source is either a multisource cobalt-60 gamma unit (the gamma knife) or a modified linear accelerator. Systems utilizing charged particles also have been described. An imaging-compatible stereotactic coordinate frame is applied to the patient's head under local anesthesia, and imaging with either a high-resolution computed tomography (CT) scan or magnetic resonance imaging (MRI) is performed. The resultant multiplanar images show the tumor's exact position in relation to other anatomic structures, as referenced by the stereotactic frame. These images are captured by a high-speed digital computer that then aids in radiation beam targeting and dosimetry to treat the tumor volume. The radiation therapist uses this digitized information to design the appropriate radiation field for tumor treatment.

Once a treatment plan has been formulated, the patient is placed into the stereotactic radiotherapy unit. The typical treatment time is 10 to 20 min. Although some patients require overnight admission, the majority go home the same day.

Targeting, Imaging and Dosimetry

The multiple radiation beams used in stereotactic radiosurgery generate a gradient radiation field that results in a high radiation dose within the target lesion (usually a tumor) and a diminished dose to surrounding structures (Figure 21–1). The center of the radiation field is called the isocenter and receives the maximal radiation dose, while a roughly elliptical distribution of radiation density surrounds the isocenter (Figure 21–2). The exact shape of this radiation field density varies depending on the particular unit utilized. Irregularly-shaped radiation fields can be created by using multiple isocenter treatment. To accomplish this, the treatment is given multiple times, and the resultant field is the sum of the multiple treatment fields. When combined, the multiple elliptical radiation fields results in a custom-shaped field suitable for use in treating an irregularly shaped tumor.

The radiation field distribution is designed so that the entire tumor can be encompassed within the 50% to 80% isodose. This means that the periphery of the lesion receives 50% to 80% of the highest central dose. The radiation gradient is quite steep at the 50% isodose, resulting in a rapid reduction in radiation dose to normal structures as a function of distance from the center of the tumor (Figure 21–3). The slope or steepness of the radiation gradient at the 50% isodose becomes shallower as the treated tumor volume increases, meaning that the surrounding normal tissues receive relatively more radiation when a large tumor is treated compared to the radiation exposure to surrounding tissues when a small tumor is treated. Therefore, from the standpoint of

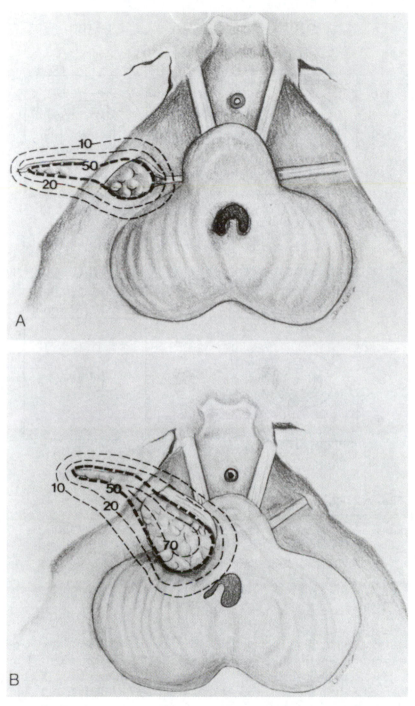

Figure 21–1. Artist's conception of typical isodose plans for small (A) and large (B) acoustic tumors. (From "Stereotactic Radiosurgery for Acoustic Tumors" by M. E. Linskey, L. D. Lunsford, J. C. Flickinger, and D. Kondziolka, 1992, *Neurosurgery Clinics of North America, 3,* p. 194. Copyright 1992 by W.B. Saunders Company. Reprinted with permission.)

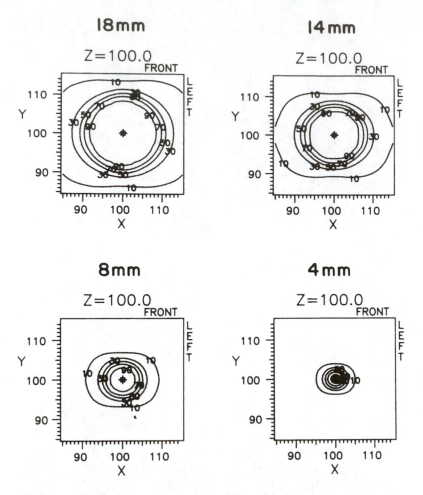

Figure 21–2. Isodose distribution for each collimator helmet in the axial plane. Larger collimator helmets result in larger volumes of treatment. (From *Radiosurgery: Baseline and Trends*, by L Steiner (Ed.), 1992, p. 59. New York: Raven Press. Copyright 1992 by Raven Press, Ltd. Reprinted with permission.)

radiation exposure alone, there is potential for higher morbidity when treating larger lesions with stereotactic radiosurgery.

The dosage used early in the experience at the Karolinska Institute was 25 to 35 Gy to the periphery, with a maximal central dose of 50 to 70 Gy. These dosages eventually were decreased to 10 to 15 Gy for the periphery and 15 to 25 Gy centrally to reduce the incidence of cranial neuropathies (Noren, Arndt,

& Hindmarsh, 1983; Noren, Greitz, Hirsch, & Lax, 1992; Noren, Greitz, Hirsch, & Lax, 1993). The University of Pittsburgh gamma knife group similarly found a high incidence of cranial neuropathies after gamma knife treatment with a peripheral dose of 20 Gy, so the marginal dosage was reduced for subsequent patients to 16 to 18 Gy (Hirsch & Noren, 1988; Linskey, Lundsford, Flickinger, & Kondziolka, 1992b)

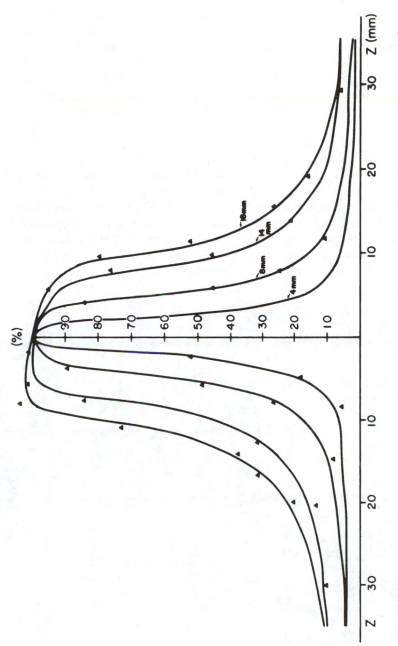

Figure 21-3. Dose profile comparison for each collimator helmet in the axial plane. The radiation dose decreases as a function of distance from the isocenter (Z=0), and the decrease is steepest between 50% and 80% of the maximal dose. (From *Radiosurgery: Baseline and Trends* by L. Steiner (Ed.), 1992, p. 58, New York: Raven Press. Copyright 1992 by Raven Press, Ltd. Reprinted with permission.)

Gamma Knife Unit

The gamma knife unit (Berk & Agarwal, 1992) provides radiation energy generated by 201 independent cobalt-60 sources housed in a shielded encasement (Figure 21–4). These cobalt-60 sources are stationed within sealed wells and require replacement periodically. The patient's head then is inserted into the unit with the appropriate collimator helmet in place over the stereotactic frame. The exact configuration of the treated volume is determined by the collimator size, the plugging pattern, multiple isodose targeting, and time of exposure with each target or "weighting".

The collimator size refers to the size of the apertures in the collimator helmet that allow radiation beams to travel to the target. The Leksell unit provides a choice of four helmets corresponding to collimator diameters of 4, 8, 14, and 18 mm. The smaller the collimator size used, the smaller the target volume. The plugging pattern can be tailored to each lesion. Specific apertures can be plugged (blocked) to create a target volume that is different in shape from the standard elliptical target volume that results if all the collimators were open. The use of multiple target points can create an overall target volume that is irregularly shaped, as discussed previously. Several target points are chosen within the lesion, and radiation beams are applied for the appropriate amount of time to each target point. Using this technique of multiple target points and weighting, a treatment volume that fits the lesion more precisely can be created, as compared to a strictly elliptical radiation field that results from the use of a single target point (Berk & Agarwal, 1992). A high-speed computer aids in designing the optimal treatment plan for each patient.

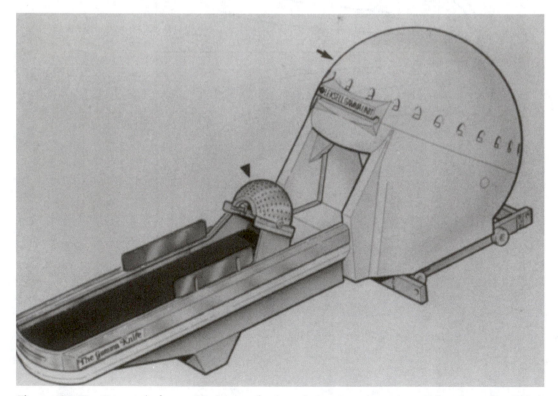

Figure 21–4. Gamma knife unit. The housing for the cobalt sources *(arrow)*, as well as the collimator helmet *(arrowhead)*, are shown.

Linear Accelerator Unit

A distinct disadvantage of the gamma knife unit is the cost of installation and the need to replace the cobalt-60 sources periodically. In addition, the gamma knife unit can be used only for stereotactic radiosurgery. Several centers with linear accelerator units have modified their units so that stereotactic radiosurgery can be performed, and some of these centers have treated acoustic neuromas (Mendenhall, Friedman, & Bova, 1994). The advantage of the linear accelera-tor is that the same unit that performs conventional external beam radiation can be used to perform stereotactic radiosurgery. In addition, there are no cobalt-60 sources that require periodic replacement. In order for the linear accelerator to provide the required mechanical aiming accuracy of 0.2 ± 0.1 mm, a series of high-precision bearings that control the position of the collimator and the stereotactic ring must be installed to prevent positioning errors due to "gantry sag" and nonisocentric couch rotation (Figure 21–5).

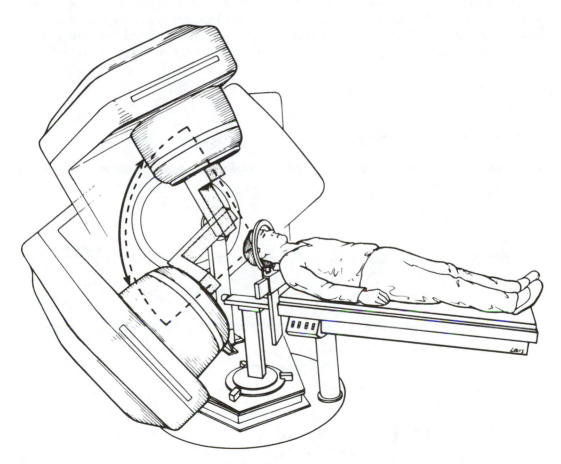

Figure 21–5. Linear accelerator unit with portable stereotactic attachment to improve on the inherent inaccuracy of the linear accelerator to allow its use in stereotactic radiosurgery. (From "Linear Accelerator Radiosurgery at the University of Florida," by W. A. Friedman, F. J. Bova, and R. Spiegelmann, 1992, *Neurosurgery Clinics of North America, 3*, p. 145. Copyright 1992 by W. B. Saunders Company. Reprinted with permission.)

The principle behind stereotactic radiotherapy utilizing either the gamma knife or the linear accelerator is the same. A defined target volume containing tumor or other lesion is exposed to a high level of radiation energy, while the dose of radiation to the surrounding tissues remains relatively low. The difference between the two modalities is in the delivery system. Whereas the gamma knife unit generates the radiation gradient field using multiple simultaneous radiation beams, the linear accelerator uses a single source that is rotated in multiple noncoplanar arcs (Figure 21–6). The size and shape of the radiation field depends on the collimator size, the number of arcs performed, the number of isocenters employed, and any modulation of the radiation beam intensity during each arc. The linear accelerator system can utilize a collimator diameter up to 35 mm, as compared to the maximum of 18 mm for the current gamma knife unit. This potentially can result in greater flexibility in treatment planning. In general, as a larger collimator size is used, a wider beam of radiation results, and a larger volume of tissue is treated per arc of radiation. Similarly, as a larger number of arcs are used, a larger volume of tissue is treated. Multiple isocenters can be used as with the gamma knife unit to encompass an irregularly shaped tumor, but the linear accelerator system can also modulate the radiation beam intensity during each arc to encompass an irregularly shaped lesion without the use of multiple isocenter dosing (Brada & Laing, 1994; Friedman, Bova, & Spiegelmann, 1992).

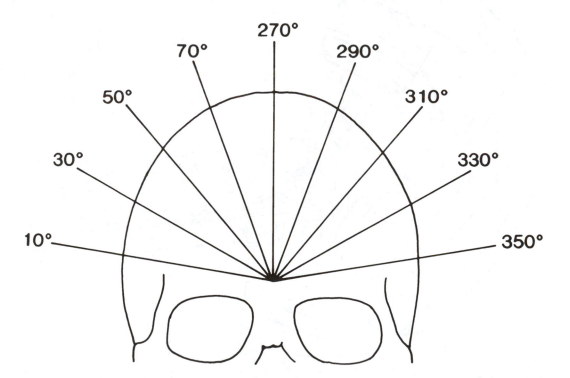

Figure 21–6. Stereotactic radiosurgery treatment utilizing the linear accelerator is delivered using up to nine noncoplanar arcs intersecting at the target. (From "Linear Accelerator Radiosurgery at the University of Florida," by W. A. Friedman, F. J. Bova, and R. Spiegelmann, 1992, *Neurosurgery Clinics of North America, 3,* p. 148. Copyright 1992 by W.B. Saunders, Company. Reprinted with permission.)

The details of patient treatment using the linear accelerator are quite similar to those of the gamma knife. A stereotactic frame is attached to the patient's head under local anesthesia, a CT or MR scan is performed, a treatment plan is prepared with the aid of a high-speed computer, and the patient is treated over the course of 15 to 20 min. The patient typically requires no overnight stay.

Patient Selection

Candidates for treatment of acoustic neuromas using stereotactic radiosurgery have included the elderly, those with bilateral tumors or tumors in only-hearing ears, those with medical contraindications to major surgery, those with recurrent tumor after surgery who wish no further surgery, and those who refuse surgery altogether, as outlined in the first article on treatment of acoustic tumors from the University of Pittsburgh radiosurgery group (Kamerer, Lunsford, & Moller, 1988). Subsequent publications continued to support this view that microsurgical removal should remain the primary treatment modality, and stereotactic radiosurgery should be reserved for those who are not good surgical candidates (Lunsford, Kamerer, & Flickinger, 1990; Linskey et al., 1992b; Lunsford & Linskey, 1992).

More recently, proponents of stereotactic radiosurgery have suggested that this treatment modality should be considered for all patients with acoustic neuromas (Noren et al., 1993; Pollock et al., 1995). Instead of radiosurgery being an alternative to surgical excision as primary therapy, they suggest that the results of radiosurgery in treating acoustic tumors are now equal to if not better than microsurgical excision, and all patients should be presented with either option as primary therapy. Needless to say, this issue has become quite controversial, and this chapter alone cannot resolve this issue. We will present the data available at present as accurately as possible, so that the reader will attain a better understanding of the issues at hand.

TISSUE INTERACTIONS

Radiobiology

The fundamental mechanism of tissue destruction in single fraction radiosurgery differs from that of multiple fraction radiotherapy. In the latter, the selective destruction of pathologic tissue depends on differences between the pathologic and normal tissues in susceptibility to radiation and efficacy of repair after radiation damage. Conversely, stereotactic radiosurgery delivers a single dose of radiation sufficient to control the growth of the tumor while sparing the normal structures from destructive doses of radiation. This differential in radiation dose is accomplished by the use of multiple beams of radiation converging at the tumor, thereby creating an energy distribution that is high within the tumor and low within the surrounding normal tissues (Larsson, 1992).

Although a multiple radiation beam targeting system can significantly reduce the amount of radiation delivered to normal tissues, the difference in radiation delivered to the tumor and the dose delivered to surrounding normal tissues depends on the tumor volume. The radiation distribution field generated by a stereotactic radiosurgery system creates a high dose at the center of the target, and a progressively smaller dose farther away from the center. The periphery of the tumor typically receives the lowest dose of radiation, and this peripheral dose in theory should determine whether adequate tumor control will be achieved. Therefore, in order to deliver an adequate tumoricidal dose, the tumor periphery must be radiated at an appropriately high level. Consequently, larger tumors require more radiation for adequate treatment, and this larger dose must pass through normal tissues to be delivered to the tumor. Another way to describe this situation is that the slope of the radiation gradient at the periphery of the treated volume is steeper when treating smaller lesions. Therefore, the treatment of larger tumors results in the exposure of surrounding normal tissues to higher radiation doses, with higher potential for morbidity. Such a relationship was confirmed in patients undergoing stereotactic radiosurgery treatment of arteriovenous malformations (Flickinger, Lunsford, & Kondziolka, 1992).

Radiation Effects on Normal Tissue

Animal studies have confirmed that discrete, radionecrotic lesions can be created within the brain to cause specific functional effects within 1 to 2 weeks after treatment with stereotactic radiosurgery. A single, central dose of 200 to 300 Gy was found to result in small, well-defined necrotic lesions 2 to 5 mm in diameter, without other histological changes in the short term (Fabricius, Larsson, Steen, & Akerman, 1962; Gale & Larsson, 1963).

In humans, early studies were performed on 21 patients who underwent gamma knife treatment for chronic pain (Dahlin et al., 1975). Acutely after a dose of 200 Gy, there was circumscribed destruction of neural tissue with only a slight cellular response at the edge of the lesion and no significant edema. There was additional degenerative and inflammatory reaction 3 to 4 weeks after irradiation. Following this stage, there was a 1-year period consisting of resorption of cellular debris, the start of glial scar formation, astrocyte proliferation around the necrotic area, and presence of occasional giant cells. Along the periphery of the radiolesion, a chronic inflammatory response developed with congested blood vessels and formation of new capillaries with endothelial thickening. More than 1 year after radiation, the inflammatory changes resolved and were replaced by prominent glial scar formation.

It is thought that stereotactic radiation therapy in the dosages used currently causes both acute and late deleterious effects. The early effects occur within the first week after treatment and, excluding acute ede-

ma, are thought to be insignificant. The late effects require months to years to develop, and include demyelinization and white matter necrosis caused by destruction of oligodendroglia and endothelial cell damage resulting in ischemia (Larsson, 1992).

Radiation Effects on Tumor

The radiation dose-survival curves of tumor cells and normal tissues in vitro have been shown to vary according to the type of tissue (Hall & Wright, 1988; Nilsson, Carlsson, & Larsson, 1980). In the treatment of malignant lesions, it is assumed that all tumor cells must be destroyed in order to obtain a cure. The effective treatment of slowly growing benign tumors may require less stringent criteria, but there are several issues to consider. Benign lesions are, in general, less susceptible to destruction by radiation. The effective control of these tumors by a single dose of radiation depends on direct cell death, as well as changes around the tumor, such as ischemia from endothelial damage. A sufficient number of cells must be destroyed eventually so that the number remaining, if any, is not adequate to regenerate a significant tumor volume. The dosage necessary to effect a cure in slowly growing neoplasms, such as acoustic neuromas, is not yet known, and a long period may be required to obtain this information.

RESULTS OF STEREOTACTIC RADIOSURGERY ON ACOUSTIC NEUROMAS

Clinical Studies

There are two groups that have reported large series of patients who underwent treatment of acoustic neuromas with the gamma knife technique. The group at the Karolinska Institute in Stockholm, Sweden, has been treating such patients since the early 1970s, and the group at the University of Pittsburgh began to treat patients in 1987. A group at the University of Florida has reported a series of patients treated with the linear accelerator radiosurgery technique.

The studies generated by these groups are summarized in Tables 21–1, 21–2, 21–3, 21–4, and 21–5. The experience of the group at the Karolinska Institute in treating patients with unilateral and bilateral acoustic neuromas is reported in Noren et al. (1983), Noren et al. (1992), and Noren et al., (1993) and are summarized in Table 21–1. Undoubtedly, the three studies report results on overlapping groups of patients, with the latest studies containing more patients. It is unclear whether the latest report includes all patients from previous reports, or whether some patients from the earlier report have been excluded. It is noteworthy that the radiation dosage was changed during the course of the latter two studies. The early patients in Noren et al. (1992) received a maximal tumor dose, ranging from 50 to 70 Gy and a minimal tumor dose ranging from 25 to 35 Gy, at the periphery. The later patients received a lower dosage: The maximal tumor dose ranged from 15 to 25 Gy, while the minimum tumor dose ranged from 10 to 15 Gy. In Noren et al. (1993), the dosage for the early patients consisted of 18 to 20 Gy to

TABLE 21–1. Reports of gamma knife radiosurgery to treat acoustic neuromas at the Karolinska Institute, Stockholm, Sweden.

	Noren et al., 1983	Noren et al., 1992	Noren et al., 1993
No. pts.	N = 14	N = 219	N = 254
No. bilat.	1	49	61
f/u	> 4 years	12–206 months	12–206 months
Max dose	50–125 Gy	15–70 Gy	15–40 Gy
Min dose	7–45 Gy	10–35 Gy	10–20 Gy
Tumor size	Mean not provided	Mean not provided	Not reported
	Range 7–30 mm	Range 4–33 mm	Mean not provided

TABLE 21–2. Reports of gamma knife radiosurgery to treat acoustic neuromas at the University of Pittsburgh.

	Flickinger et al., 1991	Linskey et al., 1992	Ogunrinde et al., 1994	Pollock et al. 1995
No. pts.	N = 85	N = 85 (87 tumors)	N = 98	N = 47
No. bilat.	N = 15	N = 14	N = 0	N = 0
Prior surgery	N = 14	N = 20	N = 23	N = 0
f/u	9–29 months	> 1 year	24–72 months	25–48 months
Max dose	24.3–50 Gy	24.3–50 Gy	24–50 Gy	25–36 Gy
Min dose	14–20 Gy	12–20 Gy	12–20 Gy	16.3–18 Gy
Tumor size	Mean 17.2 mm	Mean not reported	Mean 17.2 mm	Mean not reported
	Range 7.1–29.1 mm	Range IAC—3 cm	Range IAC—2.5 cm	Range IAC—30 mm

TABLE 21-3. Reports of linear accelerator radiosurgery to treat acoustic neuromas at the University of Florida (Mendenhall, et al., 1994).

No. pts.	N = 32
No. bilat.	N = 4
Prior surgery	N = 13
f/u	4–59 months
Max dose	Not reported
Min dose	10–22.5 Gy
Tumor size	Not reported

TABLE 21-4. Tumor Size of Acoustic Neuromas before Stereotactic Radiosurgery at the Karolinska Institute, Stockholm, Sweden.

Average Extrameatal Tumor Diameter	Noren et al., 1983		Noren et al., 1992		Noren et al., 1993	
	No.	**(%)**	**No.**	**(%)**	**No.**	**(%)**
4–15 mm	5	(36)	91	(41)	Not reported	
16–25 mm	5	(36)	98	(45)		
26–30 mm	4	(28)	30	(14)		
Total	14		219			

TABLE 21–5. Tumor size of acoustic neuromas before stereotactic radiosurgery at the University of Pittsburgh.

Average Extrameatal Tumor Diameter	Linskey et al., 1992		Ogunrinde et al., 1994	
Intracanalicular	4	(4)	6	(6.1)
<1 cm	9	(10)	9	(9.2)
1–1.99 cm	51	(55)		
1.0–2.5 cm			75	(76.5)
2–2.99 cm	26	(28)		
> 2.5 cm			8	(8.2)
>3 cm	3	(3)		
Total	93		98	

the periphery, which was reduced to 10 to 15 Gy to the periphery and 15 to 25 Gy to the center of the tumor for the later patients. In general, the later reports describe patients who received lower doses of radiation.

The University of Pittsburgh experience is reported in Flickinger et al. (1991), Linskey et al. (1992b), Ogunrinde, Lunsford, Flickinger, and Kondziolka (1994), and Pollock et al. (1995), and the characteristics of the respective study populations are listed in Table 21–2. Again, these studies undoubtedly report on overlapping groups of patients, and patients were selected in each study to elucidate specific outcomes. Flickinger et al. (1991) and Linskey et al. (1992b) represent results on a mixture of patients, including those with bilateral tumors, tumors recurrent after surgery, and various pretreatment facial nerve function. The radiation dosage for the early patients consisted of a minimum peripheral dose of 20 Gy, which apparently resulted in a high incidence of cranial nerve palsies. The later patients were treated with a peripheral dosage of 16 to 18 Gy. Ogunrinde et al. (1994) included only unilateral tumors but did include tumors recurrent after surgery.

Pollock et al. (1995) retrospectively compared two separate cohorts of patients with unilateral acoustic neuromas, including 71 patients who underwent microsurgical excision and 78 patients who underwent gamma knife radiosurgery between January 1990 and December 1991. All patients who had undergone previous tumor excision or radiation, neurofibromatosis type 2 patients, and patients with tumors larger than 3 cm in diameter were excluded, leaving 40 patients in the microsurgery group and 47 patients in the gamma knife group. The microsurgery was performed by the retrosigmoid approach using facial nerve and auditory brainstem monitoring, and excision was thought to be complete in all cases. The stereotactic radiosurgery was performed using the cobalt-60 Gamma unit with an average radiation dose to the margin of 16.3 Gy and a range of 13 to 18 Gy. The maximal tumor dose averaged 31.2 Gy, with a range of 25 to 36 Gy. The median follow-up interval was 36 months, with a range of 25 to 48 months.

The preoperative clinical characteristics of the two patient populations, including age, gender, hearing loss, tinnitus, imbalance/ataxia, vertigo, headache, balance, trigeminal symptoms, facial nerve paresis, tumor size, and tumor volume were compared and were noted to be equivalent, except for a significantly higher age of patients in the gamma knife group. The tumor size distribution for both groups is shown in Table 21–6, and were noted to be equivalent.

Mendenhall et al. (1994) presented 32 patients who underwent stereotactic radiosurgery using the linear accelerator between July 1988 and February 1993. This

TABLE 21–6. Tumor size of acoustic neuromas before microsurgery or stereotactic radiosurgery at the University of Pittsburgh (Pollock et al., 1995).

Average tumor diameter (mm)	Microsurgery (N = 40) No. of Patients (%)	Radiosurgery (N = 47) No. of Patients (%)	P Value
Intracanalicular	6 (15)	4 (9)	0.16
<10	8 (20)	5 (11)	
10–20	9 (48)	24 (51)	
20–30	7 (18)	14 (29)	
Average tumor volume (cm³)			
<1.0	22 (55)	20 (43)	0.14
1.0–4.0	11 (27)	13 (28)	
>4.0	7 (18)	14 (29)	

study also included patients with tumors recurrent after surgery and patients with bilateral tumors.

Facial Nerve Results

The consistent ability of surgeons to preserve anatomically the integrity of the facial nerve during the resection of acoustic tumors was a significant advance of the 1960s. Many believe that the introduction of facial nerve monitoring during surgery enhanced the surgeon's ability to avoid significant mechanical trauma to the facial nerve during tumor dissection. However, patients may develop deterioration of facial nerve function after acoustic neuroma surgery, particularly when the tumor is large. When anatomic integrity of the facial nerve has been preserved, this dysfunction usually resolves over a period of months to its final functional level. The House-Brackmann facial nerve grading system has been used by many authors in reporting results, and grade I to II is considered a good result.

Today, anatomic preservation of the facial nerve during surgical excision of acoustic neuromas is expected, and long-term results of facial nerve function have been excellent in the recent literature when facial nerve monitoring has been used. The most recent facial nerve results were reported by Arriaga, Luxford, Atkins, and Kwartler (1993); Silverstein, Rosenberg, Flanzer, and Seidman (1993); Uziel, Benezech, and Frerebeau (1993); and Lalwani, Butt, Jackler, Pitts, and Yingling (1994), as shown in Table 21–7. They represent surgical results on tumors of all sizes, and all cases in the latter three reports were performed utilizing facial nerve monitoring. In these monitored cases, grade I to II function was attained in 85% to 94.5% of cases overall, and results were expectedly better for the smaller tumors. The patients in the report by Arriaga et al. (1993) represent a mixture of patients, some of whom underwent surgery without facial nerve monitoring. This may explain the grade I to II result in only 74.8% of patients. Another study by Nadol et al. (1992) presented 78 patients who underwent acoustic tumor resection with 1-year follow-up. The House-Brackmann grading system was not used, but they noted normal facial nerve function at long-term follow-up in 90% of patients. All of these series contained patients who had normal preoperative facial nerve function. All were retrospective, so data were not necessarily from consecutive patients.

TABLE 21-7. Facial nerve outcomes after microsurgical excision of acoustic neuromas.

No. pts. f/u Tumor size	Arriaga et al., 1993 N = 515 1.0–7.2 years Mean 2.3 cm (0.4–6.0 cm)		Silverstein et al., 1993 N = 65 Not specified IAC to > 3 cm		Uziel et al., 1993 N = 95 >1 year IAC to > 4 cm		Lalwani et al., 1994 N = 129 >1 year IAC to > 3 cm	
Grade	No.	(%)	No.	(%)	No.	(%)	No.	(%)
I	308	(59.8)	46	(72)	86	(90.5)	—	(71)
II	77	(15.0)	8	(13)	4	(4.0)	—	(19)
III	62	(12.0)	5	(8)	2	(2.0)	—	(6)
IV	36	(7.0)	3	(5)	0	(0)	—	(2)
V	13	(2.5)	0	(0)	2	(2.0)	—	(0)
VI	19	(3.7)	2	(3)	1	(1.0)	—	(3)
I–II	354	(74.8)	54	(85)	90	(94.5)	—	(90)

As in the case with surgical treatment, facial nerve outcomes after stereotactic radiosurgery have improved over time as dosing regimens and techniques have become more refined. The majority of cranial nerve dysfunctions after stereotactic radiosurgery become manifest several months after treatment and are thought to be due to delayed demyelinating injury (Bergstrom, 1980; Larsson, 1992) that is related to the tumor volume treated which, in turn, relates to the length of nerve irradiated (Linskey, Flickinger, & Lunsford, 1993). Only one patient developed a facial paralysis within 24 hr of treatment, and this was thought to be related to acute post-irradiation edema (Linskey et al., 1992b). As mentioned in the reports by Noren et al. (1992) and Linskey et al. (1992b), a high incidence of facial nerve and other cranial nerve dysfunction was noted with the radiation dosages used early in the respective centers' experience, before the dosages were lowered. In Noren et al.'s report of 1983, showing outcomes in 14 patients, the rate of facial nerve dysfunction was 36%. A subsequent report (Noren et al., 1992) of 219 tumors in 209 patients showed a facial nerve dysfunction rate of 16%. The mean time to onset of facial nerve involvement after treatment was 7.5 months, with a range of 4 to 15 months. The facial nerve function recovered after a mean time of 6.5 months after onset, with a range of 2 to 23 months, but neither the worst facial nerve grade nor the final grade after recovery was reported. Mendenhall et al. (1994) reported that 5 out of 32 patients (16%) who underwent stereotactic radiosurgery using the linear accelerator system developed a facial nerve palsy. The worst grade was not reported, but three had partial resolution and two had no resolution.

The University of Pittsburgh group used the House-Brackmann facial nerve grading system to report their results (Table 21–8). The reports by Flickinger et al. (1991) and Ogunrinde et al. (1994) likely represent follow-up on overlapping populations of patients reported at different times. Ogunrinde

et al. (1994) reported 98 patients who underwent gamma knife radiosurgery for acoustic neuromas and obtained a minimum of 24 months follow-up. At latest examination, 62% were grade I and 12% were grade II, for an overall grade I and II outcome of 74%. The confounding factor in this analysis is that only 78% of these patients had grade I facial nerve function prior to radiosurgery, so that it is impossible to discern the outcomes in patients who had normal function prior to treatment. Most of this pretreatment facial nerve dysfunction appeared to be due to prior surgical treatment. Flickinger et al. (1991) does state that 14 out of 46 patients (30%) with normal facial nerve function prior to treatment developed a facial nerve paresis of grade II or higher, although the number recovering to normal was not stated. Furthermore, these data likely represent a mixture of both early patients who were treated with the higher dosages and who had higher rates of facial nerve dysfunction, and later patients who received reduced dosages.

The most recent results of gamma knife treatment at the University of Pittsburgh were reported by Pollock et al. (1995). In this study comparing results of gamma knife radiosurgery to retrosigmoid microsurgical tumor excision in patients with normal pretreatment facial nerve function and no prior treatment for their tumors, 40 postsurgical patients were reported with 63% grade I and 15% grade II facial nerve result at greater than 25 months follow-up, for a total grade I to II result of 78%. The 47 patients who underwent gamma knife treatment had 83% grade I and 9% grade II, for a total grade I to II result of 91%.

Although the patients from both the surgical and radiosurgical groups in this study appeared to be well matched in terms of tumor size distribution, the patients were not assigned to the two groups in a prospective randomized fashion. Therefore, it is conceivable, although unlikely, that some difference between these groups resulted in the significantly better facial nerve result in the gamma knife group. It is also unclear why

TABLE 21-8. Facial nerve outcomes after gamma knife radiosurgery to treat acoustic neuromas at the University of Pittsburgh.

Grade	Flickinger et al., 1991				Ogunrinde et al., 1994				Pollock et al., 1995			
	Pre		Post		Pre		Post		Pre		Post	
	No.	(%)	No.	(%)	No.	(%)	No.	(%)	No.	(%)	No.	(%)
I	65	(76)	52	(61)	76	(78)	61	(62)	47	(100)	39	(83)
II	7	(8)	8	(9)	6	(6)	12	(12)	0	(0)	4	(9)
III	3	(3)	9	(11)	6	(6)	14	(14)	0	(0)	3	(6)
IV	2	(2)	3	(3)	1	(1)	4	(4)	0	(0)	1	(2)
V	3	(4)	6	(6)	4	(4)	2	(2)	0	(0)	0	(0)
VI	5	(6)	7	(7)	5	(5)	5	(5)	0	(0)	0	(0)
I–II	72	(84)	60	(70)	82	(84)	73	(74)	47	(100)	43	(92)
Total	85		85		98		98		47		47	

the microsurgery group in this study had poorer facial nerve outcomes compared to other surgical studies that reported an 85% to 95% grade I to II outcome, especially since these other series did not exclude tumors larger than 3 cm in diameter (Table 21–7). It is possible, and even probable, that the tumor measurement systems used in the various studies are not uniform. However, this alone would not explain the discrepancy between the surgical group in Pollock et al. (1995) and the remainder of the surgical series in which facial nerve outcomes are remarkably similar (Lalwani et al., 1994; Nadol et al., 1992; Silverstein et al., 1993; Uziel et al., 1993).

Among the recent studies, lower rates of preservation of facial function were reported in patients who underwent tumor excision without utilizing facial nerve monitoring. Nevertheless, the remainder of facial nerve results from the most recent microsurgical reports utilizing facial nerve monitoring, excluding those of the study by Pollock et al. (1995), are similar to the most recent results with gamma knife radiosurgery at the University of Pittsburgh.

The efficacy of functional preservation of the facial nerve during acoustic tumor treatment with either microsurgery and stereotactic radiosurgery is in an evolutionary process. It is likely that, as physicians in the surgical and radiosurgical disciplines refine their techniques, rates of facial nerve functional preservation will continue to improve. In fact, Noren et al. (1993) at the Karolinska Institute reported that, in 1990, only 1 patient out of 39 (2.5%) treated with the gamma knife for acoustic neuromas developed a facial nerve paresis and, in 1991, only 1 out of 55 patients (1.8%) developed a facial nerve paresis. The tumor size distribution, radiation dosages, and follow-up times for these groups of patients were not reported, so it is difficult to place these facial nerve results in the proper perspective. It also will be important to follow these patients over time to determine the tumor regrowth and long-term cranial nerve results, especially since the radiation dosages have been decreasing.

Trigeminal Nerve

A significant incidence of trigeminal nerve dysfunction after stereotactic radiosurgery has been reported. At the Karolinska Institute, Noren et al. (1983) reported 2 out of 14 patients (14%) undergoing gamma knife therapy for acoustic neuromas who developed trigeminal nerve dysfunction 8 and 9 months after treatment. In one patient, the symptoms of facial numbness resolved over time but, in the other, a dense and permanent facial numbness resulted. This corresponds to a 7% incidence of permanent trigeminal dysfunction. In a subsequent report of 219 tumors in 209 patients, Noren et al. (1992) showed a 20% incidence of alteration of facial sensation with onset between 6 and 8 months after treatment. Overall, 8% of patients developed a permanent abnormality in facial sensation. At the University of Florida, Mendenhall et al. (1994) reported a 19% incidence of trigeminal dysfunction after treatment with linear accelerator-based radiosurgery, most of which was permanent. These results are shown in Table 21–9.

The experience with gamma knife radiosurgery at the University of Pittsburgh has been similar (Table 21–10). Flickinger et al. (1991) reported that 12 out of 42 patients (29%) developed new trigeminal neuropathies at a median interval of 7 months after treatment of acoustic tumors with gamma knife radiosurgery. Although many improved, the number of patients with permanent trigeminal dysfunction was not reported. The trigeminal dysfunction began to improve at a median of 13 months after onset, with a range of 1 to 17 months. Similarly, Linskey et al. (1992b) reported that 21 of 66 patients (32%) developed trigeminal nerve dysfunction. Only 10% of these patients resolved completely by the final follow-up, which ranged from 3 to 33

TABLE 21-9. Incidence of new trigeminal nerve dysfunction after stereotactic radiosurgery to treat acoustic neuromas.

	Noren et al., 1983 (N = 14)		Noren et al., 1992 (N = 219)		Mendenhall et al., 1994 (N = 32)	
	No.	(%)	No.	(%)	No.	(%)
Transient V	1	(7.1)	—	(12)	0	(0)
Permanent V	1	(7.1)	—	(8)	6	(19)
Total, V dusfunction	2	(14.2)	—	(20)	6	(19)

TABLE 21-10. Incidence of new trigeminal nerve dysfunction after stereotactic radiosurgery to treat acoustic neuromas at the University of Pittsburgh.

	Flickinger et al., 1991 (N = 42)		Ogunrinde et al., 1994 (N = 66)		Pollock et al., 1995 (N = 47)	
	No.	(%)	No.	(%)	No.	(%)
Transient V	—	(—)	2	(3)	—	(22)
Permanent V	—	(—)	19	(29)	—	(11)
Total, V dysfunction	12	(29)	21	(32)	—	(32)

months, so up to 29% had permanent trigeminal symptoms. As with the discussion on facial nerve outcomes, these studies represent a mixture of patients of the earlier Pittsburgh series who underwent the high dose and the later low dose of irradiation. In a more recent study, Pollock et al. (1995) reported a 32% incidence of transient fifth nerve dysfunction after gamma knife radiosurgery, compared to 22% for the surgical group. At greater than 25 months follow-up, trigeminal symptoms were present in 14% of the radiosurgery group, compared to 11% for the microsurgery group. These results are shown in Tables 21–10 (third column) and 21–11 (second column).

Unlike the ubiquitous reporting of trigeminal dysfunction in the stereotactic radiosurgery literature, the microsurgical literature does not provide much information on trigeminal nerve dysfunction. New and permanent cranial nerve V dysfunction is thought to be a rare sequela after microsurgical excision of acoustic neuromas, usually associated only with excision of very large tumors. Wiet, Kazan, Raslan, and Herzon (1986) reported that none of the 60 patients who underwent surgical excision of acoustic neuromas developed fifth nerve symptoms. Harner, Beatty, and Ebersold (1990) reported on 335 excisions in 332 patients, of

which four developed permanent facial hypesthesia. In all four cases, tumor removal had resulted in partial resection of the trigeminal nerve. Ebersold, Haner, Beatty, Harper, and Quest (1992) reported 1 patient out of 256 procedures performed on 221 patients who developed transient ipsilateral facial hypesthesia lasting for 2 months, followed by total resolution. These results are shown in Table 21–12. In a large patient survey after microsurgical excision, Parving, Tos, Thomsen, Moller, and Buchwald (1992) did not even include trigeminal symptoms as part of the data base. In fact, a review of many of the other recent reports of surgical experience with acoustic neuromas shows that very few even mention trigeminal nerve dysfunction as a complication.

In contrast, two reports showed a significant incidence of trigeminal nerve dysfunction after surgery (Table 21–11). The microsurgical arm of the study by Pollock et al. (1995) showed a 22% rate of trigeminal nerve symptoms, of which 11% was persistent at a follow-up of 2 years. Wiegand and Fickel (1989) reported the results of a survey of 541 patients who are members of the Acoustic Neuroma Society, a national support group. Of these patients, 159 (29%) reported facial paresthesia at some point after surgical excision of acoustic neuromas.

TABLE 21–11. Incidence of new trigeminal nerve dysfunction after microsurgical excision of acoustic neuroma.

No. pts. f/u Tumor size	Wiegand et al., 1989 (N = 541) Not reported Mean not reported Range < 2 cm to > 4 cm		Pollock et al., 1995 (N = 47) >2 years Mean not reported Range 0.5–3 cm	
	No.	**(%)**	**No.**	**(%)**
Transient V	—	(—)	—	(11)
Permanent V	—	(—)	—	(11)
Total, V dysfunction	159	29	—	(22)

TABLE 21-12. Incidence of new trigeminal nerve dysfunction after microsurgical excision of acoustic neuroma.

No. pts. f/u Tumor size	Wiet et al., 1986 (N = 60) Not reported Mean not reported Range IAC—>3 cm		Harner et al., 1990 (N = 335) Not reported Median 3 cm Range 0.5—6.5 cm		Ebersold et al., 1992 (N = 256) Not reported Mean not reported Range IAC—6.5 cm	
	No.	(%)	No.	(%)	No.	(%)
Transient V	0	(0)	Not reported		1	(0.4)
Permanent V	0	(0)	4	(1.2)	0	(0)
Total, V dysfunction	0	(0)	4	(1.2)	1	(0.4)

There was no information regarding permanence of the condition. Wiegand and Fickel admit in their paper that the studied population is skewed to those who had complications or poorer outcomes, as the Acoustic Neuroma Society generally attracts such patients more often than patients who had no difficulty. Indeed, the patients in this study had larger tumors on average than usually seen in most series, as only 14% of these patients had tumors smaller than 2 cm and only 35% of patients reported normal facial nerve function at the time of the survey. Furthermore, we have found that patients often confuse trigeminal and facial nerve function, especially when asked to fill out a questionnaire. Therefore, it is difficult to conclude that the 29% rate of trigeminal nerve symptoms after surgical excision of acoustic neuromas as reported by Wiegand and Finkel (1989) represents an accurate figure.

In summary, despite reports of Pollock et al. (1995) and Wiegand and Fickel (1989), it is doubtful that the rate of permanent trigeminal dysfunction after microsurgical removal of acoustic neuromas is 10% to 30%. Our own surgical experience supports the very low incidence of trigeminal nerve dysfunction described by Wiet et al. (1986), Harner et al. (1990), and Ebersold et al. (1992). Of course, it is possible that surgeons are not evaluating patients' trigeminal dysfunction postoperatively as closely as the radiosurgical groups are doing, and published rates of 0% to 1.2% incidence of trigeminal dysfunction after microsurgical excision may be underestimates. It is also possible that the discrepancy between rates of trigeminal dysfunction between microsurgical and radiosurgical groups is a reporting epiphenomenon. Perhaps the radiosurgery reports have more liberal definitions of trigeminal dysfunction. For instance, Linskey et al. (1991), at the University of Pittsburgh, reported that their criteria for trigeminal neuropathy counted any subjective facial numbness or paresthesia reported by the patient, regardless of whether or not

decreased facial sensation could be detected on neurological examination. Using these criteria, their rate of trigeminal neuropathy after gamma knife radiosurgery in 89 patients was 32%. As a result of these reporting ambiguities, it is not possible to determine if the rate of trigeminal nerve dysfunction after stereotactic radiosurgery is higher than that of surgery or if, in fact, they are comparable, as the report by Pollock et al. (1995) suggests.

Hearing Preservation

Hearing preservation utilizing both microsurgery and stereotactic radiosurgery depends to a large degree on the size of the treated tumor and the presence of neurofibromatosis type 2. The value of preserved hearing to a patient also depends on the amount of residual hearing prior to treatment and to what extent this hearing has been preserved. For instance, a pretreatment speech reception threshold (SRT) of 20 dB HL with an 80% speech discrimination score (SDS), preserved after treatment to a 30 dB HL SRT with 70% SDS, is much more meaningful than a pretreatment SRT of 80 dB HL with 20% SDS, preserved after treatment to an SRT of 90 dB HL with 10% SDS, even though both instances may provide statistically equivalent hearing preservation in certain systems of evaluation. In addition, the status of the contralateral hearing and any significant risk factors for hearing loss in the good ear are important parameters.

Relatively high rates of "hearing preservation" have been reported with the use of stereotactic radiosurgery. Noren et al. (1983) reported hearing results in the early group of patients treated with the gamma knife unit at the Karolinska Institute and showed that hearing could be saved in certain cases. Three patients had discrimination scores 50% or higher prior to treatment, and one of these patients maintained this score after treatment. There was an additional patient who had a discrimination score of 0% prior to treatment, whose score improved to 52% after treatment. All follow-up hearing evaluations were performed 4 years or more after treatment. Noren et al. (1993) reported their latest results for a group of patients with 132 tumors and pretreatment hearing better than 90 dB HL; 1 year after treatment, hearing was unchanged in 22% of the patients, slightly to moderately impaired in 55%, and severely impaired or lost in 23%. The overall rate of hearing preservation was reported to be 78%. However, it is not clear how useful this level of hearing preservation would be for the patient. Given the data as presented, we cannot determine if the hearing preserved was of any benefit to the patient in all 78% or to a smaller number of

patients who retained a more significant level of hearing after treatment.

Linskey et al. (1992b) reported on hearing preservation results after gamma knife radiosurgery for acoustic neuromas at the University of Pittsburgh. There were 86 patients with 87 tumors, and the Gardner-Robertson classification (Table 21–13) was used to evaluate hearing function. The results are shown in Table 21–14. If we assume that all of the patients with class I hearing after treatment had this hearing level prior to treatment, then 4 out of 12 (33%) retained class I hearing. Similarly, if we assume that none of the patients with class III hearing or worse improved to class II or better, then out of 20 patients with class

TABLE 21–13. Gardner-Robertson classification of hearing.

Class	Description	PTA (dB HL)	SDS
I	Good	0–30	70–100%
II	Serviceable	31–50	50–69%
III	Nonserviceable	50–90	5–49%
IV	Poor	91–max	1–4%
V	None	NR	0%

TABLE 21–14. Hearing outcomes after gamma knife radiosurgery to treat acoustic neuromas at the University of Pittsburgh (Linskey et al., 1992).

Class	HR Presurgery No.	(%)	HR Postsurgery No.	(%)
I	12	(14)	4	(5)
II	8	(9)	3	(3)
III	24	(28)	18	(21)
IV	2	(2)	3	(3)
V	41	(47)	59	(68)
Total	87		87	

I to II hearing prior to treatment, 7 (35%) retained class I to II hearing after treatment.

Pollock et al. (1995) reported on the most recent hearing preservation results after gamma knife radiosurgery for acoustic neuromas at the University of Pittsburgh. The Gardner-Robertson classification (Table 21–13) again was used to evaluate hearing function. Out of eight patients with class I or II (good or serviceable) hearing prior to gamma knife treatment, six patients (75%) retained class I or II hearing level after treatment. The audiological follow-up ranged from 27 to 38 months, with a median of 35 months. This was compared to a presumably similar cohort of 21 patients with class I or II hearing who underwent microsurgical excision, of whom only three (14%) retained class I or II hearing after treatment (Table 21–15). The tumor size distribution was similar in both groups and included tumors up to 3 cm (Table 21–6).

A comparison of hearing preservation rates after stereotactic radiosurgery and after microsurgery is difficult for two reasons. First, definitions of hearing preservation used in various series are not uniform. Second, some authors stratify results by tumor size, while others report results on all tumor sizes combined. Hearing preservation rates for patients undergoing microsurgical removal of acoustic tumors range from 20% to 50%, if the results are not stratified according to tumor size.[1] For the intracanalicular tumors, hearing preservation rates have been reported to be 43% to 82% .[2] These results vary depending on the selection criteria for hearing preservation surgery and the definition of hearing preservation.

Despite the difficulty in comparing hearing preservation rates between stereotactic radiosurgery and microsurgery for the treatment of acoustic neuromas, it appears that hearing preservation rates are of the same order of magnitude for either modality. The latest hearing results from the University of Pittsburgh (Pollock et al., 1995), citing a 75% success rate in preserving Gardner-Robertson class I to II hearing, are quite impressive, especially when compared to the 14% success rate of the surgical

TABLE 21–15. Hearing outcomes after treatment of acoustic neuromas at the University of Pittsburgh (Pollock et al., 1995).

No. pts. f/u Tumor size	Microsurgery (N = 21) >2 years Mean not reported Range IAC—3 cm	Radiosurgery (N = 8) >2 years Mean not reported Range IAC—3 cm
	Number of Patients with Class I or II	
Preoperative	21	8
Postoperative	3	6
Hearing preservation	14%	75%

---

[1]Atlas, Harvey, & Fagan, 1992; Cohen, Lewis, & Ransohoff, 1993; Fischer, Fischer, & Remond, 1992; Gantz, Parnes, Harker, & McCabe, 1986; Glasscock, Hays, Minor, Haynes, & Carrasco, 1993; Hoehmann, 1991; Nadol et al., 1992; Nedzelski, Chiong, Cashman, Stanton, & Rowed, 1994; Umezu & Alba, 1994.

[2]Brackmann, House, & Hiteselberger, 1994; Cohen et al., 1993; Ebersold et al., 1992; Gantz et al., 1986; Haines & Levine, 1993; Nadol et al., 1992; Umezu & Alba, 1994.

"control" group, and may indicate that the most recent stereotactic radiosurgery technique for unilateral tumors is superior to microsurgical excision. Only the results of Haines and Levine (1993) and Brackmann, House, and Hitselberger (1994) are comparable, but these surgical series consisted of tumors that were largely intracanalicular. One must keep in mind, however, that the number of patients in the gamma knife hearing preservation group in Pollock et al. (1995) was quite small, and hearing stability at longer follow-up is not yet available in this group of patients.

Tumor Control

A critical question regarding the efficacy of stereotactic radiosurgery in the treatment of acoustic neuromas is the control of tumor growth. Radiosurgery does not result in the physical obliteration of all tumor tissue. The tumor mass remains after treatment, and success of treatment is determined by whether tumor growth is terminated or slowed sufficiently so that surgical intervention is not required for the remainder of the patient's natural life. Patients who have undergone stereotactic radiosurgery currently require post-treatment imaging at regular intervals to follow the progression of tumor size. The time interval between scans has been increasing as more experience has been gained regarding tumor behavior after radiosurgery.

Approximately 3 to 6 months after stereotactic radiosurgery, tumors can lose central enhancement on CT or MR scanning. This finding is thought to represent central tumor necrosis and is considered a good prognostic sign for adequate tumor control. Within the first year after treatment, some tumors enlarge temporarily, then decrease in size 12 to 18 months after treatment (Noren et al., 1993). The majority of tumors either maintain the same volume or decrease in size. A small number of tumors increase in size after treatment and continue

to grow. These cases constitute treatment "failures."

Noren et al. (1993) presented the latest tumor control data on 254 patients treated with gamma knife radiosurgery for acoustic tumors at the Karolinska Institute. There was loss of contrast enhancement in 70% of cases starting 6 to 12 months after treatment. The size of unilateral tumors decreased in 55%, remained unchanged in 33%, and increased in 12%. Half of the tumors that initially grew decreased in size over the course of 12 to 18 months. Therefore, the tumor control rate was 94% for unilateral tumors in these patients who have been followed for 12 to 206 months. All tumors that increased in size after treatment did so within 5 years of treatment in this group of patients.

In the most recent report of tumor control after gamma knife treatment of acoustic neuromas at the University of Pittsburgh, Pollock et al. (1995) reported that, in 47 patients, the tumor was unchanged in 60%, decreased in 34%, and increased in 6%. The median follow-up of 24 months, with a range of 3 to 46 months, was somewhat short. In a similar cohort of 98 patients at the University of Pittsburgh, with a minimum of 2 years follow-up, Ogunrinde et al. (1994) reported a tumor growth rate of only 3%. All three of the patients with tumor growth underwent subsequent microsurgical tumor excision.

An argument that many acoustic tumors fail to grow during observation periods of up to 2 years has been made to question the true efficacy of tumor control after stereotactic radiosurgery. In fact, Bederson, von Ammon, Werner, and Yasergil (1991) found that, when tumors were followed in 70 patients without significant cranial nerve dysfunction except for eighth nerve findings, 49% had no detectable growth on CT scan during 1 year. Of these patients with no tumor growth detected within the first year, 2-year follow-up was available in 18 patients, and only one of these patients had tumor growth. Strasnick, Glasscock, Haynes,

McMenomey, and Minor (1994) reported similar results. In a response to this variable and sporadic nature of the natural rate of tumor growth, Linskey et al. (1991) performed a comparison of tumor control rates after gamma knife treatment of acoustic neuromas at the University of Pittsburgh to a historical control group of untreated tumors found in the literature. In the historical group, tumor growth occurred in 38% of 199 patients, with a mean follow-up of 2.6 years (0.24–16 years). In comparison, only 4% of 89 treated patients experienced tumor growth after a mean follow-up of 1.7 years (0.25–3 years), and the difference was statistically significant. A comparison between treated and untreated sides of neurofibromatosis type 2 patients has shown similar results (Linskey, Lunsford, & Flickinger, 1992a). Nonetheless, the issue of natural history of tumor growth in acoustic neuromas must be considered when evaluating any treatment regimen. Results can be skewed significantly by patient selection.

Cure rates after microsurgical excision of acoustic neuromas in the past decade have been considered to be quite high. Although hearing preservation surgery has been criticized for potentially sacrificing cure rates (Neely, 1984), if total microsurgical tumor removal is attained, recurrence rates have ranged from 0% to 3% (Cohen et al., 1993; Gantz et al., 1986; Glasscock et al., 1993; Harner et al., 1990; Pollock et al., 1995; Schessel, Nedzelski, Kassel, & Rowed, 1992), and many of these recurrences have been attributed to tumor remnants of the lateral internal auditory canal after retrosigmoid approaches (Thedinger, Whittaker, & Luetje, 1991). In a series of 3,000 patients who underwent translabyrinthine removal of acoustic neuromas, Slattery and Brackmann (1995) reported a recurrence rate of 0.2%. Most recurrences are reported after near-total or subtotal excisions, which represent a small minority of all surgical cases, and range, in these cases, from 13% to 22% (Cohen et al., 1993; Harner et al., 1990; Wazen, Silverstein, Norrell, & Besse, 1985). Recurrences have been reported up to 18 years after the prima-

ry surgery (Beatty, Ebersold, & Harner, 1987).

It is clear that surgical therapy, even with attempted hearing preservation, offers an exceedingly high rate of cure after treatment of acoustic neuromas. The 6% recurrence rate reported by the Karolinska Institute group (Noren et al., 1993) and the 3% to 6% recurrence rate reported by the Pittsburgh group (Pollock et al., 1995; Ogunrinde et al., 1994) may be slightly higher than surgical results but are still somewhat comparable. However, there are several issues of concern regarding tumor growth control after stereotactic radiosurgery. First, long-term follow-up data spanning 10 to 20 years is not available for most patients. Although the data from Noren et al. (1993) suggests that 5-year tumor control means a cure, we do not know if these tumors will begin to grow again after 20 years of a quiescent period. If this occurs in a significant number of patients, stereotactic radiosurgery would be a less attractive option for the treatment of younger patients. Second, the radiation dose has been reduced over time, both at the Karolinska Institute and at the University of Pittsburgh, in order to reduce the rate of cranial nerve dysfunction after treatment. Therefore, the longest follow-up is available only for those patients who received the higher doses. The true tumor control rates for the lower doses used today are not known, and only long-term follow-up in these patients will provide the answer. Finally, more information regarding outcomes and sequelae after surgical excision of acoustic tumors after failure of stereotactic radiosurgery will be needed. If outcomes in such patients are poor, any real difference in tumor control rates between radiosurgery and standard surgical treatment will require close scrutiny.

Surgical Excision after Tumor Recurrence

There have been only anecdotal reports on outcomes after surgical treatment of acoustic neuromas that recur after treatment with stereotactic radiosurgery. We are aware of two patients at the University of Pittsburgh who underwent surgical excision of acoustic tumors recurrent after stereotactic radiation, and both were technically difficult due to significant fibrosis around the tumor with obliteration of tissue planes between tumor and cranial nerves and between tumor and brainstem. Both patients had grade VI facial nerve paralysis and ipsilateral anacusis after surgery. However, one of these patients had a malignant schwannoma, which likely contributed significantly to the difficulty in managing this case.

Slattery and Brackmann (1995) reported five patients, two with neurofibromatosis type 2 (NF-2) and three with unilateral acoustic tumors, who underwent stereotactic radiosurgery utilizing various techniques and subsequently developed tumor regrowth requiring surgical excision. The details of the dosages and technology used were not indicated. They found that tumor removal from the facial nerve was difficult in all cases because of the lack of an adequate dissection plane between the nerve and tumor, presumably due to radiation-induced fibrosis. The facial nerve anatomically was preserved in three patients, but all five patients did not recover any facial nerve function postoperatively. All patients also were deaf on the affected side, so the translabyrinthine approach was used. Of the two NF-2 patients who underwent simultaneous auditory brainstem implantation (ABI), one gained no benefit whatsoever, and the other was stimulated successfully initially but required explantation because of infection at the percutaneous plug. The low success rate in hearing rehabilitation with the ABI after radiosurgery is thought to be due to difficulty in proper electrode array placement resulting from radiation-induced distortion of brainstem anatomy. Dysfunction of the auditory pathways due to radiation also is possible, but this etiology is still speculative.

For now, reports of treating recurrent tumor after stereotactic radiosurgery continue to be anecdotal. In general, these patients seemed to be difficult to treat surgically and had poorer rates of cranial nerve preserva-

tion. It is possible that we are being made aware preferentially of those cases that have been most difficult. A true evaluation of outcomes in such patients will have to await further experience and reporting.

Neurofibromatosis 2

Neurofibromatosis type 2 (NF-2) is caused by a defect located in chromosome 22 and usually is characterized by bilateral acoustic neuromas or the presence of other central nervous system neoplasms. The diagnostic criteria for NF-2 include the presence of bilateral acoustic tumors or the combination of a first degree relative having NF-2 and either a unilateral acoustic neuroma or two of the following: neurofibroma, meningioma, glioma, schwannoma, or juvenile posterior subcapsular lenticular opacity. The treatment of patients with bilateral acoustic neuromas has been problematic, because hearing preservation rates have been lower than in those with unilateral tumors after microsurgical excision. Hearing loss after treatment is devastating especially in these patients, who face eventual bilateral anacusis. In addition, facial nerve preservation rates have been poorer, and tumor control rates have been lower compared to those with unilateral tumors. The lower rates of functional cranial nerve preservation and cure rates after surgery in patients with NF-2 have been attributed to the more aggressive and invasive nature of the tumors. These tumors also tend to grow faster than their unilateral counterparts and affect patients at an earlier age, commonly during the second decade of life.

Stereotactic radiosurgery has been used to treat patients with acoustic tumors due to NF-2. Noren et al. (1993) reported that, at the Karolinska Institute, the tumor control rate in these patients was 84%. Facial and trigeminal dysfunction and hearing results after gamma knife radiosurgery in these patients were not reported. Linskey et al. (1992a) reported on the University of Pittsburgh experience in treating 17 patients with bilateral acoustic neuromas. Of 10 patients who had at least a 1 year follow-up, 10% of tumors increased in size. Of 13 patients with normal facial function prior to treatment, four patients (31%) developed a new facial nerve palsy 1 day to 11 months after treatment. The distribution of final facial nerve grades was not reported. There were five patients with Gardner-Robertson class I or II hearing prior to treatment, and none retained this hearing level after treatment. However, 4 of 12 patients (33%) with class III to IV pretreatment hearing retained some hearing after treatment. Even this relatively poor hearing level may be important in a patient who may be deaf on the contralateral side. The incidence of new trigeminal nerve symptoms after treatment was 27%, with onset ranging from 3 to 6 months. Facial nerve results in these patients were not reported.

Surgical hearing preservation rates in NF-2 patients have been variable. Glasscock et al. (1993) reported on 25 operative cases with attempted hearing preservation in NF-2 patients with tumors smaller than 1.5 cm. Most patients had Gardner-Robertson class I hearing level preoperatively. The short-term hearing preservation rate, defined as classes I through III, was 44%, which dropped to 24% with follow-up of 1 to 12 years. Doyle and Shelton (1993) reported their experience with 13 middle fossa excisions performed on 10 patients with NF-2 for tumors up to 2 cm. Of 10 patients with class I to II hearing preoperatively who underwent total tumor removal, 4 (40%) retained class I to II hearing postoperatively when evaluated up to 1 year after treatment. Of the 12 cases of total tumor removal, 67% retained measurable hearing (I-IV). Facial nerve function was House-Brackmann grade I in eight patients (80%) and grade III in two patients (20%). Recurrent tumor was noted in 18% of the 10 cases of total resections.

Briggs, Brackmann, Baser, and Hitselberger (1994) recommended that stereotactic surgery should not be considered primary therapy for acoustic tumors in patients with NF-2. The reasons for their recommenda-

tion were that the long-term tumor control rate after stereotactic radiosurgery is not yet known, and the long-term hearing results are worse than those after microsurgical excision. The authors also cited a 34% incidence of facial nerve dysfunction after stereotactic radiosurgery. Furthermore, their experience with surgical removal of acoustic tumors that recur after stereotactic radiosurgery has been complicated due to radiation-induced fibrosis. They also cited one case in which an auditory brainstem implantation (ABI) for hearing rehabilitation could not be done because of fibrosis and anatomic distortion in the region of the lateral recess where the electrode array needs to be placed. As a result of the poor results of ABI after treatment of acoustic tumors with stereotactic radiosurgery, these previously irradiated patients currently are excluded as candidates for ABI.

Hearing results and facial nerve preservation rates are poorer for NF-2 patients, compared to those with unilateral tumors using either microsurgery or stereotactic radiosurgery. The comparison of efficacy between the two treatment modalities is difficult for patients with unilateral tumors, but it is even more difficult for NF-2 patients, because there is less information available. Gamma knife radiosurgery appears to provide a short-term tumor control rate of 90%. Long-term facial nerve outcomes are unknown, and hearing preservation at significant levels has not been demonstrated and appears to be worse than after surgery, although data are still sparse. Patients with NF-2 who are considering stereotactic radiosurgery to treat their acoustic tumors should be aware of these uncertainties in order to make an informed decision.

COMPLICATIONS

There have been no reports of meningitis, wound infection, cerebrospinal fluid leak, pulmonary complications, myocardial infarction, or acute neurologic deficit other than cranial nerve dysfunction directly attributable to stereotactic radiosurgery. In addition, there have been no reports of sixth nerve palsy or lower cranial nerve palsies reported, although these sequelae usually occur only in the surgical treatment of very large acoustic tumors. Dysfunction of the facial nerve, trigeminal nerve, and hearing apparatus already have been discussed. Other complications associated with stereotactic radiosurgery will be discussed as follows.

Hydrocephalus

The development of communicating hydrocephalus requiring shunt surgery after stereotactic radiosurgery has been reported (Thomsen, Tos, & Borgesen, 1990), and is thought to result from high CSF protein levels. Noren et al. (1983) reported that 2 of 14 patients (14%) required a ventriculovenous shunt after gamma knife radiosurgery. In a subsequent report, Noren et al. (1993) reported that 3% of patients required a shunt procedure after gamma knife radiosurgery.

At the University of Pittsburgh, Linskey et al. (1992b) reported that 4.5% of 89 patients whose tumors did not grow after gamma knife radiosurgery required a ventriculoperitoneal (VP) shunt for hydrocephalus presenting 5 to 16 months after treatment. However, in a subsequent report of 47 patients undergoing gamma knife treatment (Pollock et al., 1995), six patients (12.8%) required a VP shunt. These patients had larger than average tumors and had evidence of ventricular enlargement prior to treatment.

In comparison, the incidence of hydrocephalus requiring a shunt after surgical excision of acoustic neuromas ranges from 0.7% to 1.7% (Table 21–16). Since the occur-

TABLE 21-16. Rates of complications after acoustic neuroma surgery.

Complication	Incidence (%)
Cerebrospinal leak	2.6–15.0
Severe headache	0.4–14.3
Bacterial meningitis	0.7–7.0
Pulmonary complications	0.6–2.7
Lower cranial nerve palsy	0–3.1
Ataxia	1.7–1.9
Urinary tract infection	0–1.9
Hydrocephalus	0.7–1.7
Death	0.6–1.7
Cerebrovascular accident	0–1.7
Sixth nerve palsy	1.2–1.6
Cardiac complications	0–0.4
Intracranial bleed	0.4–0.6
Deep venous thrombosis	0.4–0.6
Wound complication	0–0.7

Note: Data compiled from Cohen et al., 1993; Ebersold et al., 1992; Mangham, 1988; Wiet et al., 1986.

rence of hydrocephalus after surgery is so low in patients with tumors of all sizes, including those larger than 3 cm, it is clear that stereotactic radiosurgery results in a higher incidence of hydrocephalus, especially for the larger tumors.

Possible Long-Term Cerebral Effects

Irradiation of the brain has been known to produce demyelinization and endothelial damage. There has been concern that patients undergoing stereotactic radiotherapy will develop complications related to these changes. However, there have not been any long-term debilitating symptoms that can be attributed to these effects. Patients do develop changes within the brainstem detectable on MR scans as high signal intensity changes on T2 weighted images. Linskey et al. (1991) reported that eight patients (9%) treated at the University of Pittsburgh's gamma knife unit developed these changes in the cerebellar peduncle, the pons, or both within 5 to 15 months of treatment. CT scans were less sensitive and detected these changes in only two out of these eight patients, but the changes that were visible appeared as hypodense regions. Some of these changes reverted to normal on follow-up scan at 14 and 19 months in two patients. However, these radiological changes did not correlate with the development of worsening balance function. These changes also did not correlate with tumor size, tumor margin dose, or maximum tumor dose. The proposed etiology of these changes is edema, although demyelinization, ischemic injury, and radionecrosis are also possible (Linskey et al., 1992b). The long-term significance of these changes is unclear, and long-term follow-up will be needed to evaluate the effects of these brainstem changes.

Other Complications

Acute complications after stereotactic radiosurgery include nausea and vomiting in 21% of cases and transient headache in 11%, both of which have been adequately treated with a single 40 mg intravenous dose of methylprednisolone, mild analgesics, and antiemetics (Lunsford & Linskey, 1992).

Persistent complications include balance dysfunction, which was reported at the University of Pittsburgh in 31% and occurred 3 to 17 months after treatment, vertigo in 4%, nausea in 4%, and chronic headaches in 5% (Linskey et al., 1992b). At the Karolinska Institute, chronic balance dysfunction was reported in 8% of patients (Noren et al., 1993). The mechanism of the balance dysfunction is unknown, as MRI changes within the brainstem after treatment did not correlate with balance symptoms. Possible etiologies include edema, radiation injury, ischemic injury to the middle cerebellar peduncle, or direct vestibular neurotoxic effect of radiosurgery. The incidence of persistent ataxia and dysequilibrium after acoustic neuroma surgery is thought to be very low, unless the patient experienced significant symptoms prior to treatment. However, because of the lack of data regarding the severity of balance dysfunction in patients after stereotactic radiosurgery, it is impossible to compare balance outcomes between the two modalities.

Comparison to Surgical Complications

The acute surgical and medical complications that may result from resection of acoustic neuromas can be life-threatening, but such devastating sequelae have become rare. Surgical mortality rates for recent series of acoustic neuroma patients have ranged from 0% to 1.7% (Cohen et al., 1993; Ebersold et al., 1992; Mangham, 1988; Wiet et al., 1986). Rates of other post-surgical complications from these large surgical series are listed in Table 21–16. Excluding headache, ataxia, and hydrocephalus, stereotactic radiosurgery is not associated with any of these surgical complications. Although most patients recover fully after the majority of surgical complications, a small number of patients have permanent sequelae. Finally, although the surgical mortality rate is very low, there is still a chance of death resulting from a surgical complication.

OUR EXPERIENCE

Gamma Knife Treatment

We have referred 14 patients from the Department of Otolaryngology—Head and Neck Surgery to the gamma knife unit at the University of Pittsburgh during the past 8 years for treatment of acoustic neuromas. The reasons for the use of gamma knife, rather than surgery, included advanced patient age, the presence of medical conditions that made surgery too risky, and patient preference. One of these patients was treated recently and does not have follow-up data, leaving 13 patients with a minimum of 6 months follow-up for discussion. The radiation dosage that patients received was re-

duced between 1991 and 1992, so the data are presented both combined and separated into two groups, the early group having received greater than or equal to 15 Gy to the periphery and a later group having received less than 15 Gy to the periphery. All peripheral doses were at or above 50% of the maximal dose. Two of the patients had bilateral acoustic tumors that were diagnosed when the patients were in their 70s.

Table 21–17 shows the patient characteristics including age, tumor size, and follow-up intervals. The main difference between the two groups is that the early group has a much longer follow-up interval, as expected. The size of the tumor was determined by the medial to lateral dimension of the tumor, including both the internal auditory canal and cerebellopontine angle components (IAC+CPA) on either MRI or CT scan. During the follow-up interval, none of the tumors increased in size (Table 21–18). Overall, 62% remained unchanged and 38% decreased in size. Interestingly, a higher percentage of tumors decreased in size in

TABLE 21–17. Characteristics of gamma knife patients followed at the Department of Otolaryngology, University of Pittsburgh.

	All Patients	*≥15 Gy[a]* *(Early)*	*<15 Gy[b]* *(Late)*
Dates of Rx	1987–1994	1987–1991	1992–1994
Number	13	7	6
Average age	72.5 years	71.3 years	74.0 years
Age range	67–79 years	67–78 years	67–79 years
Average tumor size (IAC+CPA)	2.1 cm	1.9 cm	2.3 cm
Tumor size range	1.2–3.2 cm	1.2–3.2 cm	1.2–2.9 cm
Average f/u	13 months	35 months	11 months
Range f/u	6–60 months	20–60 months	6–18 months

[a] ≥15 Gy marginal dose.
[b] <15 Gy marginal dose.
* (Atlas et al., 1992; Cohen et al., 1993; Fischer et al., 1992; Gantz et al., 1986; Glasscock et al., 1993; Hoehmann, 1991; Nadol et al., 1992; Nedzelski et al., 1994; Umezu, & Aiba, 1994)
§ (Brackmann et al., 1994; Cohen et al., 1993; Ebersold et al. 1992; Gantz et al., 1986; Haines & Levine, 1993; Nadol et al., 1992; Umezu, & Aiba, 1994)

TABLE 21–18. Change in tumor size in gamma knife patients followed at the Department of Otolaryngology, University of Pittsburgh.

	All Patients	**≥15 Gy[a]** **(Early)**	**<15 Gy[b]** **(Late)**
Average f/u	13 months	35 months	11 months
Range f/u	6–60 months	20–60 months	6–18 months
Increased	0 (0%)	0 (0%)	0 (0%)
Unchanged	8 (62%)	3 (43%)	5 (83%)
Decreased	5 (38%)	4 (57%)	1 (17%)

[a] ≥15 Gy marginal dose
[b] <15 Gy marginal dose
* (Atlas et al., 1992; Cohen et al., 1993; Fischer et al., 1992; Gantz et al., 1986; Glasscock et al., 1993; Hoehmann, 1991; Nadol et al., 1992; Nedzelski et al., 1994; Umezu, & Aiba, 1994)
§ (Brackmann et al., 1994; Cohen et al., 1993; Ebersold et al. 1992; Gantz et al., 1986; Haines & Levine, 1993; Nadol et al., 1992; Umezu, & Aiba, 1994)

the earlier group (57%), as compared to the later group (17%). This may be a result of the lower radiation dose utilized or the shorter follow-up times in the later group, as some tumors do not shrink until a year after treatment.

The incidence of dysequilibrium after gamma knife radiosurgery is shown in Table 21–19. Overall, 8% of patients experienced transient dysequilibrium, 38% developed long-term dysequilibrium, and 8% had an episode of acute vertigo which resolved. Most patients who experienced balance difficulties after treatment had some balance symptoms prior to treatment, but the numbers above represent subjective worsening of symptoms. The dysequilibrium symptoms were not quantified using any scoring system. Interestingly, the patients in the early group had a much higher incidence of balance problems after treatment, and only one of the six patients in the later group developed this problem. Again, this could represent an effect of the lower radiation dosage in the later group or the fact that the patients in the later group have not been followed long enough to develop dysequilibrium at the rate seen in the early group.

The incidence of facial and trigeminal nerve dysfunction after gamma knife treatment is shown in Table 21–20. Overall, none of the patients developed transient facial nerve palsy, but 2 patients out of 13 (15%) developed a permanent House-Brackmann grade III/VI palsy. Both patients were in the early group, leading to an incidence of facial nerve dysfunction in the early group of 29% and an incidence of 0% in the late group. Trigeminal dysfunction was noted transiently in two patients (15%) and permanently in two patients (15%), for a total incidence of any trigeminal dysfunction of 30%. Again, the rate of trigeminal dysfunction was higher in the early group (43%) compared to the late group (17%). This trend for improved preservation of cranial nerve function with lower radiation dosages is consistent with the reports by Noren et al. (1993) and Lunsford and Linskey (1992). It also is possible that the incidence of cranial nerve palsy is so low in the late group because three out of these six patients have follow-up times of only 6 months, and cranial neuropathies after stereotactic radiosurgery can present first more than 6 months after treatment.

Only two of our patients had Gardner-Robertson hearing level of I to II prior to treatment, and one patient retained this level of hearing after treatment. A large num-

TABLE 21–19. Dysequilibrium in gamma knife patients followed at the Department of Otolaryngology, University of Pittsburgh.

	All Patients		≥15 Gy[a] (Early)		<15 Gy[b] (Late)	
	N = 13		N = 7		N = 6	
Transient	1	(8%)	1	(14%)	0	(0%)
Permanent	5	(38%)	4	(57%)	1	(17%)
Decreased	1	(8%)	1	(14%)	0	(0%)

[a] ≥15 Gy marginal dose
[b] <15 Gy marginal dose
[*] (Atlas et al., 1992; Cohen et al., 1993; Fischer et al., 1992; Gantz et al., 1986; Glasscock et al., 1993; Hoehmann, 1991; Nadol et al., 1992; Nedzelski et al., 1994; Umezu, & Aiba, 1994)
[§] (Brackmann et al., 1994; Cohen et al., 1993; Ebersold et al. 1992; Gantz et al., 1986; Haines & Levine, 1993; Nadol et al., 1992; Umezu, & Aiba, 1994)

TABLE 21–20. Cranial nerve dysfunction in gamma knife patients followed at the Department of Otolaryngology, University of Pittsburgh.

	All Patients		≥15 Gy[a] (Early)		<15 Gy[b] (Late)	
	N = 13		N = 7		N = 6	
Transient VII	1	(0%)	0	(0%)	0	(0%)
Permanent VII[c]	2	(15%)	2	(29%)	0	(0%)
Transient V	2	(15%)	1	(14%)	1	(17%)
Permanent V	2	(15%)	2	(29%)	0	(0%)

[a] ≥ 15 Gy marginal dose
[b] < 15 Gy marginal dose
[c] < Both patients with House-Brackmann grade 3/6
[*] (Atlas et al., 1992; Cohen et al., 1993; Fischer et al., 1992; Gantz et al., 1986; Glasscock et al., 1993; Hoehmann, 1991; Nadol et al., 1992; Nedzelski et al., 1994; Umezu, & Aiba, 1994)
[§] (Brackmann et al., 1994; Cohen et al., 1993; Ebersold et al. 1992; Gantz et al., 1986; Haines & Levine, 1993; Nadol et al., 1992; Umezu, & Aiba, 1994)

ber of our patients (54%) had class V hearing prior to treatment. Therefore, there were too few patients with adequate pretreatment hearing to report hearing results.

Only one patient (8%) in our series developed hydrocephalus requiring a VP shunt. This patient underwent gamma knife radiosurgery to treat a 2.1 cm unilateral acoustic neuroma. The maximal dose was 27.5 Gy, and the peripheral dose was 14 Gy. She developed hydrocephalus with ataxia, mental status changes, and bladder incom-

petence 6 months after treatment, which resolved over time after the shunting procedure. The tumor size remains unchanged at 23 months.

Tumor Regrowth after Gamma Knife Treatment

In addition to patients referred to the gamma knife unit at the University of Pittsburgh, we have been involved in the treatment of two patients with acoustic neuromas who underwent stereotactic radiosurgery at the University of Pittsburgh and developed symptomatic tumor regrowth requiring surgical excision.

The first patient is a 65-year-old male who presented with progressive left hearing loss, tinnitus, gait instability, and left facial numbness. Facial nerve function was normal, and the hearing on the left consisted of a pure tone average (PTA) of 70 dB HL and SDS of 28%. Work-up led to a diagnosis of left acoustic neuroma, which on MRI at the time measured 1.8 cm (IAC+CPA). The patient refused surgery and elected to undergo gamma knife radiosurgery at the University of Pittsburgh. He was treated with a maximal dose of 40 Gy, with a peripheral dose of 20 Gy at the 50% isodose. The patient's tumor appeared to have no growth for the first 6 months after treatment, although his gait ataxia did not improve. The facial numbness did appear to improve, but 7 months after treatment, he developed a grade II/VI left facial nerve palsy and recurrence of facial numbness. The discrimination had been reduced to 0% by this time. Repeat scans suggested that the tumor may have increased in size and ventriculomegaly was present. The patient underwent a ventriculoperitoneal shunt for ataxia and mental confusion at 16 months, which improved his symptoms. By 3 years after treatment, the left facial nerve palsy had progressed to grade IV/VI, and the patient was having considerable difficulty with his balance. Repeat scans confirmed that the tumor had continued to grow, so he underwent microsurgical excision of the recurrent tumor through a retrosigmoid approach.

At surgery, the tumor was noted to be densely adherent to the brainstem and to the facial nerve, making dissection of tumor away from these structures difficult. The facial nerve was left intact anatomically by leaving a firmly adherent, small tumor residual. The lower cranial nerves were dissected free more easily. Postoperatively, the patient had a grade VI/VI facial nerve

paralysis, and developed left lower cranial nerve palsies with recurrent aspiration necessitating insertion of a gastric tube.

The second patient is a 44-year-old man who presented with gradual right hearing loss with tinnitus. The facial nerve was normal, and hearing on the right consisted of a PTA of 42 dB HL and SDS of 96%. An MRI showed a 3.0 cm tumor (IAC+CPA). The patient refused surgery and underwent gamma knife radiosurgery at the University of Pittsburgh with a maximal dose of 34 Gy and a peripheral dose of 17 Gy at the 50% isodose. The patient had no complications and enjoyed normal facial and trigeminal nerve function, as well as his pretreatment hearing level for the next 6 years. Serial scans showed that the tumor size was stable, and there was decreased contrast enhancement centrally. After 3 years, the tumor decreased in size. Six years after treatment, he developed a rapidly progressive right facial nerve palsy and deterioration in hearing. A repeat scan revealed regrowth of the tumor to 3.4 cm with homogeneous enhancement. Facial nerve function was noted to be grade III/VI. There was mild facial hypesthesia and no residual hearing. Microsurgical tumor removal was recommended, and the patient agreed to proceed.

The retrosigmoid approach was used for exposure. The tumor was noted to be hard and fibrotic, measured approximately 4 cm, and displaced the fifth nerve superiorly and the lower cranial nerves inferiorly. Total tumor removal was achieved with great difficulty. The facial nerve was left anatomically intact but could be stimulated only at the internal auditory canal. Postoperatively, the patient's facial nerve function was VI/VI and, therefore, he underwent gold weight insertion into the right upper eyelid. The postoperative course was complicated by CSF rhinorrhea that was controlled with lumbar drainage.

The histology of this tumor was consistent with a malignant schwannoma, characterized by high cellularity, nuclear atypism, areas of necrosis, and high mitotic activity.

This is a rare tumor that has been reported several times in the past (Best, 1987; Han et al., 1992; Kudo, Matsumoto, & Terao, 1983). This particular case is thought to have been a malignant tumor that was controlled partially by gamma knife radiosurgery but regrew after 6 years, although malignant transformation of an initially benign schwannoma is an unlikely possibility. It is the only tumor to date that has grown after 5 years of apparent growth control. An interval MR scan 6 weeks after surgery revealed no tumor residual, but a scan at 12 weeks revealed a 4 cm recurrent tumor. The patient is scheduled for tumor re-excision.

Summary of Our Experience

The outcomes of patients who underwent gamma knife radiosurgery for whom we have been involved in treating have been quite consistent with the data found in the literature. The tumor control, facial nerve, trigeminal nerve, and dysequilibrium results have been similar to reported findings. The two cases of recurrent tumor after gamma knife treatment are anecdotal, but these represent the only cases we have encountered so far.

CONCLUSION

Stereotactic radiosurgery is a potent addition to the arsenal of therapeutic modalities available for the treatment of acoustic neuromas. It offers potential tumor control without the need for an intracranial procedure with its attendant acute morbidities and cost. Patients return to their baseline activity level within a matter of days after treatment. There are no serious acute sequelae after stereotactic radiosurgery, and the facial nerve morbidity appears similar to those of surgical series. However, there are several unresolved issues regarding long-term outcomes data. Fifth nerve morbidity after radiosurgery appears much higher than in surgical series, but this issue has not been studied intensely in the surgical literature. There may be apparent differences due to variations in reporting criteria for trigeminal dysfunction. Hearing results after stereotactic radiosurgery overall appear to be at least as good as, if not better than, surgical excision but, again, it is difficult to compare directly the hearing results between the two modalities because of differences in reporting methods. Hearing results in patients with neurofibromatosis type 2 after stereotactic radiosurgery have not been good and may be worse than hearing results after surgery, but radiosurgical series for NF-2 patients have limited numbers of patients. There have been no reports containing substantial data regarding facial nerve and trigeminal nerve outcomes after stereotactic radiosurgery in patients with NF-2.

The incidence of hydrocephalus requiring a shunt after stereotactic radiosurgery appears to be significantly higher than that seen after surgical excision of acoustic neuroma. This complication is more common after treatment of larger tumors that may impinge on the fourth ventricle and aqueduct, so patients with large tumors are not good candidates for treatment by stereotactic radiosurgery. The long-term tumor control rate is a significant, unresolved issue, relating to the fact that, if stereotactic radiosurgery is to be offered to younger patients with a life expectancy exceeding 10 to 20 years, good tumor growth control beyond this time frame must be obtained. Although there are a few patients with follow-up as long as 20 years, more data are needed, especially in those patients receiving the lower doses that were administered starting in the late 1980s at the Karolinska Institute and in the early 1990s at the University of Pittsburgh. Currently, there are no adequate follow-up data to inform patients regarding long-term tumor control, and patients electing stereotactic radiosurgery over surgical resection need to understand this fact. In addition, surgery for tumor regrowth after stereotactic radiosurgery has been noted to be difficult, and preservation of facial nerve function has been problematic in certain cases, although there have been only a few reports of such cases. In NF-2 patients, prior treatment with radiosurgery currently is an exclusionary criterion for auditory brainstem implantation should their tumors grow and require excision.

Finally, the long-term effects of stereotactic radiosurgery on brainstem function are unknown. The possibility of tumor induction after radiosurgery also exists, although there has not been a confirmed case of this to date during 26 years of treatment. Stereotactic radiosurgery offers a noninvasive alternative for the treatment of acoustic neuromas and offers potential cost-effectiveness and lack of acute morbidity. Physicians treating patients with acoustic tumors should know about this treatment modality, its known potential morbidities, and the uncertainties of long-term tumor control and long-term morbidity. The physician and the fully informed patient then can proceed with the treatment program that is optimal for that individual.

REFERENCES

Atlas, M. D., Harvey, C., & Fagan, P. A. (1992). Hearing preservation in acoustic neuroma surgery: A continuing study. *Laryngoscope, 102,* 779–783.

Arriaga, M. A., Luxford, W. M., Atkins, J. S., Kwartler, J. (1993). Predicting long-term facial nerve outcome after acoustic neuroma surgery. *Archives of Otolaryngology—Head and Neck Surgery, 108,* 220–224.

Beatty, C. W., Ebersold, M. J., & Harner, S. G. (1987). Residual and recurrent acoustic neuromas. *Laryngoscope, 97,* 1168–1171.

Bederson, J. B., von Ammon, K., Werner, W. W., & Yasergil, M. G. (1991). Conservative treatment of patients with acoustic tumors. *Neurosurgery, 28,* 646–651.

Bergstrom, R. (1980). Changes in peripheral nerve tissue after irradiation with high energy protons. *Acta Radiologica: Therapy, Physics, Biology, 58,* 301–312.

Berk, H. W., & Agarwal, S. K. (1992). Physical aspects of radiosurgery with the gamma knife. In L. Steiner (Ed.), *Radiosurgery: Baseline and trends* (pp. 49–62). New York: Raven Press.

Best, P. V. (1987). Malignant triton tumor in the cerebellopontine angle. *Acta Neuropathologica, 74,* 92–96.

Brackmann, D. E., House, J. R., & Hitselberger, W. E. (1994). Technical modifications to the middle fossa craniotomy approach in removal of acoustic neuromas. *American Journal of Otology, 15,* 614–619.

Brada, M., & Laing, R. (1994). Radiosurgery/ stereotactic external beam radiotherapy for malignant brain tumours: The Royal Marsden Hospital experience. *Recent Results in Cancer Research, 135,* 91–104.

Briggs, R. J. S., Brackmann, D. E., Baser, M. E., & Hitselberger, W. E. (1994). Comprehensive management of bilateral acoustic neuromas. *Archives of Otolaryngology—Head and Neck Surgery, 120,* 1307–1314.

Cohen, N. L., Lewis, W. S., & Ransohoff, J. (1993). Hearing preservation in cerebellopontine angle tumor surgery: The NYU experience 1974–1991. *American Journal of Otology, 14,* 423–433.

Dahlin, H., Larsson, B., Leksell, L., Rosander, K., Sarby, S., & Steiner, L. (1975). Influence of absorbed dose and field size on the geometry of radiation-surgical brain lesion. *Acta Radiologica: Therapy, Physics, Biology, 14,* 139–144.

Doyle, K., J., & Shelton, C. (1993). Hearing preservation in bilateral acoustic neuroma surgery. *American Journal of Otology, 14,* 562–565.

Ebersold, M. J., Harner, S. G., Beatty, C. W., Harper, C. M., & Quast, L. M. (1992). Current results of the retrosigmoid approach to acoustic neurinoma. *Journal of Neurosurgery, 76,* 901–909.

Fabricius, E., Larsson, B., Steen, L., & Akerman B. (1962). Observations on pigeons with prethalamic radiolesions in the nervous pathways from the telencephalon. *Acta Physiologica Scandanavica, 56,* 286–298.

Flickinger, J.C., Lunsford, L. D., Coffey, R. J., Linskey, M. E., Bissonette, D. J., Maitz, A. H., & Kondziolka, D. (1991). Radiosurgery of acoustic neurinomas. *Cancer, 67,* 345–353.

Flickinger, J.C., Lunsford, L. D., & Kondziolka, D. (1992). Assessment of integrated logistic tolerance predictions for radiosurgery with the gamma knife. In L. Steiner (Ed.), *Radiosurgery: Baseline and trends* (pp. 15–22). New York: Raven Press.

Fischer, G., Fischer, C., & Remond, J. (1992). Hearing preservation in acoustic neurinoma surgery. *Journal of Neurosurgery, 76*, 910–917.

Friedman, W. A., Bova, F. J., & Spiegelmann, R. (1992). Linear accelerator radiosurgery at the University of Florida. *Neurosurgery Clinics of North America, 3*, 141–166.

Gale, C. C., & Larsson, B. (1963). Radiation-induced "hypophysectomy" and hypothalamic lesions in lactating goats. *Acta Physiologica Scandanavica, 59*, 299–318.

Gantz, B. J., Parnes, L. S., Harker, L. A., & McCabe, B. F. (1986). Middle cranial fossa acoustic neuroma excision: Results and complications. *Annals of Otology, Rhinology, and Laryngology, 95*, 454–459.

Glasscock, M. E., Hays, J. W., Minor, L. B., Haynes, D. S., & Carrasco, V. N. (1993). Preservation of hearing in surgery for acoustic neuromas. *Journal of Neurosurgery, 78*, 864–870.

Haines, S. J., & Levine, S. C. (1993). Intracanalicular acoustic neuroma: Early surgery for preservation of hearing. *Journal of Neurosurgery, 79*, 515–520.

Hall, E. J., & Wright, E. A. (1988). Radiation response characteristics of human cells in vitro. *Radiation Research, 114*, 415–424.

Han, D. H., Kim, D. G., Chi, J. G., Park, S. H., Jung, H.-W., & Kim, Y. G. (1992). Malignant triton tumor of the acoustic nerve. *Journal of Neurosurgery, 76*, 874–877.

Harner, S. G., Beatty, C. W., & Ebersold, M. J. (1990). Retrosigmoid removal of acoustic neuroma: Experience 1978–1988. *Archives of Otolaryngology—Head and Neck Surgery, 103*, 40–45.

Hirsch, A., & Noren, G. (1988). Audiological findings after stereotactic radiosurgery in acoustic neurinomas. *Acta Oto-laryngologica, 106*, 244–251.

Hoehmann, D. (1991). Pre- and postoperative hearing thresholds and brainstem responses in patients with acoustic neuroma: Follow-up study using the middle fossa approach. *American Journal of Otology, 12*, 172–178.

House, W. F. (1964). Evolution of transtemporal bone removal of acoustic tumors. *Archives of Otolaryngology, 80*, 731–742.

Kamerer, D. B., Lunsford, L. D., & Moller, M. (1988). Gamma knife: An alternative treatment for acoustic neurinomas. *Annals of Otology, Rhinology, and Laryngology, 97*, 631–635.

Kudo, M., Matsumoto, M., & Terao, H. (1983). Malignant nerve sheath tumor of acoustic nerve. *Archives of Pathology and Laboratory Medicine, 107*, 293–297.

Lalwani, A. K., Butt, F. Y. S., Jackler, R. K., Pitts, L. H., & Yingling, C. D. (1994). Facial nerve outcome after acoustic neuroma surgery: A study from the era of cranial nerve monitoring. *Otolaryngology—Head and Neck Surgery, 111*, 561–570.

Larsson, B. (1992). Radiobiological fundamentals in radiosurgery. In L. Steiner (Ed.), *Radiosurgery: Baseline and trends* (pp. 3–14). New York: Raven Press.

Leksell, L. (1971). A note on the treatment of acoustic tumours. *Acta Chirurgica Scandanavica, 137*, 763–765.

Linskey, M. E., Lunsford, L. D., & Flickinger, J. C. (1991). Neuroimaging of acoustic nerve sheath tumors after stereotactic radiosurgery. *American Journal of Neuroradiology, 12*, 1165–1175.

Linskey, M. E., Lunsford, L. D., & Flickinger, J. C. (1992a). Tumor control after stereotactic radiosurgery in neurofibromatosis patients with bilateral acoustic tumors. *Neurosurgery, 31*, 829–839.

Linskey, M. E., Lunsford, L. D., Flickinger, J. C., & Kondziolka, D. (1992b). Stereotactic radiosurgery for acoustic tumors. *Neurosurgery Clinics of North America, 3*, 191–205.

Linskey, M. E., Flickinger, J. C., & Lunsford, L. D. (1993). Cranial nerve length predicts to the risk of delayed facial and trigeminal neuropathies after acoustic tumor radiosurgery. *International Journal of Radiation Oncology, Biology, Physics, 25*, 227–233.

Lunsford, L. D., Kamerer, D. B., & Flickinger, J. C. (1990). Stereotactic radiosurgery for acoustic neuromas. Commentary. *Archives of Otolaryngology—Head and Neck Surgery, 116*, 907–909.

Lunsford, L. D., & Linskey, M. E. (1992). Stereotactic radiosurgery in the treatment of patients with acoustic neuroma. *Otolaryngologic Clinics of North America, 25*(2), 471–491.

Mangham, C. (1988). Complications of translabyrinthine vs. suboccipital approach for acoustic tumor surgery. *Archives of Otolaryngology—Head and Neck Surgery, 99*, 396–400.

Mendenhall, W. M., Friedman, W. A., & Bova, F. J. (1994). Linear accelerator-based radiosurgery for acoustic schwannomas. *International*

Journal of Radiation Oncology, Biology, Physics, 28, 803–810.

Nadol, J. B. Jr, Chiong, C. M., Ojemann, R.G., McKenna, M. J., Martuza, R. L., Montgomery, W. W., Levine, R. A., Ronner, S. F., & Glynn, R., J. (1992). Preservation of hearing and facial nerve function in resection of acoustic neuroma. *Laryngoscope, 102*(10), 1153–1158.

Nedzelski, J. M., Chiong, C. M., Cashman, M. Z., Stanton, S. G., & Rowed, D. W. (1994). Hearing preservation in acoustic neuroma surgery: Value of monitoring cochlear nerve action potentials. *Archives of Otolaryngology— Head and Neck Surgery, 111*, 703–709.

Neely, J. G. (1984). Is it possible to totally resect an acoustic tumor and conserve hearing? *Archives of Otolaryngology—Head and Neck Surgery, 92*, 162–167.

Nilsson, S., Carlsson, J., & Larsson, B. (1980). Survival of irradiated glia and glioma cells studied with a new cloning technique. *International Journal of Radiation Biology & Related Studies in Physics, Chemistry, & Medicine, 37*, 267–279.

Noren, G., Arndt, J., & Hindmarsh, T. (1983). Stereotactic radiosurgery in cases of acoustic neuroma: Further experiences. *Neurosurgery, 13*, 12–22.

Noren, G., Greitz, D., Hirsch, A., & Lax, I. (1992). Gamma knife radiosurgery in acoustic neuroma. In L. Steiner (Ed.), *Radiosurgery: Baseline and trends* (pp. 141-148). New York: Raven Press.

Noren, G., Greitz, D., Hirsch, A., & Lax, I. (1993). Gamma knife surgery in acoustic neuroma. *Acta Neurochirgica Supplementum, 58*, 104–107.

Ogunrinde, O. K., Lunsford, L. D., Flickinger, J. C., & Kondziolka, D. (1994). Facial nerve preservation and tumor control after gamma knife radiosurgery of unilateral acoustic tumors. *Skull Base Surgery, 4*, 87–92.

Parving, A., Tos, M., Thomsen, J., Moller, H., & Buchwald, C. (1992). Some aspects of life quality after surgery for acoustic neuroma. *Archives of Otolaryngology—Head and Neck Surgery, 118*, 1061–1064.

Pollock, B. E., Lunsford, L. D., Kondziolka, D., Flickinger, J. C., Bissonette, D. J., Kelsey, S. F., & Jannetta, P. J. (1995). Outcome analysis of acoustic neuroma management: A comparison of microsurgery and stereotactic radiosurgery. *Neurosurgery, 36*, 215–229.

Schessel, D. A., Nedzelski, J. M., Kassel, E. E., & Rowed, D. W. (1992). Recurrence rates of acoustic neuroma in hearing preservation surgery. *American Journal of Otology, 13*, 233–235.

Slattery, W. H., & Brackmann, D. E. (1995). Results of surgery following stereotactic irradiation for acoustic neuromas. *American Journal of Otology, 16*, 315–319.

Silverstein, H., Rosenberg, S. I., Flanzer, J., & Seidman, M. D. (1993). Intraoperative facial nerve monitoring in acoustic neuroma surgery. *American Journal of Otology, 14*(6), 524–532.

Strasnick, B., Glasscock, M. E., Haynes, D., McMenomey, S. O., & Minor, L. B. (1994). The natural history of untreated acoustic neuromas. *Laryngoscope, 104*, 1115–1124.

Thedinger, B. S., Whittacker, C. K., Luetje, C. M. (1991). Recurrent tumor after a suboccipital removal. *Neurosurgery, 29*, 681–687.

Thomsen, J., Tos, M., & Borgesen, S. E. (1990). Gamma knife: Hydrocephalus as a complications of stereotactic radiosurgical treatment of an acoustic neuroma. *American Journal of Otology, 11*, 330–333.

Umezu, H., & Aiba, T. (1994). Preservation of hearing after surgery for acoustic schwannomas: Correlation between cochlear nerve function and operative findings. *Journal of Neurosurgery, 80*, 844–848.

Uziel, A., Benezech, J., & Frerebeau, P. (1993). Intraoperative facial nerve monitoring in posterior fossa acoustic neuroma surgery. *Archives of Otolaryngology—Head and Neck Surgery, 108*, 126–134.

Wazen, J., Silverstein, H., Norrell, H., & Besse, B. (1985). Preoperative and postoperative growth rates in acoustic neuromas documented with CT scanning. *Archives of Otolaryngology— Head and Neck Surgery, 93*, 151–155.

Wiegand, D. A., & Fickel, V. (1989). Acoustic neuroma—The patient's perspective: Subjective assessment of symptoms, diagnosis, therapy, and outcome in 541 patients. *Laryngoscope, 99*, 179–187.

Wiet, R. J., Kazan, R. P., Raslan, W., & Herzon, G. D. (1986). Complications in the approach to acoustic tumor surgery. *Annals of Otology, Rhinology, and Laryngology, 95*, 28–31.

Index